Baillière's Midwives' Dictionary

11TH EDITION

Denise Tiran MSc RM RGN ADM PGCEA

Director, Expectancy Ltd, Croydon; Honorary Lecturer,
University of Greenwich, London, UK

with a contribution from

Amanda Sullivan BA(Hons) PGDip PhD
RM RGN

Consultant Midwife, Nottingham University Hospitals NHS Trust,
Nottingham, UK

BAILLIÈRE
TINDALL

ELSEVIER

D0767767

Edinburgh London New York Oxford Philadelphia St Louis Sydney Toronto 2008

BAILLIÈRE
TINDALL
ELSEVIER

An imprint of Elsevier Limited

© 1997, 2008 Elsevier Limited. All rights reserved.

The right of Denise Tiran to be identified as author of this work has been asserted by her in accordance with the Copyright, Designs and Patents Act 1988.

First edition 1951
Sixth edition 1976
Seventh edition 1983
Eighth edition 1992
Ninth edition 1997
Tenth edition 2003
Eleventh edition 2008
 Reprinted 2008

ISBN: 978 0 7020 2884 7

British Library Cataloguing in Publication Data
A catalogue record for this book is available from the British Library

Library of Congress Cataloging in Publication Data
A catalog record for this book is available from the Library of Congress

Note

CONTENTS

Since publication of the last edition of *Baillière's Midwives' Dictionary*, the midwifery profession has faced many new challenges. In Western countries increasingly defensive obstetrics and a rise in caesarean sections has had a considerable impact on midwifery practice, while science and technology developments have expanded the range of investigative procedures and treatments for infertility, miscarriage and congenital abnormality, leading to improved obstetric and perinatal outcomes. The migration of populations across international borders has also proved a challenge to which midwives have risen admirably but about which they are still learning. In developing countries the pandemic nature of HIV/AIDS and the fact that, still, many childbearing women do not have ready access even to clean water, let alone to adequate facilities in the event of obstetric emergencies, remain issues of major concern. Conversely, an increased global focus on safe motherhood has facilitated new initiatives, which are bringing together qualified professionals, traditional attendants and consumers in a spirit of shared ideals, hopes and resources.

Midwives continue to be in a uniquely privileged position to assist in enhancing and improving the care of mothers and babies at local, regional, national and international levels. However, in order to achieve positive results it is essential that midwives develop and maintain a high standard of evidence-based knowledge and competence, through pre-registration and continuing education, professional debate and research. Even the most experienced of midwives needs access to resources to facilitate this process, particularly as the midwifery profession now has so many areas of specialism within it. No single midwife can expect to know everything, but it is necessary to know where to find solutions to unanswered questions or to be able to double-check facts in a hurry. *Baillière's Midwives' Dictionary* attempts to provide one quick reference source, which can be used by students and lecturers in the classroom and by qualified midwives in clinical practice, wherever they may be.

Acknowledgements

As always, I would like to thank everyone at Elsevier Ltd for the invitation to revise the world-famous *Baillière's Midwives' Dictionary*. I would particularly like to express my gratitude to Dr Amanda Sullivan, Consultant Midwife and Interim Deputy Director of Nursing at Nottingham University Hospital NHS Trust, who has revised all the antenatal terms and provided many new definitions of contemporary investigative tests. Thanks also go to Dr Kevin O'Craft, Prenatal Cytogeneticist at Nottingham University Hospital NHS Trust, for supplying the karyotype image and Dr Tony Hitch and Gemma Purcell, biochemists at Nottingham University Hospital NHS Trust, for their extremely helpful advice and information regarding biochemical testing in pregnancy. Once again I am grateful to retain the contribution from Dr Richard Mainwaring Burton, Queen Mary's Sidcup NHS Trust, in Appendix 2 on normal blood and urine values and tests. I would also like to thank the numerous student and qualified midwives I have met while teaching and lecturing around the country who have provided feedback on the previous editions of the *Dictionary* and helped to focus my thoughts on what was required in this revision.

Finally, as ever, my personal thanks go to my wonderful son, Adam, now 17 and about to embark on his own career journey, and to my new partner, Harry, whose specialist expertise in physiology has been a tremendous professional help. Their unfailing love and support, not only while working on the *Dictionary* but in everything else, are the very foundations of my life.

London, 2007

Denise Tiran
www.expectancy.co.uk

abdomen cavity between diaphragm and pelvis, lined by peritoneum; contains stomach, intestines, liver, gallbladder, spleen and pancreas, kidneys, suprarenal glands and ureters. The urinary bladder and uterus become abdominal organs when distended in pregnancy. *Pendulous a.* anterior abdominal wall hangs down over the pubis. *Scaphoid a.* sunken abdomen in low-birthweight babies, due to shrinkage of liver and spleen *in utero*.

Abdomen

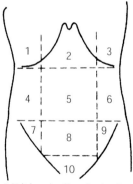

1, Right hypochondrium; **2,** epigastrium; **3,** left hypochondrium; **4,** right lumbar region; **5,** umbilical region; **6,** left lumbar region; **7,** right iliac fossa; **8,** hypogastrium; **9,** left iliac fossa; **10,** suprapubis.

abdominal concerning the abdomen.

abdominal enlargement during pregnancy the abdomen becomes progressively larger as the uterus increases in size; it is visible externally mainly from about 16 weeks' gestation. Excess enlargement may be due to multiple pregnancy, polyhydramnios, uterine FIBROIDS or abnormal ovum development (hydatidiform mole).

abdominal examination systematic examination of the mother's abdomen by visual inspection, for shape, scars, STRIAE GRAVIDARUM, skin tension and contour, and symphysis–fundal distance measurement, by gentle PALPATION and by AUSCULTATION. The uterus is palpable above the symphysis pubis from 12 weeks' gestation, increasing steadily in size until term. Fetal growth is estimated by measuring the symphysis–fundal distance in centimetres and plotting this on a growth chart to detect deviations in growth rate. PRESENTATION is assessed by palpation after 36 weeks and may need to be confirmed by an ultrasound assessment. The fetal heart is auscultated with a Pinard's stethoscope or electric monitor for rate, rhythm and regularity, and should be differentiated from the uterine SOUFFLE. Postnatally the abdomen is palpated to monitor uterine INVOLUTION, to assess that the uterus is regaining its non-pregnant size and position and to elicit deviations from normal such as constipation or urinary retention.

abdominal pain minor abdominal discomfort in pregnancy is common as a result of growth, stretching and alteration in position, but severe pain may be due to THREATENED ABORTION, ECTOPIC PREGNANCY, uterine FIBROIDS, TORSION or ABRUPTIO PLACENTAE.

1

abdominal palpation *See* ABDOMINAL EXAMINATION.

abdominal pregnancy ECTOPIC PREGNANCY in which the fertilised ovum embeds in the abdominal cavity.

abdominal striae *See* STRIAE GRAVIDARUM.

abdominal wall structure covering the abdominal organs, i.e. skin, fat, fascia, muscles and peritoneum. *A. w. defects* neonatal defects that develop *in utero*, usually requiring immediate surgical intervention, e.g. EXOMPHALOS and GASTROSCHISIS.

abduct to draw away from an axis or the median plane.

abduction drawing away from the centre.

aberrant wandering or deviating from the normal site or course.

ABO blood groups blood groups are classified according to whether they contain agglutinogens A, B, A and B (AB) or none (O). Serum may contain antibodies, anti-A agglutinins, anti-B agglutinins or both; blood given in transfusion must not contain the same antibodies as the recipient's blood group (e.g. a group A person must not receive group B blood, which contains anti-A agglutinins) or a fatal reaction will occur. Group AB individuals have no agglutinin or antibody in the serum so can receive blood from any group, i.e. they are *universal recipients*; group O individuals have no agglutinogens so their blood can be given to anyone, i.e. they are *universal donors*. *See also* RHESUS FACTOR.

ABO incompatibility occurs in about one in 200 pregnancies when the maternal blood group is O, the serum containing anti-A and anti-B antibodies. If the fetus is group A, B or AB, an antibody differing immunologically from normal anti-A and anti-B may cross the placenta and cause haemolysis in the neonate, even in a first baby. Jaundice appears within 24 hours of birth but is usually mild. The bilirubin level rises very rapidly but anaemia is less obvious. The COOMBS' TEST is usually negative, unlike in Rhesus incompatibility. The jaundice is treated with phototherapy or, in severe cases, by exchange transfusion. *See also* ABO BLOOD GROUPS, ISOIMMUNISATION and RHESUS FACTOR.

abort to bring to a premature end, especially a pregnancy; to check the course of a process or disease.

abortifacient any means used to cause abortion, including chemical and surgical methods.

abortion expulsion from the uterus of products of conception before 24 weeks of pregnancy, the fetus not being delivered alive. *Therapeutic a.* induced abortion in accordance with the 1967 Abortion Act; the 1991 Amendments to the Act permit termination after 24 weeks' gestation in certain circumstances. Before 12 weeks' gestation, abortion is usually performed by vacuum extraction or dilatation and curettage; later, drugs, e.g. prostaglandins, are used. *Spontaneous a.* may be due to a blighted ovum, such as a HYDATIDIFORM or VESICULAR MOLE, or a CARNEOUS MOLE, which may result in a MISSED ABORTION. ECTOPIC PREGNANCY also usually results in miscarriage. Abortion may be COMPLETE or INCOMPLETE; some women suffer HABITUAL ABORTION. Treatment aims primarily to prevent complications such as haemorrhage and sepsis. *See also* THREATENED ABORTION and INEVITABLE ABORTION.

abrachia congenital absence of arms.

abrasion cut or scratch on the skin. *Neonatal a.* skin damage, often IATROGENIC, caused by trauma during delivery from forceps blades, vacuum extraction cups, electrodes or scalpels.

abreaction reliving an experience so that previously repressed associated emotions are released.

abruptio tearing asunder. *A. placentae or placental abruption* partial or complete separation of the placenta from its site, usually in the upper uterine segment, after 24 weeks of pregnancy, causing pain and haemorrhage. *See* PLACENTA.

abscess localised accumulation of pus in a space or cavity. *Bartholin's a.* in Bartholin's gland, near the orifice of the vagina; *breast a.* in the breast; *pelvic a.* in the pouch of Douglas.

abuse misuse, maltreatment or excessive use. *See* CHILD ABUSE. *Substance a.* use of substances including illegal drugs or misuse of prescribed drugs.

acardiac twin twin that develops without a viable cardiac structure; life is maintained *in utero* via the placental circulation of the other viable twin.

acceleration of labour *See* AUGMENTATION OF LABOUR.

accessory extra or supplementary. *A. auricles* are commonly found immediately anterior to the ear.

accidental antepartum haemorrhage term previously used for ABRUPTIO PLACENTAE.

accountable liable to be held responsible for a course of action.

accreditation process of evaluation of an institution or individual to obtain official recognition of standards set against agreed criteria, e.g. education. *A. of prior learning* system in which credit is awarded towards a current programme of study for courses or modules that have been previously completed. *A. of prior experiential learning* credit is awarded towards a current programme of study for previously acquired professional experience that has not been formally assessed; this may entail completing a PROFESSIONAL DEVELOPMENT PORTFOLIO.

accreta morbid attachment. *Placenta a.* placenta attached to the uterine muscle because of a deficiency of decidua basalis.

acetabulum cup-shaped socket in the pelvic innominate bone into which the head of the femur fits.

acetoacetic acid a product of abnormal fat metabolism, occurring in diabetic and dehydrated mothers.

acetone by-product of acetoacetic acid. Produced in abnormal amounts in uncontrolled diabetes mellitus and metabolic acidosis. Its characteristic 'pear drops' smell may be noticed on the mother's breath or in the urine.

acetonuria ketones in the urine.

acetylcholine chemical transmitter released by some nerve endings at the synapse between one neuron and the next, or between a nerve ending and the effector organ it supplies. These nerves are cholinergic, e.g. parasympathetic nerves and lower motor neurons to skeletal muscles. Acetylcholine is rapidly destroyed by cholinesterase.

achlorhydria absence of hydrochloric acid in the gastric juice; associated with conditions such as pernicious anaemia and stomach cancer.

achondroplasia failure to form cartilage. Autosomal dominant genetic condition causing dwarfism, usually as a result of a new MUTATION; characterised by shortening of the long bones, with development of very short limbs and a large head, but normal trunk and mentality.

aciclovir antiviral agent used to treat herpes simplex, orally or by intravenous infusion.

acid substance that will form a salt when combined with an alkali; turns blue litmus paper red. Acids assist in the chemical processes required by body tissues; a stable balance between acids and bases is essential for life. *Hydrochloric a.* colourless compound of hydrogen and chlorine, present in gastric juice; can cause MENDELSON'S SYNDROME if inhaled. *See also* ACID–BASE BALANCE.

acid–base balance state of equilibrium between acidity and alkalinity of body fluids; also called hydrogen ion (H^+) balance. The positively charged H⁺ is the active constituent of all acids. Most of the body's metabolic processes produce acids as their end products, but alkaline body fluid is required as a medium for vital cellular activities; therefore, chemical exchanges of H⁺ must occur continuously to maintain equilibrium and an optimal pH (H⁺ concentration) of between 7.35 and 7.45.

acidaemia an alteration, due to acid accumulation, in the pH (acidity) of the blood, normally slightly alkaline. Occurs in hyperemesis gravidarum and diabetes mellitus or in labour if the woman is dehydrated and tissue perfusion is poor. *Fetal or neonatal a.* may occur as a result of HYPOXIA, leading to coma and death if untreated.

acidosis pathological accumulation of acid or depletion of the alkaline reserve (bicarbonate content) in blood and body tissues, characterised by an increase in hydrogen ion concentration (decrease in pH to below 7.30). adj. *acidotic. Metabolic a.* acidosis resulting from accumulation in the blood of ketoacids (derived from fat metabolism) at the expense of bicarbonate, thus diminishing the body's ability to neutralise acids. Occurs in diabetic ketoacidosis, lactic acidosis and failure of renal tubules to reabsorb bicarbonate. *Respiratory a.* acidosis resulting from ventilatory impairment and subsequent accumulation of carbon dioxide in the blood, which unites with water to form carbonic acid. Occurs with severe birth asphyxia and other neonatal respiratory conditions. In the mother it occurs with either an acute obstruction of the airways or a chronic condition involving the respiratory organs. *See also* ACIDAEMIA.

acinus minute hollow structure, lined by secreting cells, with a duct. The acini in the breast secrete milk. Sometimes called alveoli. pl. *acini.*

acquired immune deficiency syndrome (AIDS) severe progressive disease caused by the human immunodeficiency virus and manifesting as fever, weight loss, diarrhoea and lymphadenopathy. Opportunistic infections such as cytomegalovirus, herpes simplex, *Mycobacterium tuberculosis* and *Pneumocystis carinii* eventually lead to death, as will tumours such as lymphomas and Kaposi's sarcoma. *See also* HUMAN IMMUNODEFICIENCY VIRUS.

acromegaly chronic disease involving enlargement of the bones and tissues of the hands, feet and face, a result of over-functioning of the pituitary gland leading to hypersecretion of growth hormone; often caused by a pituitary tumour.

acromion process of the scapula, forming the point of the shoulder.

acrosome cap-like membrane-bound structure covering the anterior part of the spermatozoon's head; contains enzymes involved in penetration of the ovum.

active management of labour obstetric intervention to prevent prolonged labour and its complications. First-stage delay may be diagnosed from the PARTOGRAM and may be accelerated by artificial rupture of membranes and/or oxytocic infusion; the midwife's responsibilities include monitoring progress and carrying out medical instructions for the care of these women. *A. m. of third stage of labour* involves administration of an oxytocic injection (e.g. Syntometrine 1 mL) to facilitate placental separation, either with crowning of the head or delivery of the anterior shoulder; placental separation occurs within 2.5 minutes, and the midwife can then deliver the placenta and membranes manually, e.g. by CONTROLLED CORD TRACTION.

active transport movement of ions or molecules across cell membranes and epithelial layers, usually against a concentration gradient, resulting directly from expenditure of metabolic energy; process of maintaining normal differences in electrolytic composition between intracellular fluids. Differs from simple diffusion or osmosis in that it requires expenditure of metabolic energy.

acupressure component of Chinese medicine in which pressure is applied to various points on the body to stimulate or sedate internal energies. A more contemporary form is the Japanese technique of SHIATSU. Acupressure has been used successfully to treat nausea and vomiting in pregnancy and relieve pain in labour. *See also* ACUPUNCTURE.

acupuncture component of traditional Chinese medicine based on the principle that the body has energy lines, or meridians, running through it from top to toe. In optimum health – body, mind and spirit – this energy flows along the meridians unimpeded but ill health or physical, psychological or spiritual stresses, including pregnancy, cause the energy flow to become unbalanced, resulting in blockages or excesses of energy at certain points. Application of fine needles to the specific acupuncture points aims to rebalance the energy flow and assist in returning the person to full health. Acupuncture has been used to treat a variety of disorders of pregnancy, relieve pain in labour and for Caesarean section anaesthesia.

acute developing rapidly and running a short course; the reverse of chronic.

acute fatty liver of pregnancy (AFLP) acute yellow atrophy; rare complication of pregnancy of unknown aetiology, characterised by rapid progressive atrophy of the liver with massive fatty necrosis and a mortality rate of over 80%. Typically, an obese woman presents with third-trimester vomiting, headache, malaise, drowsiness, tender, but not enlarged, liver and jaundice; concomitant hypertension

and symptoms of fulminating pre-eclampsia can mask the diagnosis; liver enzymes are slightly raised, hypoglycaemia and renal failure follow quickly. Fatty infiltration of the liver is seen on ULTRASOUND or COMPUTED TOMOGRAPHY; liver biopsy is contraindicated because of the risk of coagulopathy. Management involves correction of any coagulopathy and immediate delivery of the baby, preferably vaginally, although Caesarean section may be safer for the baby.

acute inversion of the uterus turning inside out of the uterus, a rare, serious complication of labour, caused by mismanagement of the third stage of labour or occasionally occurring spontaneously. Sudden profound maternal shock is accompanied by severe abdominal pain, bleeding, if the placenta is wholly or partially separated, palpation of a concave-shaped fundus in the abdomen or no uterus felt at all if inversion is complete, and the presence of the uterus in the cervix or vagina, felt on examination or visible at the vulva. The foot of the bed should be raised to relieve tension and alleviate shock, and the midwife should urgently call for the doctor who will attempt to replace the uterus by applying pressure to the lower segment near the cervix and working upwards to the fundus. If replacement of a totally inverted uterus is not possible it should be gently placed inside the vagina to reduce traction on the fallopian tubes and ovaries. Severe shock is treated by replacing fluids and blood and administering a narcotic analgesic; a general anaesthetic is then given to enable manual replacement of the uterus or, alternatively, the hydrostatic method may be used. If all attempts fail, a hysterectomy will be required.

acute renal failure sudden, severe, but reversible, interruption of kidney

5

function, usually a complication of another disorder such as haemorrhage or shock. OLIGURIA (diminished secretion of urine) occurs accompanied by other symptoms related to fluid and electrolyte imbalance, anaemia, hypertension and uraemia. Dialysis is required to monitor fluid and electrolyte imbalances until kidney function improves.

adactylia, adactyly congenital absence of fingers or toes.

adaptation the ability to overcome difficulties and adjust oneself to changing circumstances. Neuroses and psychoses are often associated with failures of adaptation.

addict person exhibiting addiction.

addiction physiological or psychological dependence on some agent, e.g. alcohol or drugs, with a tendency to increase its use.

adduct to draw towards a centre or median line.

adduction the art of adducting; the state of being adducted.

adherent placenta placenta that is firmly attached to the uterine wall, which fails to separate during the third stage of labour. *See* PLACENTA, PLACENTA ACCRETA, PLACENTA PERCRETA.

adhesion union between two surfaces that are normally separated, usually due to inflammation when fibrous tissue forms, e.g. peritonitis may cause adhesions between organs. Possible cause of intestinal obstruction or of infertility, by occlusion of the lumen in the fallopian tubes.

adipose tissue *See* TISSUE.

adnexa appendages. *Uterine a.* the ovaries and fallopian tubes.

adnexal mass enlarged area between uterus and ovaries; suggests ECTOPIC PREGNANCY if viewed on first-trimester ultrasound, especially if there is fluid in the pouch of Douglas and no visible intrauterine pregnancy; may also be due to physiological follicular cysts, corpus luteal cysts or tumours.

adolescence developmental stage from puberty to the cessation of physical growth.

adoption legal procedure by which responsibility for a child is transferred from the natural parents to adopting parents. The Adoption Act 2002 details how and when an adoption can take place and who can adopt; local authorities offer advice, social work support and may act as an adoption agency; private and charitable adoption organisations registered with the local authority are also available.

adrenal pertaining to the adrenal (suprarenal) glands, two complex endocrine glands, situated one at the upper pole of each kidney. *Congenital a. hyperplasia* congenital autosomal recessive condition in which the adrenal glands overproduce androgens because of a deficiency of the 21-hydroxylase enzyme, necessary for normal production of steroids from cholesterol, and causing rapid salt loss; characterised by ambiguous genitalia.

adrenaline (epinephrine) one of several hormones secreted by the adrenal medulla that help to regulate the sympathetic nervous system; a powerful vasopressor that increases blood pressure, heart rate, cardiac output and glucose release from the liver. Adrenaline can also be produced synthetically. An increase in adrenaline secretion as a result of a tumour (PHAEOCHROMOCYTOMA) is a very rare condition that causes acute hypertension and can occur in pregnancy; diagnosis is made by measuring VANILLYLMANDELIC ACID (VMA) via a 24-hour urine collection – VMA is an excretory product of the catecholamines and its levels are raised in phaeochromocytomas.

adrenocorticotrophic hormone (ACTH) hormone of the anterior pituitary gland that stimulates the adrenal cortex.

adult respiratory distress syndrome condition resulting from severe hypovolaemic shock, in which the mother has impaired gaseous exchange, reduced oxygen and increased carbon dioxide levels, alveolar collapse and pulmonary oedema, leading ultimately to respiratory failure.

aerobe organism requiring air or free oxygen to sustain life.

aerobic requiring air or free OXYGEN to grow and multiply.

aetiology the science of causes, e.g. of disease.

afebrile without fever.

affective pertaining to emotional tone or feeling. *A. disorder* mental disorder characterised by mood disturbance accompanied by either manic or depressive symptoms or both, e.g. bipolar disorder (manic-depressive illness), major depression, cyclothymic disorder and dysthymic disorder (depressive neurosis).

afferent towards the centre. *A. nerve* sensory nerve fibre carrying impulses from the periphery to the central nervous system.

affiliation order court order by which an absent father is required to make regular payments towards his child's maintenance.

afibrinogenaemia absence of fibrinogen in the blood; more usually HYPOFIBRINOGENAEMIA. Acquired hypofibrinogenaemia is usually secondary to DISSEMINATED INTRAVASCULAR COAGULATION (DIC).

afterbirth lay term for the placenta and membranes expelled from the uterus after the birth of the baby.

aftercoming head fetal head (coming after the trunk) in a breech delivery. *See* BREECH.

afterpains painful uterine contractions occurring in the early puerperium, common in multiparous women and frequently felt during breastfeeding. Severe and persistent afterpains may indicate that a blood clot, membrane or fragment of placenta has been retained in the uterus.

agenesis absence of an organ as a result of non-appearance of its primordium in the embryo.

agglutination aggregation of separate particles into clumps or masses. 1. the clumping together of red blood corpuscles in serum, as may occur if incompatible cells are transfused. Agglutination of sensitised red blood cells by urine reveals the presence of chorionic gonadotrophin (hCG) in a pregnancy test. 2. the clumping together of platelets as a result of the action of platelet agglutinins. 3. the clumping of bacteria when brought into contact with specific immune serum.

agglutinin substance that reacts with an AGGLUTINOGEN and causes agglutination to occur.

agglutinogen substance that stimulates a specific agglutinin to cause agglutination.

agnathia failure of development of the jaw.

air atmosphere surrounding the earth, mainly composed of two gases: OXYGEN (approximately 21%) and NITROGEN (approximately 79%). *A. hunger* deep, sighing respiration occurring when the body's OXYGEN supply is depleted, as in severe haemorrhage or shock.

airway 1. passage by which air enters the lungs. 2. mechanical device used for securing unobstructed respiration during general anaesthesia or other occasions when the patient is not ventilating or exchanging gases properly.

ala wing, e.g. the sacral ala. pl. *alae.*

alanine aminotransferase liver function test assessed in mothers with pre-eclampsia or HELLP SYNDROME.

alba, albicans white. *Linea a.* white line in the midline of the abdomen in Caucasians.

albumin any protein that is soluble in water and moderately concentrated salt solutions and is coagulable by heat. *Serum a.* plasma protein formed principally in the liver. Albumin is responsible for colloidal osmotic pressure of the blood; has an important role in regulating exchange of water between plasma and interstitial compartment (space between the cells). Reduced albumin in the plasma leads to increased flow of water from the capillaries into the interstitial compartment, causing increased tissue fluid, leading to oedema if severe. Albumin is also a transport protein carrying fatty acids, bilirubin, drugs and some hormones.

albuminuria presence in the urine of albumin, usually serum albumin; occurs in renal or severe cardiac disease and some pregnancy complications.

alcohol in pregnancy expectant mothers should restrict alcohol intake, especially in the first trimester. High alcohol consumption may lead to low-birthweight babies, neonatal feeding and sleeping problems and/or fully developed FETAL ALCOHOL SYNDROME.

aldosterone one of the hormones of the adrenal cortex, which help to regulate electrolyte and water balance by promoting retention of sodium (and, therefore, of water) and excretion of potassium; the retention of water increases plasma volume and blood pressure. Its secretion is stimulated by angiotensin II.

Alexander technique method of psychophysical re-education by which people learn better use of their bodies, involving postural realignment and physical and psychological relaxation methods, usually taught as a series of 20–30 lessons. The technique can be used to relieve problems in pregnancy such as persistent backache.

alimentary pertaining to nutrition. *A. tract* the passage through which the food passes from mouth to anus.

alkalaemia increased alkalinity or pH of the blood, caused either by an overdose or accumulation of alkaline substances or by an excessive loss of acids, e.g. by vomiting.

alkali substance capable of uniting with an acid to form a salt, turning red litmus paper blue. Alkalis form carbonates and combine with fatty acids to form soaps and help to maintain normal functioning of body chemistry. *See also* ACID–BASE BALANCE *and* BASE. *A. reserve* ability of the combined buffer systems of the blood to neutralise acid. The pH of the blood is normally slightly alkaline, between 7.35 and 7.45. Because the principal buffer in the blood is bicarbonate, the alkali reserve is essentially represented by the plasma bicarbonate concentration; however, haemoglobin, phosphates and other bases can also act as buffers. Lowered alkali reserve means a state of acidosis; an increased reserve indicates alkalosis. Alkali reserve is measured by the combining power of carbon dioxide, i.e. the amount of carbon dioxide that can be bound as bicarbonate by the blood.

alkaline (adj.), pertaining to alkali. *Serum a. phosphatase* measure of liver function; in pregnancy, levels rise progressively and are approximately double the non-pregnant levels by late pregnancy; the upper limit of normal is three times greater than the non-pregnant range.

alkaloids organic nitrogenous substances that form the active principle of certain drugs, e.g. morphine, atropine and strychnine.

alkalosis pathological condition resulting from accumulation of base or from loss of acid without comparable loss of base in the body fluids; characterised by decreased hydrogen ion concentration (increased pH). Alkalosis is the opposite of ACIDOSIS.

allantois membranous sac projecting from ventral surface of the embryo, which eventually helps to form the placenta.

allele one of two or more alternative forms of a gene at the same site in a chromosome, which will determine alternative characters in inheritance.

all-fours position position that the mother may assume in the second stage of labour; has been shown to increase the pelvic outlet, facilitating normal delivery.

alloimmunisation immune response to donated blood, bone marrow or a transplanted organ; Rhesus-negative pregnant women with a Rhesus-positive fetus can become alloimmunised following a sensitising event, e.g. antepartum haemorrhage or miscarriage through development of antibodies that target the foreign material, causing haemolytic disease of the newborn.

alpha-adrenergic mechanism autonomic nerve pathway mechanism through which excitatory responses occur as a result of the release of adrenergic substances such as adrenaline (epinephrine) and noradrenaline (norepinephrine).

alpha fetoprotein (AFP) plasma protein produced by the fetal liver, gastrointestinal tract and in the YOLK SAC; crosses from fetal into maternal circulation via the placenta, therefore maternal blood can be screened for fetal anomalies. Raised levels indicate open neural tube or abdominal wall defects; low levels are associated with chromosomal anomalies, e.g. EDWARD'S SYNDROME (trisomy 18) and DOWN'S SYNDROME (trisomy 21). AFP levels for Down's syndrome are assessed in the second trimester in conjunction with HUMAN CHORIONIC GONADOTROPHIN (HCG) and UNCONJUGATED OESTRIOLS (UE$_3$); levels are also dependant on gestation, number of fetuses, maternal weight and diabetes mellitus. AFP is undetectable in children over 1 year but production is re-stimulated in certain liver diseases, e.g. tumour or viral hepatitis.

alpha thalassaemia *See* THALASSAEMIA.

alternative medicine form of medicine different from conventional health care focusing on the inter-relationship between body, mind and spirit. More commonly termed COMPLEMENTARY MEDICINE.

alveolus any hollowed-out structure, e.g. tooth socket, air sac in the lungs, or acinus as in the breasts. pl. *alveoli*.

ambient surrounding or prevailing.

ambivalence the property of having equal power in two directions or on both sides at the same time. In psychiatry, having equally strong opposing emotions, such as love and hate for the same person.

ambulatory walking.

amelia developmental anomaly with absence of the limbs.

amenorrhoea absence of menstruation. *Primary a.* absence of menstruation in a post-pubertal woman who has never menstruated. *Secondary a.* cessation of menstrual periods in a woman who has previously menstruated. The commonest cause is pregnancy, but stress, environment or disease may also contribute to the condition.

amino acids organic substances derived from proteins, essential to human nutrition.

aminophylline alkaloid from camellia, which relaxes plain muscle spasm of the bronchioles and coronary arteries, given by mouth, intravenously or as a suppository; useful in treating asthma and heart failure.

ammonia alkaline gas formed by decomposition of proteins, amino acids and other nitrogen-containing substances. Converted to urea in the liver.

Amnihook instrument for performing an AMNIOTOMY.

9

amniocentesis antenatal extraction of AMNIOTIC FLUID from the intrauterine cavity by insertion of a fine-gauge needle through the mother's abdomen under continuous ultrasound guidance. Desquamated fetal cells from skin and gastrointestinal and urinary tracts can be isolated from the sample to assess fetal KARYOTYPE and detect inherited genetic disorders; to determine fetal BILIRUBIN levels when fetal HAEMOLYTIC disease from ALLOIMMUNISATION is suspected; or as a therapeutic procedure to drain POLYHYDRAMNIOS, to prolong the pregnancy and reduce maternal discomfort. A 1% risk of miscarriage from amniocentesis is dependent on the operator. Rhesus-negative mothers may require anti-D immunoglobulin.

amniocytes desquamated fetal cells in amniotic fluid from fetal skin and respiratory and urinary tracts; can be isolated and cultured or multiplied with molecular techniques such as FLUORESCENCE *IN SITU* HYBRIDISATION (FISH) or POLYMERASE CHAIN REACTION (PCR) to determine the fetal KARYO-TYPE and for genetic analysis.

amnion the innermost membrane enveloping the fetus and producing and enclosing the liquor amnii. *A. nodosum* nodular condition of the fetal surface of the amnion, as in oligohydramnios; may be associated with absence of fetal kidneys.

amnionicity presence/absence of AMNION for each fetus in MULTIPLE PREGNANCY; diamniotic twins each have an amnion and amniotic cavity, but these are shared by monoamniotic twins and the risk of entangled umbilical cords increases fetal morbidity and mortality rates.

amnioscope endoscope that allows observation of the fetus and amniotic fluid directly through the intact amniotic sac.

amnioscopy endoscopic examination of the amniotic sac and fluid to determine whether the LIQUOR AMNII is MECONIUM stained; largely superseded by CARDIOTOCOGRAPHY and ultrasound assessment.

amniotic band syndrome neonatal condition in which the baby is born with limb reduction abnormalities, due to possible rupture of the amnion during pregnancy, which then wraps around a developing limb and causes necrosis, strangulation and/or amputation.

amniotic cavity cavity enclosing the embryo, from which the amnion forms.

amniotic fluid fluid contained in the amniotic sac, also called LIQUOR AMNII, surrounding and swallowed by the fetus. It is secreted from the cells of the amnion, transudate from fetal vessels in the cord and placenta and from maternal vessels in the decidua. This normally clear, straw-coloured fluid is 99% water, 1% solids (proteins, carbohydrates, lipids, phospholipids, electrolytes, urea, uric acid, creatinine, pigments, enzymes, placental hormones, desquamated cells, lanugo, vernix caseosa and increasing amounts of urine from the fetus). The fluid allows the fetus to move freely, equalises pressure and temperature, acts as a shock absorber and provides some fetal nutrition. The amount varies from 500 mL to 1500 mL at term; an excess is called POLYHYDRAMNIOS and an abnormally small amount is OLIGOHYDRAMNIOS.

amniotic fluid embolism entry of amniotic fluid into the maternal circulation via the sinuses of the placental site; the term embolism is a misnomer. Rare cause of collapse in labour or of HYPOFIBRINOGENAEMIA. *See also* ANAPHYLACTOID SYNDROME OF PREGNANCY.

amniotic fluid index (AFI) measurement of amniotic fluid volume; fluid depth is measured in the four uterine quadrants and added together to estimate the total; measurement of below 5 cm indicates OLIGOHYDRAMNIOS and above 25 cm indicates POLYHYDRAMNIOS.

amniotic sac bag of amnion or fetal membrane that contains the fetus, suspended in amniotic fluid.

amniotomy surgical rupture of the amniotic sac for induction or acceleration of labour. With the mother in the lithotomy or dorsal position, the midwife or obstetrician performs an examination *per vaginam*; the forewaters are ruptured by passing an instrument through the cervix and piercing the membranes, whilst taking care not to damage the fetal presenting part. Straight or curved Kocher's forceps may be used or a specially designed AMNIHOOK. Occasionally, it is necessary to rupture the membranes so that the amniotic fluid can be observed or to prevent the risk of cord prolapse when the cord is presenting below the fetal part. Rarely, a hindwater rupture may be performed. *See also* Appendix 3.

amoxicillin a penicillin analogue similar in action to ampicillin but more efficiently absorbed from the gastrointestinal tract, therefore requiring less frequent dosage and not as likely to cause diarrhoea. Given orally, 250 mg three times daily.

ampicillin broad-spectrum synthetic penicillin that is active against many of the Gram-negative pathogens in addition to the usual gram-positive ones that are affected by penicillin. May be given orally, 250–500 mg four times daily, or intramuscularly or intravenously, 0.5–1.0 g in one dose. Useful in treating neonatal listeriosis.

ampulla dilated end of a canal, e.g. of a fallopian tube.

amyl nitrite vasodilator given by inhalation for angina pectoris and to relieve muscular spasm in CONSTRICTION RING.

anaemia reduction in the number of red blood cells, or amount of haemoglobin present in them, resulting from haemorrhage, excessive breakdown of red blood cells or failure to manufacture red blood cells. *Iron deficiency a.* most common type, often related to poor nutrition; iron supplementation may be given to women with a low serum ferritin; intramuscular or intravenous iron may be required in severe cases; blood transfusion may be given to prevent intrapartum complications, such as major haemorrhage. Anaemia that fails to respond to iron therapy may be MEGALOBLASTIC ANAEMIA, caused by folic acid deficiency. *Physiological a.* apparent anaemia in which the mother's red blood cell count is reduced but remains within acceptable limits; caused by the HAEMODILUTION that occurs normally in pregnancy. *See also* SICKLE CELL ANAEMIA.

anaerobe micro-organism that does not require free oxygen for its existence, e.g. *Clostridium welchii.*

anaesthesia state in which the whole body (*general a.*) or part of it (*local* or *regional a.*) is insensible to pain, feeling or sensation, induced to permit surgical or other painful procedures.

anaesthetic agent that induces anaesthesia. A general anaesthetic renders the patient unconscious; a local anaesthetic induces anaesthesia of a particular part of the body.

anal pertaining to the anus. *A. atresia* absence or closure of the anal opening, an occasional congenital defect found in the neonate.

analgesia insensibility to pain.

analgesic agent capable of inducing analgesia; a pain-relieving drug.

anaphylactoid syndrome of pregnancy rare but potentially fatal condition associated with AMNIOTIC FLUID EMBOLISM in which the presence of amniotic fluid in the maternal circulation triggers an anaphylactoid response, characterised initially by pulmonary vasospasm causing hypoxia, hypotension, pulmonary oedema and cardiovascular collapse, followed by the development of left ventricular failure, uncontrollable haemorrhage and coagulation disorder, with a high risk of maternal morbidity and mortality.

anaphylaxis unusual or exaggerated allergic reaction (often within seconds) to foreign proteins or other substances, e.g. drugs (antibiotics, local anaesthetics, codeine, insulin, adrenocorticotrophic hormone, enzymes); diagnostic agents (iodinated X-ray contrast media); biological fluids used to provide immunity (vaccines, antitoxins, gamma globulin); protein foods; the venom of bees, wasps, and hornets; pollens and moulds. Symptoms, caused by histamine release, include bronchospasm, peripheral vasodilatation, increased capillary permeability and constriction of bronchioles and bronchi. Adrenaline (epinephrine) should be administered immediately to produce bronchodilatation, reduce laryngeal spasm and elevate blood pressure, followed by steroid therapy to counteract histamine effects by decreasing capillary permeability; intravenous fluids and plasma aim to restore intravascular fluid volume and pressor agents [dopamine, noradrenaline (norepinephrine) and isoprenaline] and increase and maintain blood pressure. adj. *anaphylactic.*

anastomosis communication between two vessels or other structures, either natural or established operatively. pl. *anastomoses.*

androgens any steroid hormone that promotes male characteristics, i.e. androsterone and testosterone. adj. *androgenic.* Androgenic hormones, manufactured mainly by the testes under stimulation from the PITUITARY GLAND, are responsible for growth and development of the penis, scrotum, secondary sexual characteristics and muscle and bone.

android male-like, masculine. *A. pelvis* see PELVIS.

anembryonic pregnancy blighted ovum; pregnancy with no visible embryo in the gestation sac; occurs with early embryonic death although the trophoblast continues to develop; common cause of miscarriage. Diagnosis can only be made when the gestation sac mean diameter is larger than 20 mm; must be differentiated from a viable pregnancy that is too small to visualise the fetal pole.

anencephaly gross congenital malformation, incompatible with life, in which the cranial vault and the cerebral hemispheres fail to develop. Usually diagnosed antenatally by ultrasound scan but, if undetected, it may cause primary face presentation in labour.

aneuploidy having an incorrect number of chromosomes, including monosomy (missing chromosome in a pair) or trisomy (extra chromosome in a pair, such as trisomy 21 or DOWN'S SYNDROME).

angina pectoris severe chest pain and constriction, often radiating down the left arm, caused by inadequate blood flow to the heart.

angiography radiography of vessels of the body after introduction into them of a suitable contrast medium.

angioma tumour composed of blood vessels, e.g. a naevus on the skin.

angiotensin vasoconstrictor principle formed in the blood when RENIN is released from the kidney. Its vasopressor action raises blood pressure and diminishes fluid loss in the kidney by restricting blood flow. *A. converting enzyme (ACE) inhibitors* drugs used to control hypertension, but contraindicated in pregnancy because of the possible risks of teratogenesis.

angular pregnancy implantation of fertilised ovum in the angle where the fallopian tube enters the uterus.

anhydramnios absence of amniotic fluid.

ankylosis abnormal fixation or union of bones forming an articulation and resulting in a stiff joint. Ankylosis of the sacrococcygeal joint is a rare cause of obstructed delivery.

anococcygeal pertaining to the anus and coccyx. *A. body* mass of muscular and fibrous tissue between the anus and coccyx; part of the insertion of the levator ani muscles.

anode positive electrode to which negative ions are attracted. adj. *anodal.*

anodyne agent that relieves pain.

anomaly marked deviation from normal. *A. scan* ultrasound scan to detect fetal structural anomalies, usually performed between 18 and 21 weeks' gestation although may be undertaken in the first trimester; involves examination of the central nervous system (skull, brain, spine), thorax, heart, abdomen, urogenital tract, skeleton, extremities and face.

anorexia loss of appetite for food. *A. nervosa* complete lack of appetite with extreme emaciation. May be a cause of subfertility, because ovulation usually ceases.

anovular absence of ovulation.

anoxia the state of being deprived of OXYGEN. *See also* ASPHYXIA.

anoxic relating to or affected with anoxia.

antacid substance that neutralises acid, e.g. magnesium trisilicate.

ante- prefix meaning 'before'.

anteflexion bending forwards, e.g. of the body of the uterus on the cervix.

antenatal before birth. *A. care* care provided by midwives and obstetricians during pregnancy to ensure that fetal and maternal health are satisfactory, to enable early detection and treatment of any deviations from normal. Psycho-emotional preparation of the parents for labour and parenthood and health education are also included.

antepartum before parturition, i.e. birth. *A. haemorrhage* bleeding from the genital tract at any time after the 24th week of pregnancy until the baby is born, caused by PLACENTA PRAEVIA, ABRUPTIO PLACENTAE or incidental causes, e.g. cervical polyps or erosion, vaginitis or, rarely, carcinoma. The midwife should call a doctor, maintain records of observations, administer analgesia, take blood for cross-matching and provide support. An internal examination should *never* be performed.

anterior before, in front of.

anteroposterior from front to back.

anteversion turning forwards, e.g. of the uterus in relation to the vagina.

anthropoid man-like, e.g. anthropoid apes, man-like apes. *A. pelvis see* PELVIS.

anti- prefix meaning 'against', 'opposite'.

antibiotic pertaining to antibiosis, therefore destructive to life. Antibiotic drugs are drugs derived from living micro-organisms, which destroy or inhibit the growth of pathogenic bacteria.

antibody specific substance formed in the body that counteracts the effects of antigens or bacterial toxins. Antibodies, the effectors of the immune response, can be transferred passively from one individual to another, as in, for example, the transfer of maternal antibodies across the placental barrier to the fetus, which has not yet developed a mature immune system. The developmental process of antibody production is usually completed a few months after birth.

anticardiolipin antibodies (ACAs) antiphospholipid antibodies that can cause hypercoagulation; strongly associated with venous and arterial thrombosis, thrombocytopenia and recurrent fetal loss; often occur with other autoimmune disorders, e.g. systemic lupus erythematosus; in pregnancy, may react against the trophoblast, causing subplacental clots that interfere with placentation, leading to placental thrombosis and resulting in growth restriction or fetal loss. *See also* ANTIPHOSPHOLIPID ANTIBODIES.

anticoagulant agent that prevents or delays the clotting of blood, e.g. heparin.

anticonvulsant drug that prevents fits or convulsions, e.g. phenobarbital.

anti-D immunoglobulin globulin derived from human plasma, which contains antibodies to red cell Rhesus factor D. Intramuscular injection into the deltoid muscle (rather than into the gluteal region), to facilitate absorption, is offered routinely to Rhesus-negative woman at 28 and 34 weeks' gestation to prevent Rhesus D sensitisation; also given following any potentially sensitising incident, e.g. stillbirth, abortion or amniocentesis; administered again within 72 hours of delivery if the baby is Rhesus positive.

antidepressant effective against depressive illness; a drug used for relief of symptoms of depression.

antidiuretic 1. pertaining to or causing suppression of the rate of urine secretion. 2. an agent that causes suppression of urine formation. *A. hormone (ADH)* vasopressin; a hormone that suppresses the secretion of urine, with a specific effect on the epithelial cells of the renal tubules, stimulating the reabsorption of water independently of solids and resulting in concentration of urine. Secreted by the hypothalamus but stored and released by the posterior lobe of the PITUITARY GLAND, it also has vasopressor activity.

antidote agent that counteracts the effect of poison.

antiemetic drug that prevents or alleviates nausea and vomiting.

antigen any substance that, on introduction into the body, brings about immunity by stimulating antibody production.

antihistamine group of drugs that block tissue receptors for histamine, used to treat various allergic conditions and in the treatment of hyperemesis gravidarum.

antihypertensive effective against hypertension; agent that reduces high blood pressure. Some, for example methyldopa (Aldomet), act on alpha-adrenergic mechanisms in the central or sympathetic nervous system to reduce peripheral vascular resistance. Vasodilators act directly on the arterioles to produce the same effect. Beta-blockers, such as propranolol (Inderal), act at beta-adrenergic receptors in the heart and kidneys to reduce cardiac output and renin secretion.

antiphospholipid antibodies these autoimmune antibodies cause abnormal coagulation and thrombosis, including anticardiolipin antibodies and lupus anticoagulant; associated with fetal loss, poor placentation, thrombosis and autoimmune thrombocytopenia; if untreated in pregnancy there is a risk of preterm labour, pregnancy-induced hypertension, maternal thrombosis and fetal and maternal mortality, but aspirin and heparin greatly improve pregnancy outcomes; antenatal care should be given in a specialist obstetric–haematology clinic.

antiretroviral therapy (ART) drug therapy that attacks a retrovirus, particularly valuable in treating those with HUMAN IMMUNODEFICIENCY VIRUS and ACQUIRED IMMUNE DEFICIENCY SYNDROME. *Highly active ART (HAART)* combines three different types of drugs that attack the virus at different stages of replication. ART therapy in pregnancy reduces the risk of vertical transmission to the fetus.

antiseptics agents used to prevent sepsis, i.e. infection.

antiserum serum derived from the blood of an animal or human with a disease and having properties that are antagonistic to the bacteria producing the disease. pl. *antisera*.

antispasmodic relieving spasm.

antithrombin any naturally occurring or therapeutically administered substance that neutralises the action of thrombin and thus limits or restricts blood coagulation.

antithromboplastin any agent or substance that prevents or interferes with the interaction of blood clotting factors as they generate prothrombinase (thromboplastin).

antitoxin antibody produced to neutralise a bacterial toxin. Serum from animals immunised with the specific antitoxin is used in the prevention and treatment of DIPHTHERIA and TETANUS.

anuresis retention of urine in the bladder.

anuria failure of the kidneys to secrete urine, which may complicate severe concealed haemorrhage from abruptio placentae, eclampsia and septic abortion, and lead to bilateral cortical necrosis of the kidney.

anus extremity of the alimentary canal through which the faeces are discharged. *Imperforate a.* one that, owing to congenital defect, is not patent.

Anusol rectal cream or suppositories used to relieve pain associated with haemorrhoids.

aorta the large artery proceeding from the left ventricle of the heart. *Abdominal a.* that part of the vessel in the abdomen. *Arch of the a.* the curve of the aorta over the heart. *Thoracic a.* the part of the aorta that passes through the chest.

aperient drug that stimulates bowel action.

Apert's syndrome congenital abnormality in which there is fusion at birth of all the cranial sutures in addition to syndactyly (webbed fingers).

Apgar score scoring system devised by Dr Virginia Apgar to assess the condition of a baby during its first few minutes of life so that severe asphyxia neonatorum can be diagnosed and treated at once. *See also* ASPHYXIA NEONATORUM *and* Appendix 1.

aphtha whitish spots caused by the fungus *Candida albicans*; THRUSH. pl. *aphthae*.

aphthous vulvitis infestation of the vulva with thrush (*Candida albicans*).

APL principle chorionic gonadotrophin, the anterior pituitary-like hormone of the placenta.

aplastic relating to any structure with incomplete or defective development.

apnoea absence of breathing. Apnoeic periods occur in newborn infants in whom the respiratory centre is immature or depressed. *A. monitors* are designed to give an audible signal when a certain period of apnoea has occurred.

aponeurosis flat sheet of fibrous connective tissue attaching muscle to bone or other tissues.

apoplexy sudden failure of cerebral function as a result of haemorrhage from, or thrombosis of, a cerebral vessel, characterised by coma, stertorous breathing and degrees of paralysis.

appendicitis inflammation of the vermiform appendix. Uncommon and much more dangerous in pregnancy because the appendix is drawn up in the abdomen and the inflammatory process can spread more readily.

appendix vermiformis vermiform appendix; a worm-like tube with a blind end, projecting from the caecum in the right iliac region.

Apresoline *See* HYDRALAZINE.

Aquanatal exercises form of ante- and postnatal exercises in water enabling women to tone muscles, keep fit and meet other expectant and new mothers, and offered in some areas as an additional option for preparation for labour. Classes are usually conducted in a local public swimming pool by an experienced instructor with a midwife in attendance.

aqueduct canal for the passage of fluid. *A. of Sylvius* canal leading from the third to the fourth ventricle of the brain; stenosis may cause hydrocephalus. Obstruction of the absorption of cerebrospinal fluid occurs after meningitis or subarachnoid haemorrhage.

arachnoid web-like membranous middle covering of the brain between the dura mater and the pia mater. The cerebrospinal fluid circulates in the subarachnoid space beneath it.

arbor vitae literally, the tree of life. 1. the tree-like appearance of white matter in the cerebellum. 2. the appearance of the folds of columnar epithelium lining the cervix uteri.

arborescent branching like a tree.

arcuate arched, bow-shaped. *A. ligament* strong ligament stretching across the subpubic arch of the pelvis.

arcus tendineus a thickening, generally known as the 'white line', in the pelvic fascia, which gives rise to part of the levator ani muscle.

areola pigmented area surrounding the nipple, which darkens during pregnancy. The lacteal sinuses lie under this area of the breast.

arnica homeopathic remedy used to prevent and treat bruising, shock and trauma, useful postnatally to ease perineal discomfort. One 30 C strength tablet should be taken within an hour of delivery, followed by one tablet three times daily for 3 days; arnica cream is useful for bruised buttocks but should not be applied directly over open wounds, e.g. episiotomy suture lines.

aromatherapy complementary therapy using highly concentrated essential plant oils, administered by massage, in the bath, by inhalation or in compresses, douches, pessaries and creams, with therapeutic properties attributed to various chemicals; essential oils should rarely be applied neat to the skin nor administered orally; many are contraindicated in pregnancy and labour as they may cause adverse maternal or fetal effects; avoid all essential oils during the first trimester unless under expert supervision; should not be used on babies under 3 months as the antibacterial action of all oils may interfere with full development of the immune system. Midwives must be properly trained to use aromatherapy.

artefact artificially produced lesion.

arterial pertaining to the arteries.

arteriography radiography of an artery or arterial system after injection of contrast medium into the bloodstream.

arteriole small artery.

arteriosclerosis hardening and thickening of artery walls as a result of atheromatous plaques deposited on the inner surface; causes ischaemia of organs or tissues and leads to hypertension and ultimately degeneration of internal organs associated with old age or chronic disease.

artery vessel that carries blood from the heart to some other part of the body.

arthritis inflammation affecting a joint.

artificial feeding 1. feeding via orifices other than the mouth, e.g. gastrostomy, jejunal, nasal, oesophageal and rectal feeding, which may be used to feed preterm or sick babies. 2. in reference to the feeding of infants, giving food other than human milk.

artificial insemination means of achieving conception by mechanically inserting viable semen into the vagina; this may be either semen produced by the partner (AIH; artificial insemination by husband) or semen from a known or more usually an unknown donor (AID; artificial insemination by donor). In the first instance the partner may legally adopt the baby, whereas in the latter the donor has no legal rights over the child, nor responsibility for his or her upbringing.

artificial respiration maintenance of respiration by any artificial means. As a first aid measure, mouth to mouth (or mouth to mouth and nose in babies) can be used once the airways have been cleared of mucus and other debris. Administration of OXYGEN and mechanical methods of maintaining respiration may be necessary in severe cases. *See also* Appendix 7.

artificial rupture of membranes (ARM) aseptic procedure performed *per vaginam* to induce or accelerate labour progress.

ascites accumulation of free fluid in the peritoneal cavity, rarely seen in pregnancy. In the fetus or neonate, ascites is associated with HYDROPS FETALIS.

aseptic free from pathogenic bacteria.

asexual without sexual organs.

asphyxia suffocation. *A. neonatorum* failure of the baby to breathe at birth; deficiency of oxygen in the blood and an increase in carbon dioxide in the blood and tissues. *See also* APGAR SCORE, Appendix 1.

aspiration the withdrawing of fluid or air from a cavity by suction. *Meconium a.* fetal inhalation of meconium-stained liquor; the hypoxic fetus then passes meconium into the amniotic fluid. Premature inhalation before or immediately following delivery draws the meconium-stained fluid into the lungs where it causes chemical pneumonitis and plugging of the airways. The obstruction produces areas of consolidation and underaeration, as well as hyperinflation, contributing to meconium aspiration syndrome. Suction under direct vision and intubation by an experienced paediatrician at birth, if possible before the baby breathes, may prevent this. *Chorionic villus a.* sample of the chorionic villi aspirated by a syringe or suction pump, either *per vaginam* or transabdominally under ultrasound guidance, towards the end of the first trimester. The sample may be used for DNA analysis, chromosomal analysis or to aid diagnosis of some inborn errors of metabolism. *Vacuum a.* removal of uterine contents by application of a vacuum through a hollow curette or a cannula introduced into the uterus – a method of termination of early pregnancy.

aspirator any apparatus for withdrawing air or fluid from a cavity of the body.

assessment critical analysis and judgement of the status or quality of a particular condition, situation or subject. The initial stage in a process approach to midwifery care, followed by planning, implementation and evaluation of care.

assimilation process whereby food is changed into body tissue.

assimilation pelvis variation in normal development of the sacrum. *High a. p.* the last lumbar vertebra is fused into the sacrum, the pelvis is deep and there may be funnelling and associated difficulty in labour. *Low a. p.* the first sacral vertebra assumes the characteristics of a lumbar vertebra, the pelvis is shallow and the condition does not affect labour.

asthma allergic disease marked by recurrent attacks of paroxysmal dyspnoea, with wheezing, cough and sense of suffocation, triggered by foreign proteins causing smooth muscle spasm in the bronchioles.

Astrup machine apparatus for ascertaining the pH value of the blood.

asymmetrical unequal size or shape of two normally similar structures or of two halves of a structure. *A. growth restriction* fetal growth restriction due to reduced placental nutrition, in which head circumference measurements are within normal limits but abdominal circumference (measured at the level of the liver) is on a lower centile; growth of vital organs is maintained but subcutaneous fat deposition and glycogen storage in the liver stops; sometimes called 'late onset' growth restriction; not to be confused with growth restriction in which the fetal head is small but abdominal growth is conserved. *A. pelvis* pelvis with one side distorted because of disease, injury or congenital maldevelopment. *A. tonic neck reflex* neonatal reflex assessed as part of the examination of the newborn; with the baby in the supine position, the limbs should extend on the side of the body to which the head is turned, whereas those on the opposite side flex.

asymptomatic bacteriuria presence of $>10^5$ bacteria/mL in midstream urine specimen without symptoms suggestive of infection; women are screened in early pregnancy and treated as necessary as it may cause pyelonephritis and preterm labour.

asynclitism parietal presentation of the fetal head in which the transversely placed sagittal suture lies close to the symphysis pubis or sacrum; a sideways rocking mechanism of fetal descent during labour in a flat pelvis. In *anterior a.* the anterior parietal bone moves down behind the symphysis pubis until the parietal eminence enters the brim. The movement is then reversed and the head rocks back until the posterior parietal bone passes the sacral promontory. In *posterior a.* the movements are reversed, with the posterior parietal bone negotiating the sacral promontory before the anterior parietal bone passes behind the symphysis pubis. *See* SYNCLITISM.

atelectasis incomplete expansion of the lung. *Primary a.* present from the moment of birth. *Secondary a.* may occur as a result of aspiration of meconium, infected liquor, vaginal discharge or, more rarely, maternal blood. The failure of all or part of the lungs to expand; it results from respiratory obstruction or weakness of the respiratory muscles at birth, especially in the preterm baby.

athetosis condition marked by involuntary movements of the limbs. Seen in children who have suffered intracranial birth trauma or kernicterus.

atlas first cervical vertebra, articulating with the occipital bone of the skull.

atonic pertaining to atony. *A. uterus* uterus lacking efficient muscle tone, either during labour or in the early puerperium.

atony lack of muscle tone.

atresia absence of the opening of a natural canal, e.g. of the oesophagus or vagina; usually a congenital malformation.

atrial pertaining to the atrium. *A. fibrillation* a cardiac arrhythmia marked by rapid randomised contractions of the atrial myocardium, causing a totally irregular, often rapid, ventricular rate. *A. septal defect* a congenital heart defect in which there is persistent patency of the atrial septum as a result of the failure of the foramen ovale to close.

atrium chamber of the heart, formerly called 'auricle'. pl. *atria*.

atrophy wasting of any part of the body as a result of cell degeneration, because of disuse, lack of nourishment or lack of nerve supply.

atropine active principle of belladonna; alkaloid that depresses salivation and respiratory tract secretions, relaxes muscular spasm, accelerates heart rate and dilates pupils; used before administration of general anaesthesia.

attitude relationship of fetal parts – head, spine and limbs – to each other; normally one of flexion but may be deflexed or extended when the position of the occiput is not anterior.

atypical varying from the normal pattern.

audit means of evaluating care, management and organisation to ensure quality and cost-effectiveness. *Clinical a.* usually a cyclical event in which every aspect of health care can be examined and, if necessary, changes made to improve relevant aspects.

auditory concerning the hearing sense. *A. response cradle* device used to screen infants for impairment of hearing. A set of headphones is used to play noises to the baby and a computer analyses the baby's movements in response to the sounds.

augment to increase, enhance or accelerate. *Augmentation of labour* acceleration of a labour that has been diagnosed as not progressing adequately. This may be done by performing AMNIOTOMY or by the intravenous administration of an oxytocic drug such as Syntometrine.

aura premonition that often precedes an epileptic fit but not an eclamptic fit. *See* ECLAMPSIA.

aural pertaining to the ear.

auricle 1. external portion of the ear. 2. former term for either of the two atria or upper chambers of the heart.

auscultation method of examining the internal organs by listening to the sounds that they give out. Auscultation of the FETAL HEART SOUNDS is performed during pregnancy and labour using a Pinard's stethoscope, Doppler ultrasound or cardiotocography.

autistic withdrawn; describes a child with what is referred to as the triad of impairment, i.e. difficulties with language and communication, social relationships and emotional understanding.

autoclave strongly built and hermetically sealed apparatus that uses steam at high pressure to sterilise equipment.

autogenous generated within the body and not acquired from external sources.

autoimmune disease disease caused by the immunological action of an individual's own cells or antibodies on components of the body.

autoinfection self-infection, i.e. infection transferred from one part of the body to another by fingers, towels, etc.

autolysis self-digestion; the breakdown of tissue, as in uterine INVOLUTION during the puerperium. Surplus muscle is broken down into simple substances, absorbed into the bloodstream and excreted in the urine.

automated auditory brainstem response test (AABR) one of two tests in the Newborn Hearing Screening Programme; records brain activity in response to clicking sounds via sensors placed on the baby's head; babies who fail to respond to this test are referred for a full auditory diagnostic assessment.

autonomic self-governing. *A. nervous system* sympathetic and parasympathetic systems, which control involuntary muscle.

autonomy self-governing, independent. Midwives' professional autonomy means that they are personally responsible for their own actions and are legally permitted to oversee the total care of women with normal pregnancies and labours.

autopsy post-mortem examination.

autosomal dominant inheritance pattern of inheritance of autosomal (non-sex) chromosomes; inheritance of (dominant) altered genes from one parent causes the related disorder to be expressed; there is a 50% chance of inheriting the altered genes and disorder; such disorders include achondroplasia, Huntingdon's chorea and myotonic dystrophy. *See also* AUTOSOMAL RECESSIVE INHERITANCE.

autosomal recessive inheritance pattern of inheritance of autosomal (non-sex) chromosomes, expressed only when two altered genes are inherited together, one from each parent, both of whom are normally healthy; carriers inherit one healthy and one altered set of genes; there is a 25% chance of inheriting the disorder if both parents are carriers.

autosome any chromosome other than the X or Y sex chromosomes.

avascular not vascular; bloodless.

avitaminosis state resulting from vitamin deficiency.

axilla the armpit. pl. *axillae*.

axillary pertaining to the axilla. *A. tail of Spence* a process of mammary tissue extending to the axilla.

axis 1. an imaginary line passing through the centre of a body. 2. the second cervical vertebra. *a. of the birth canal/pelvis* imaginary line representing the course taken by the fetus in its passage through the pelvic canal, downwards and backwards through the pelvic brim and major part of the cavity, then, at the level of the ischial spines, turning through a right angle to proceed downwards and forwards. *See also* PELVIS. pl. *axes*.

axis traction forceps obstetric forceps designed to allow traction to be applied in the line of the pelvic axis when the head is above the level of the pelvic outlet; rarely used now.

azoospermia absence of spermatozoa in semen.

Babinski's reflex (sign) normal neonatal reflex, triggered by stroking the sole of the foot, in which the large toe bends upwards instead of downwards; flexion develops later when the infant learns to walk.

Baby Friendly Initiative (BFI) World Health Organization (WHO) and United Nations Children's Fund (UNICEF) campaign to ensure that all mothers are facilitated to breastfeed to enable them to benefit from the health and social advantages. The WHO/UNICEF initiative, Ten Steps to Successful Breastfeeding, offers health professionals an inexpensive, effective means by which to promote breastfeeding and an award incentive: a hospital that implements all 10 steps and achieves a 75% breastfeeding rate is awarded a Global Award; one that implements all 10 steps and achieves a 50–75% breastfeeding rate is awarded the UK Standard; a Certificate of Commitment is given when a hospital is working towards the 10 steps.

Ten steps to successful breastfeeding

- Breastfeeding policy available and communicated to all staff.
- All health-care staff trained to implement the policy.
- All pregnant mothers informed of the benefits and management of breastfeeding.
- Mothers assisted to commence breastfeeding within half an hour of delivery.
- Education of mothers regarding breastfeeding and maintenance of lactation even when separated from their babies.
- Neonates to be given only breast milk unless medically necessary.
- Provide 24-hour rooming in.
- Encourage on-demand breastfeeding.
- No teats or dummies to be given to breastfeeding babies.
- Establish breastfeeding support groups.

Bach flower remedies system of complementary medicine devised by Dr Edward Bach and based partly on homeopathic principles, in which remedies made from plants are used to treat emotional and psychological disorders. There are 38 flower remedies plus RESCUE REMEDY. *See also* HOMEOPATHY.

bacille Calmette–Guérin (BCG) vaccine used for inoculation against tuberculosis, given during the first week of life to infants of tuberculous mothers.

bacilluria presence of bacilli in urine.

bacillus general term for any rod-shaped organism, mostly gram-negative except for *Koch's b.* and *Döderlein's b.*, which are Gram-positive (*see* GRAM STAIN). pl. *bacilli*.

backache exaggerated lumbar lordosis as a result of increased progesterone and relaxin levels in pregnancy frequently causes backache. Postural correction, wearing a lumbar support and/or physiotherapy, osteopathy, chiropractic or learning the ALEXANDER TECHNIQUE may help.

backwards displacement of the uterus *See* RETROVERSION of the uterus.

bacteraemia presence of bacteria in blood.

bacteraemic shock *See* ENDOTOXIC SHOCK.

bacteria microscopic unicellular organisms, universally distributed. As part of the normal flora (commensals) they are beneficial to health, e.g. DÖDERLEIN'S BACILLUS. Pathogenic bacteria that enter the tissues cause disease by producing *toxins*, resulting in inflammation or the formation of granulomas, or by inducing a hypersensitivity reaction. Bacteria are classified as Gram-positive or Gram-negative based on their reaction to the Gram stain. Aerobic bacteria require oxygen; anaerobes only grow in the absence of OXYGEN; facultative anaerobes adapt to either environment. *Exotoxins* are extremely potent poisons produced by some Gram-positive bacteria. *Endotoxins* cause hypotension, fever, disseminated intravascular coagulation and shock. Other toxins include haemolysins and leucocidins, which destroy red and white blood cells respectively; kinases, which lyse blood clots; and enzymes, which attack tissue. sing. *bacterium*.

bacterial vaginosis (BV) vaginal flora overgrowth, e.g. of *Gardnerella vaginalis*, causing vaginal discharge with characteristic fishy odour; not a sexually transmitted infection but may be triggered by increased sexual activity, stress, other infections and use of perfumed feminine hygiene products; occurs in 15–29% of pregnant women; linked to pelvic inflammatory disease, preterm labour, recurrent urinary tract infections, postpartum infection, and uterine infections following termination, surgery or insertion of intrauterine contraceptive device; treated with antibiotics, e.g. metronidazole. Formerly known as gardnerella.

bacteriological examination microscopic examination of body fluids or tissues to identify bacteria.

bacteriology science of the study of bacteria.

bacteriophage virus that infects bacteria.

bacteriostatic able to prevent multiplication of bacteria.

bacteriuria bacteria in the urine, of significance when there are 10^5 organisms/mL. *Asymptomatic b.* occurs in 5% of pregnant women; if untreated this can progress to pyelonephritis.

bag of membranes amnion and chorion containing amniotic fluid and fetus; bag of waters, amniotic sac.

ballottement literally, bouncing. Tapping a structure in fluid, e.g. the fetus in the amniotic sac, causes it to rebound against the examining fingers. *Internal b.* elicited by inserting two fingers *per vaginam* at about 16–18 weeks of pregnancy to tap the fetus, causing it to float away and quickly return to the examining fingers. *External b.* elicited during an examination *per abdomen* when the head is not engaged; the fetal head is tapped sharply on one side, floats away and is then felt to return against the examining fingers.

Bandl's ring extreme thickening of the RETRACTION RING of normal labour, occurring when labour is obstructed; palpable as a transverse ridge across the abdomen; a sign of imminent uterine rupture.

barbiturates large group of hypnotic drugs, derivatives of barbituric acid. They should be avoided, except when required as anticonvulsants, as dependence and tolerance occur readily.

Barlow's test neonatal test to diagnose congenital dislocation of the hip (CDH), a modification of Ortolani's test. The baby lies on his back with feet pointing towards the examiner who grasps each leg with knees and hips flexed, places the middle fingers of each hand over the greater trochanter and the thumb of each hand on the inner aspect of the thigh. The thighs are abducted and the middle finger of each hand pushes the greater trochanter forward; if the hip is dislocated the femoral head will 'click' as it enters the acetabulum; the femoral head can be displaced backwards out of the acetabulum by exerting slight pressure when the hips are flexed and adducted (Barlow's sign).

Barr body small dark-staining body seen in the nucleus of normal female cells, often obtained from a smear of the buccal cavity and examined microscopically.

barrier contraception mechanical barrier to prevent sperm from entering cervical canal, e.g. diaphragm.

barrier nursing precautions taken by staff to prevent infection from one mother spreading to other mothers and/or staff, which normally involves caring for the mother and/or baby in a separate room or cubicle. Staff wear gowns, gloves, masks, goggles and overshoes when caring for the mother/baby. *Reverse b. n.* aims to protect the patient from external infection, e.g. after organ transplantation.

bartholinitis inflammation of one or both BARTHOLIN'S GLANDS, producing an abscess or cyst.

Bartholin's glands two glands situated in the labia majora, with ducts opening in the vagina, just external to the hymen; they produce the secretion that lubricates the vulva.

basal body temperature temperature of the body at rest. In natural family planning it is taken on waking before any activity or after at least an hour's rest.

basal metabolic rate (BMR) the minimum heat produced by a person at rest who has fasted for 18 hours; test to measure the amount of oxygen consumed, expressed as a percentage above or below the norm; in pregnancy the BMR is increased by about 30%.

base 1. lowest part or foundation. *B. of the fetal skull* consists of two temporal, one ethmoid and one sphenoid bone, and part of the OCCIPUT, firmly fused together. 2. main ingredient of a compound. 3. the non-acid part of a salt; a substance that combines with acids to form salts, essential for maintaining normal ACID–BASE BALANCE; excess concentration leads to ALKALOSIS and the pH rises.

basophil leucocyte that has an affinity for basic dyes.

battledore placenta placenta with the umbilical cord attached to the margin instead of the centre. *See also* PLACENTA.

Battledore placenta

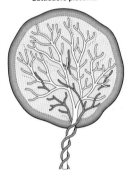

Bell's palsy facial paralysis caused by oedema of facial nerve. Occasionally occurs temporarily in pregnancy.

Benedict's qualitative reagent solution containing sodium carbonate, sodium citrate and copper sulphate, used to detect glucose and other reducing substances in urine or stools.

Benefits Agency organisation working on behalf of the Department of Work and Pensions; assesses the need for financial support and provides payments, exemption certificates and loans as appropriate; responsible for administration of maternity benefits.

benzodiazepines group of drugs with similar molecular structure, including the sedative-hypnotics (antianxiety agents), e.g. chlordiazepoxide, diazepam, oxazepam, flurazepam, clorazepate, and the anticonvulsant clonazepam. Prolonged use of these drugs may cause dependence.

bereavement loss through death or separation, or loss of previous good health, wealth or position, which produces a psychological reaction with 'stages' of anger, denial, disbelief and, finally, acceptance.

beta- β, second letter of Greek alphabet; used to denote the second position in a classification system. *B.-adrenergic receptors* specific sites in cells that respond to adrenaline (epinephrine). *B.-blocker* drug (e.g. antihypertensive drugs) that blocks the action of adrenaline at beta-adrenergic receptors on cells of effector organs; neonatal hypoglycaemia and bradycardia can occur if they are used in late pregnancy. *B. haemolytic streptococcus* virulent streptococcus capable of haemolysing erythrocytes, causing serious infection in neonates. *B. thalassaemia* see THALASSAEMIA.

betamethasone sodium phosphate a synthetic glucosteroid, the most active of the anti-inflammatory steroids; may be administered intramuscularly, 24 mg in divided doses, in women threatening preterm delivery before 34 weeks' gestation to decrease risk of respiratory distress syndrome by inducing increased lecithin levels in the baby.

bi- prefix meaning 'two'.

bicarbonate salt of carbonic acid (H_2CO_3) in which one hydrogen atom has been replaced by a base, e.g. sodium bicarbonate, $NaHCO_3$, used to correct ACIDAEMIA.

bicornuate having two horns. *B. uterus* congenital malformation in which the uterine body (corpus) is partially or completely divided vertically; normal pregnancy and labour are possible but may be associated with persistent malpresentation and retained placenta.

bidet low narrow basin on a stand with running water used for washing the perineum and external genitalia.

bifid cleft into two parts or branches. In SPINA BIFIDA the spinous processes of one or more vertebrae fail to unite and remain divided.

bifidus factor present in human milk; promotes growth of Gram-positive bacteria in gut flora, particularly *Lactobacillus bifidus*, which prevents multiplication of pathogens.

bifurcation fork or separation into two branches; may occur in the uterus because of abnormal fetal development, leading to inability to carry a pregnancy successfully to term.

bilateral pertaining to both sides.

bile dark green substance secreted by liver cells, stored in the gallbladder and passed into the intestine, where it assists digestion by emulsifying fats and activating lipase. *B. ducts* ducts through which the bile passes from the liver and gallbladder to the intestine. *B. pigments* BILIRUBIN and BILIVERDIN.

biliary pertaining to the bile duct.

bilirubin bright yellow/orange bile pigment, resulting from the breakdown of haemoglobin; it is fat soluble and unconjugated until rendered water soluble, i.e. conjugated, by the liver, when it is excreted as stercobilin in the faeces. If this process fails at any point, bilirubin passes into the skin and sclera, and JAUNDICE or ICTERUS results.

bilirubinometer instrument for measuring the serum bilirubin concentration.

biliverdin green bile pigment, oxidised form of bilirubin.

Billings' method method of family planning in which the woman is taught to recognise changes in cervical mucus occurring 3–4 days before ovulation in order to avoid intercourse around that time. The mucus increases in amount and becomes thinner in consistency to facilitate the passage of spermatozoa through the cervix. When used in conjunction with monitoring of body temperature it is known as the symptothermal method.

bimanual using both hands. *B. examination* examination of the pelvic cavity, in which one hand is on the abdomen and the other has one finger in the rectum or one or two fingers in the vagina. *B. compression of the uterus* manoeuvre to arrest severe postpartum haemorrhage after delivery of the placenta when the uterus is atonic. The right hand is introduced into the vagina and closed to form a first, which is pressed into the anterior vaginal fornix. The left hand, on the abdominal wall, pulls the uterus forwards so that the anterior and posterior walls are pressed firmly together, enabling direct pressure to be applied to the placental site to stop the bleeding.

Bimanual compression of the uterus

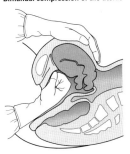

binovular developing from two ova. In binovular twin pregnancy two complete gestation sacs, each with fetus, placenta, chorion and amnion, develop in the uterus together. Also termed *dizygotic, dichorionic* or *fraternal* twins. The infants may be of the same or different sexes and like or unlike each other in appearance, as with any siblings who are not twins. About five times more common than uniovular twins.

biochemical screening tests that screen for conditions or diseases through analysis of biochemical markers; in pregnancy maternal serum screening may be used to screen for fetal Down's syndrome or inherited metabolic disorders; the newborn blood-spot screening test relies on biochemical MARKERS to identify babies with conditions such as cystic fibrosis.

biochemistry chemistry of living matter.

biophysical profile assessment of fetal well-being, based on fetal adaptations to declining placental function in the presence of fetal growth restriction or maternal disease; assesses fetal body or limb movements, tone, breathing movements, amniotic fluid volume and cardiotocograph and gives each a score of 0 or 1, with a healthy fetus achieving a score of 5.

biopsy observation of living matter. Removal of tissue from the body for microscopic examination and diagnosis.

biorhythm any cyclic biological event affecting daily life, e.g. menstrual cycle, sleep pattern.

biparietal diameter (BPD) measurement of the distance between the two parietal eminences of the fetal skull. Assessed in pregnancy using ULTRASOUND to confirm gestational age; accurate to within a week. When the BPD has passed through the maternal pelvic brim the head is engaged. CROWNING occurs when the BPD distends the vulva during delivery and the fetal head no longer recedes between contractions. *See* ENGAGEMENT.

biparous giving birth to two infants at the same time, i.e. twins.

bipolar relating to two poles or ends, and used in reference to the fetus and the parturient uterus. *B. disorder* (formerly manic depression) psychiatric disorder in which the person experiences elevated and depressive mood states leading to impaired functioning, including changes in sleep patterns, activity levels and cognitive functioning; may be accompanied by psychosis; women with bipolar disorder have a 50% chance of developing PUERPERAL PSYCHOSIS.

birth canal bony and soft tissue structures through which the fetus must pass to be born. *See* PELVIS.

birth centre environment where women can give birth with a focus on supporting normal birth with less medical intervention; may be freestanding or adjacent to a hospital maternity unit

birth certificate statement issued by the registrar for births, marriages and deaths for the district in which the baby is born, which certifies details of parentage, name and sex of child, and date and place of birth. This certificate must be obtained by the parents or, failing them, anyone present at the delivery within 42 days of birth in England (21 days in Scotland). It gives legal status to the child and is necessary before Child Benefit can be paid. A birth certificate is issued to any baby born alive, irrespective of the period of gestation. A stillbirth certificate is issued for babies of 24 weeks maturity or longer who did not breathe or show other signs of life after complete expulsion from the mother.

birth control prevention or avoidance of conception.

birth injury trauma to the baby sustained during birth. *See* HAEMORRHAGE,

CEPHALHAEMATOMA *and* ERB'S PARALYSIS.

birth mark congenital skin blemish or spot, usually visible at birth or soon after. *See also* NAEVUS.

birth, notification of someone present or in attendance at a birth, or within 6 hours afterwards, must notify the Director of Public Health about the birth within 36 hours (Public Health Act, 1936); usually undertaken by the midwife in attendance.

birth plan plan prepared by the expectant mother, usually in conjunction with her partner and midwife, which records her preferences for care during and after labour.

birth rate the number of births during one year per 1000 total estimated mid-year population (crude birth rate), per 1000 estimated mid-year female population (refined birth rate), or per 1000 estimated mid-year female population of child-bearing age, i.e. between the ages of 15 and 45 (true birth rate).

birth, registration of either parent must register the birth within 42 days at the registrar's office in the district in which the birth took place (21 days in Scotland). Failure to do so incurs a fine. The responsibility rests with the midwife if the parents default.

birthweight weight of a baby immediately following delivery, providing a baseline for assessing future development and used for national statistics; average birthweight in the UK for a healthy baby born at term is currently 3.5 kg.

birthing chair chair on which to give birth; combines advantages of an upright position with good visibility and access for the midwife during delivery; some delivery beds convert into a chair. Disadvantages are a higher mean blood loss and increased incidence of postpartum haemorrhage, but tilting the chair to 40° to the vertical immediately before delivery and during the third stage of labour may reduce these risks.

birthing room room, usually for normal labour and delivery, furnished comfortably and in a home-like way.

birthing stool stool on which a mother sits to give birth.

bisacodyl oral aperient or suppository used to combat constipation.

bisacromial diameter diameter measured between the acromion processes on the shoulder blades. The fetal measurement is about 12 cm.

bisexual 1. hermaphrodite. Having gonads of both sexes. 2. indicates the sexual preference of an individual for intimate contact with others of both sexes.

Bishop's score method of assessing the favourability of the cervix before induction of labour.

bitemporal the diameter measured between the most distant points of the coronal suture; on the fetal skull it measures 8.2 cm.

bitrochanteric diameter diameter measured between the greater trochanters of the femora; approximately 10 cm on the fetus; the diameter that engages in breech presentation.

bladder reservoir for urine, of obstetrical importance because of its position in front of the uterus and vagina. Pressure on the bladder from the enlarging uterus, or the presenting part, once engaged near term, may cause frequency of micturition. A retroverted uterus may incarcerate the bladder, leading to urinary retention between 12 and 20 weeks of pregnancy. Bladder distension during labour may inhibit uterine action and may lead to delay or haemorrhage.

blastocyst very early pregnancy about a week after conception; the outer layer (trophoblast) develops into the placenta and chorion; the inner cell mass, projecting into the cavity, develops into the fetus and amnion.

Bishop's score for assessing favourability of cervix before induction

CRITERIA	SCORE			
	0	1	2	3
CERVIX				
Dilatation (cm)	Closed	1–2	3–4	5+
Length (cm)	3	2	1	0
Consistency	Firm	Medium	Soft	
Position	Posterior	Central	Anterior	
HEAD				
Station (in cm) above ischial spines	−3	−2	−1	0

Score of 5 or below: in a primigravida this is unfavourable. Ripeness of the cervix is encouraged by the insertion of prostaglandin E_2 (Prostin E_2) in the form of a vaginal pessary on the evening before induction. Score of 6 or more: indicates a favourable cervix for induction.

blastoderm germinal cells of the embryo consisting of three layers – ectoderm, mesoderm, endoderm.

bleeding time the time required for a small inflicted wound to cease bleeding, normally 3–4 minutes.

blighted ovum anembryonic pregnancy.

BLISS (Baby Life Support Systems) charitable organisation that raises money for equipment for babies requiring special and intensive care in neonatal units.

blister collection of serum between the epidermis and the true skin. The appearance of watery blisters on the body of an infant within the first 3 weeks of life may be a sign of PEMPHIGUS NEONATORUM.

block 1. obstruction or stoppage. 2. regional anaesthesia. *Epidural b.* anaesthesia produced by injection of local anaesthetic between the vertebral spines and beneath the ligamentum flavum into the extradural space. It is widely used for the relief of pain in labour. *Paracervical b.* anaesthesia of the inferior hypogastric plexus and ganglia produced by injection of local anaesthetic into the lateral fornices of the vagina. *Pudendal b.* anaesthesia produced by blocking the pudendal nerves, accomplished by injection of local anaesthetic into the tuberosity of the ischium. *See also* EPIDURAL ANALGESIA, PARACERVICAL BLOCK, PUDENDAL BLOCK.

blood fluid circulating through the heart and blood vessels, supplying oxygen and nutritive material to all parts of the body and removing waste products, etc., essential for maintaining fluid balance. Blood is composed of fluid plasma (55%) and blood cells and platelets (45%) suspended in the fluid. *Plasma* consists of 92% water, 7% proteins and less than 1% inorganic salts, organic substances other than proteins, dissolved gases, hormones, antibodies and enzymes. Plasma from which fibrinogen has been removed is called serum. *Blood cells and platelets* include erythrocytes (red blood cells), which carry oxygen via haemoglobin from the lungs to the tissues, leucocytes (white blood cells), the body's primary defence against infection, and platelets (thrombocytes), which initiate blood clotting by adhering to the edges of injured tissue and creating a matrix on which the clot forms. There are approximately $4.2-5.4 \times 10^{12}$ erythrocytes/L in the average female adult; $5-10 \times 10^9$ leucocytes/L, although this number greatly increases when infection is present; and about $150-400 \times 10^9$ platelets/L. *Fresh b.* is useful in cases of active sepsis or haemolytic disease, or to replace blood lost through haemorrhage. *Stored b.* is kept for up to 3 weeks at 4°C and is useful for all emergency cases of haemorrhage.

blood clotting coagulation. *See* CLOTTING.

blood count *See* Appendix 2.

blood gas analysis laboratory studies of arterial and venous blood to measure oxygen and carbon dioxide levels, pressure or tension, and hydrogen ion concentration (pH). Blood gas analysis determines P_aO_2 – partial pressure (P) of oxygen (O_2) in arterial blood (a); SaO_2 – percentage of available haemoglobin saturated (Sa) with oxygen (O_2); P_aCO_2 – partial pressure (P) of carbon dioxide (CO_2) in arterial blood (a); pH – the extent to which the blood is alkaline or acidic; HCO_3 – the level of plasma bicarbonate, an indicator of the metabolic acid–base status.

blood grouping *See* ABO BLOOD GROUPS.

blood pressure (BP) pressure or force exerted by the blood against the blood vessel walls, generally referring to arterial blood pressure; determined by the pumping action of the heart, resistance to arteriole blood flow, elasticity of the artery walls, blood and extracellular fluid volume, and blood viscosity. It is measured in the brachial artery with a sphygmomanometer. *Systolic b.p.* the maximum pressure during contraction of the ventricles; *diastolic b. p.* pressure in the vessel when the ventricles are at rest. The midwife should assess the mother's blood pressure at every antenatal appointment and refer to the obstetrician if the systolic pressure rises above 130 mmHg or the diastolic pressure rises above 90 mmHg or more than 15 mmHg above the first-trimester baseline reading.

blood products products derived from blood that may be issued for immediate use, e.g. red cells, platelets; frozen down in their natural state for later use, e.g. fresh frozen plasma (FFP); or pooled and concentrated to achieve therapeutic levels, e.g. factor VIII concentrate to treat haemophilia. Most units of blood are issued for transfusion as packed red cells; the supernatant fluid (plasma) contains platelets, white cells, coagulation factors and plasma proteins, including immunoglobulin.

blood sugar concentration of sugar in blood, most commonly glucose; recorded in millimoles per litre (mmol/L). Adult non-pregnant values are between 3.3 and 5.3 mmol/L, and pregnant values are between 3.3 and 6.1 mmol/L. Neonatal concentrations may be much lower: 2.2–5.3 mmol/L. *See also* HYPOGLYCAEMIA.

blood transfusion introduction of blood from a donor to the circulation of a recipient.

blood urea proportion of urea in blood, normally between 2.5 and 5.8 mmol/L (15–35 mg/100 mL); in pregnancy the level is lowered to between 2.3 and 5.0 mmol/L (14–30 mg/100 mL).

blood volume total quantity of blood in the body, the regulation of which is affected by the intrinsic mechanism for fluid exchange at the capillary membranes and by hormonal influences and nervous reflexes that affect the excretion of fluids by the kidneys. A rapid fall in blood volume, as in haemorrhage, reduces cardiac output and causes SHOCK; an increase in blood volume, as in retention of water and salt in the body because of renal failure, causes increased cardiac output, which eventually increases arterial blood pressure. Blood volume can be assessed via an intravascular catheter, e.g. CENTRAL VENOUS PRESSURE catheter, which measures pressure in the right atrium, or via a Swan–Ganz catheter, which measures pressure on both sides of the heart.

'blues' normal physiopsychological adaptation to the early postnatal period in which the mother experiences labile emotions, thought to be mainly caused by fluctuating hormone levels as her body reverts to the non-pregnant state; usually occurs between 3 and 7 days postnatally but may last longer; the midwife should ensure that the mother has adequate psychosocial support and that her condition does not become so protracted that she is at risk of developing more serious psychological problems.

body mass index (BMI) weight in kilograms divided by height (metres) squared. A BMI of 20–25 is normal; below 20 is underweight; over 25 is overweight.

bone marrow substance in the hollow cavities of bones. *Red b. m.* in trunk and skull bones only, forms all red and white blood cells except some lymphocytes. *Yellow fatty b. m.* in the long bones of adults is not normally concerned with blood formation.

booking the initial appointment of a pregnant woman with a midwife to arrange antenatal and labour care, discuss any issues of concern and begin to develop a working relationship, held in the mother's home, general practitioner's surgery, health centre or hospital antenatal clinic. A detailed history is taken of the mother's personal and family medical, surgical, obstetric and social history and baseline observations of weight, urinalysis and blood pressure are recorded; blood is taken for a variety of tests.

booking visit first antenatal appointment to introduce the expectant mother to the maternity service and enable her to obtain information about the pregnancy and birth, as well as enabling the midwife to take a full personal social, psychological and medical history, initiate relevant tests and investigations and discuss the parents' options for care.

borborygmus rumbling sound produced by flatus in the intestine.

bottle feeding *See* ARTIFICIAL FEEDING.

bougie flexible instrument made of plastic or gum elastic, used to dilate a stricture, e.g. in the oesophagus, urethra or vagina.

bowel the intestine. *B. sounds* sounds caused by the propulsion of intestinal contents through the lower alimentary tract; absence of bowel sounds indicates decreased or absent peristaltic movement, as occurs in paralytic ileus and advanced intestinal obstruction following abdominal surgery, e.g. Caesarean section.

Bowman's capsule commencement of the kidney nephron, which surrounds a tuft of renal capillaries – the *glomerulus*. Filtration takes place from the blood into the TUBULE; also called glomerular capsule.

Boyle's anaesthetic machine continuous- flow anaesthetic machine that supplies oxygen and nitrous oxide, together with cyclopropane, halothane and other anaesthetic agents as required.

brachial relating to the arm. *B. artery* continuation of the axial artery along the inner side of the upper arm. *B. plexus* nerve plexus situated just above the clavicle and in the root of

the neck, formed by anterior primary rami of the fifth, sixth, seventh and eighth cervical spinal nerves and first thoracic nerve; may be damaged during birth by forcible widening of the angle between the head and shoulders during a breech delivery or by a vertex presentation with shoulder dystocia. ERB'S PARALYSIS or KLUMPKE'S PARALYSIS may result.

brachydactylia abnormally short fingers.

bradycardia abnormally slow heart beat with a pulse rate of less than 60 beats per minute or, in the fetus, a heart rate of less than 100 beats per minute.

bradykinin peptide formed by degradation of protein by enzymes; a powerful vasodilator that causes contraction of smooth muscle.

brain highly specialised area of the central nervous system within the cranium. *See also* FALX CEREBRI *and* TENTORIUM CEREBELLI.

brain death irreversible coma.

brain scanning imaging technique used to detect brain abnormalities, e.g. neonatal intraventricular haemorrhage.

bran husk of grain, high in roughage and B vitamins, frequently recommended to relieve antenatal constipation but should only be used in conjunction with a greatly increased fluid intake.

Brandt–Andrews manoeuvre method of delivering the membranes and placenta after separation and descent into the vagina, now superseded by CONTROLLED CORD TRACTION.

brassiere (bra) garment to support the breasts to prevent overstretching of the ligaments of Astley Cooper; pregnant women should be encouraged to wear a well-fitting, supportive brassiere with wide shoulder straps; postnatally, front-opening brassieres large enough for the lactating breasts should be advised.

Braxton Hicks contractions painless, irregular uterine contractions occurring during pregnancy, named after the obstetrician who first described them, which improve blood flow to the placenta and fetus; the intensity, frequency and regularity increase as pregnancy progresses. Sometimes mistaken for true labour or referred to as 'false labour'.

breast mammary glands, normally two in number, situated on the anterior chest wall over the second to the sixth ribs and separated from the chest wall by a layer of loose connective tissue. *See diagram. B.feeding* mothers should be encouraged to breastfeed their babies unless there are strong medical or social reasons for not doing so; midwives should ensure adequate antenatal preparation and provide practical and emotional support to facilitate the mother to establish breastfeeding.

breast milk substance secreted from the breasts via the nipples, consisting first of COLOSTRUM, then, once lactation is established, of foremilk, a high volume of relatively low fat milk, followed by hindmilk, a lower volume of milk with up to five times more fat than foremilk; contains fats, fatty acids, carbohydrates, proteins, vitamins, minerals and trace elements, plus a number of anti-infective factors including immunoglobulins, lysozymes, lactoferrin, bifidus, hormones and growth factors. *B. m. substitutes* infant formulae, usually made from modified cow's milk, with strict regulations as to the permitted constituents specified in the Infant Formula and Follow-on Formula Regulations 1995; formulae may be whey dominant, in which the ratio of proteins approximates to the whey–casein ratio in human milk, or casein dominant, which forms relatively indigestible curds in the stomach, intended to make the baby feel satisfied but which places greater metabolic demands on the baby.

breast pump suction apparatus used to withdraw milk from the breast, with a vacuum created by hand pressure on

Anatomy of the breast

Groups of acini (milk-producing cells) surrounded by contractile myoepithelial cells within the alveoli

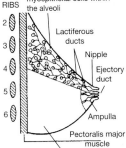

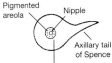

15–20 lobes separated by fibrous tissue

Pigmented areola

Nipple

Axillary tail of Spence

15–20 Montgomery's tubercles (sebaceous ducts)

a rubber bulb or by an electrical pump.

breech the buttocks. *B. presentation* longitudinal lie with fetal buttocks presenting in the lower uterine pole, as a result of pelvic, uterine, fetal or incidental causes; approximately 2.5% incidence at term. Abdominally the fetal head is palpated in the fundus; vaginally the buttocks, anal orifice, genitalia or feet are palpated; diagnosis is confirmed on ultrasound; changing the presentation with EXTERNAL VERSION or MOXIBUSTION may be attempted. *B. delivery* fetal dangers include intracranial haemorrhage, hypoxia, fractures, dislocations and soft tissue injuries; episiotomy is performed in second stage before the anterior buttock is delivered to minimise compression on the aftercoming fetal head; the feet are guided over the perineum and a loop of cord is pulled down to prevent traction on the umbilicus. If the arms are flexed, the shoulders are delivered with the next contraction; extended arms are delivered using LÖVSET'S MANOEUVRE. Once the trunk and shoulders are born, the baby is allowed to hang by his/her own weight (BURNS–MARSHALL TECHNIQUE) for about 1 minute, to aid flexion and descent of the head. When the hair line appears at the vulva the baby is held firmly by the ankles and the trunk is raised in a wide arc up and over the mother's abdomen. The MAURICEAU–SMELLIE–VEIT MANOEUVRE is used when the head is extended and fails to descend.

bregma anterior fontanelle, a kite-shaped membranous area in the head of the fetus and infant at the junction of the frontal, coronal and sagittal sutures. *See also* FETAL SKULL.

brim of the pelvis pelvic inlet. *See* PELVIS.

British Pharmacopoeia (BP) official publication containing lists of drugs and other medicinal substances in use in the UK, with details of preparation, dosages and methods of administration; compiled under the auspices of the General Medical Council and regularly revised and updated.

broad ligaments two folds of peritoneum, continuous with the perimetrium, extending to the pelvic sides; containing fallopian tubes, parametrium, ovarian blood and lymph vessels, uterine nerves and ureters.

bromethol basal anaesthetic.

bromocriptine dopamine agonist, a derivative of ergot alkaloids used to inhibit prolactin secretion and suppress lactation. Given orally, 2.5 mg on day

Types of breech presentation

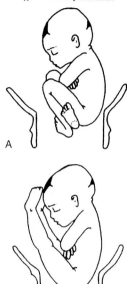

A, with flexed legs; B, with extended legs.

1, followed by 2.5 mg twice daily for 14 days.

bronchopulmonary dysplasia chronic respiratory condition occurring in babies who have been ventilated for long periods or who have needed prolonged oxygen therapy, which causes serious disruption of lung growth and patches of collapse and fibrosis, found on examination of radiographs and lung specimens. Ventilation and supplementary oxygen for several weeks or even months is required to keep the arterial oxygen tension above 55 kPa.

bronchus one of the main branches of the trachea. pl. *bronchi.*

brow presentation cephalic presentation with the attitude of the fetal head midway between flexion and extension; presenting mentovertical diameter of 13.0–13.75 cm is larger than that of the average pelvis, leading to obstructed labour. Causes include an android pelvis, in which the biparietal diameter impacts in the sacrocotyloid diameter of the pelvis, causing head extension, and fetal conditions, e.g. hydrocephaly or anencephaly. Occurs in approximately one in 1000–1500 labours. Abdominally the fetal head will be high above the pelvic brim; vaginally the head will not be felt, but occasionally the bregma and orbital ridges can be felt. Caesarean section is usually required or, if not feasible, vaginal manipulation to flex the head to a vertex presentation or to extend it further into a face presentation, with forceps then being applied. Internal podalic version and breech delivery may also be attempted.

brown fat thermogenic adipose tissue containing a dark pigment, arising during embryonic life between the shoulder blades, behind the sternum, in the neck and around the kidneys and suprarenal glands; utilised by the neonate for production of heat as required.

Brushfield's spots grey or yellow spots in the irises of the eyes of children with Down's syndrome.

buccal smear scrapings from the buccal mucosa that are examined microscopically to study BARR BODIES.

buffer chemical substance that, when present in a solution, helps to resist a change in pH. *Bicarbonate b.* the principal buffering system in the blood, involving bicarbonate ions and carbon dioxide.

bulbocavernosus muscles two perineal muscles surrounding the vaginal introitus with a weak sphincter-like action.

bulla blister. pl. *bullae.*

bupivacaine hydrochloride (Marcain) local analgesic drug used for epidural, intrathecal and para-cervical analgesia. Duration of action 2–4 hours; may cause hypotension. Dose –0.25%, 0.5% or 0.75%.

Burns–Marshall technique one method for delivering the fetal head in breech delivery. Once the trunk is delivered, the baby hangs by its own weight to aid flexion and descent of the head; when the hair line appears at the vulva the head is at the outlet; it is delivered by raising the trunk, holding the baby's ankles and exerting slight traction, and carrying the trunk through a wide arc up and over the mother's abdomen. The perineum is retracted exposing the baby's nose and mouth, enabling clearing of the airway and oxygen administration; birth of the head is completed slowly, usually with obstetric forceps applied to the aftercoming head.

Brow presentation

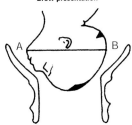

A–B, mentovertical diameter 13.5 cm.

cabergoline contemporary drug of choice for women with anovulatory hyperprolactinaemia; preferred to bromocryptine as it has significantly less side effects.

caecum 1. first or proximal part of the large intestine, forming a dilated pouch distal to the ileum and proximal to the colon, and giving off the vermiform appendix. 2. any blind pouch.

Caesarean section obstetric operation to extract the fetus from the uterus through an incision in the abdominal and uterine walls after 24 weeks of pregnancy, performed for cephalopelvic disproportion; grade III or IV placenta praevia; placental abruption to deliver a live fetus; first-stage fetal distress; failure to progress, especially with malpresentation or malposition; serious maternal medical conditions; and preterm delivery when the extrauterine environment is deemed to be safer for the fetus than the intrauterine environment. *Lower segment C. s. (LSCS)* involves a horizontal incision in the lower uterine segment to reduce the risks of uterine rupture during a subsequent labour. *Classical C. s.* involves a vertical incision in the body of the uterus, the scar of which is more likely to rupture in subsequent pregnancies. The midwife assists with pre- and postoperative care and observations; she may also be required to assist the anaesthetist or attend the mother throughout the operation if regional anaesthesia is used; act as the scrub nurse or 'runner' in theatre; or receive the baby and provide immediate resuscitative care to the infant. *See also* Appendix 3 (Figure 7).

calcaneum, calcaneus bone of the foot forming the heel.

calcification deposit of lime in any tissue, sometimes found in a mature or postmature placenta.

calcium chemical element, the most abundant mineral in the body, which, in combination with phosphorus, forms calcium phosphate, the dense, hard material of the bones and teeth. Calcium is an important cation (positively charged ion) in intra- and extracellular fluid, essential for normal blood clotting, maintenance of a normal heart beat and initiation of neuromuscular and metabolic activities; in pregnancy women should be encouraged to eat foods containing calcium, which is found in milk, cheese and green vegetables and may be given in vitamin form; vitamin D is essential for its absorption. Tetany resulting from hypocalcaemia may occur in newborn babies. Symbol Ca.

calculus stone formed in the gallbladder, bile duct, kidney or ureter.

Caldicott guardian named member of an NHS Trust responsible for agreeing and reviewing internal protocols governing protection and use of patient-identified information by staff within the health-care system; protocols must meet national requirements and be monitored regularly.

Caldwell–Moloy classification classification of female pelves as gynaecoid, android, anthropoid and platypelloid. *See* PELVIS.

calipers compasses for measuring diameters and curved surfaces, e.g. of the fetal skull.

callus 1. tissue that grows around fractured ends of bone and develops into new bone to repair the injury. 2. localised hyperplasia of the horny layer of the epidermis caused by pressure or friction.

calorie unit of heat, the amount needed to raise the temperature of 1 g of water by 1°C. Used to measure body heat and energy needs in food; 1 g of carbohydrate or protein gives 4 kcal and 1 g of fat gives 9 kcal; during pregnancy and lactation the mother needs about 2500 kcal/day; a full-term infant needs 110 kcal/kg body weight/day after the fourth day of life. The SI counterpart of this unit is the JOULE (J), which equals 4.2 cal.

cancer general term to describe malignant growths. *See* CARCINOMA.

Candida genus of yeast-like fungi, commonly part of the normal flora of the mouth, skin, intestinal tract and vagina, but which may also cause infections. *See also* CANDIDIASIS. *C. albicans* pathogen that causes thrush infection.

candidiasis mucous membrane infected with *Candida albicans*, particularly affecting the vagina, skin, mouth or nails, but may also invade the bronchi and lungs and can become systemic.

Canesten *See* CLOTRIMAZOLE.

cannula tube for insertion into a cavity or blood vessel; during insertion its lumen is usually occupied by a trocar.

capillary hair-like. 1. minute vessels connecting arterioles and venules, with semipermeable walls to facilitate interchange of various substances between the blood and tissue fluid. 2. minute vessels of the lymphatic system. *C. haemangiomata* strawberry marks.

caput head. *C. succedaneum* oedematous swelling formed on the fetal head by pressure from the dilating cervical os, which, after rupture of the forewaters, restricts the venous return in the superficial tissues. It is present before delivery but disperses within a few hours; it pits on pressure, can cross suture lines when present on the scalp

Caput succedaneum

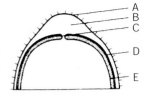

A, skin; **B,** subcutaneous tissue; **C,** aponeurosis; **D,** periosteum; **E,** bone.

and is found over the face or buttocks if these are the presenting parts. Bruising may also be a feature. *See also* CEPHALHAEMATOMA.

carbimazole antithyroid drug used to treat thyrotoxicosis; antenatal administration may cause fetal hypothyroidism.

carbohydrate food composed of carbon, hydrogen and oxygen (CHO); sugar, starch and cellulose foods that provide heat and energy; 1 g of carbohydrate yields 17 kJ (4 kcal); may be stored in the body as glycogen for future use or, in excessive amounts, as fats.

carbon dioxide (CO_2) gas present in minute quantities in the atmosphere and formed in the body tissues by the oxidation of carbon and excreted by the lungs; used with oxygen to stimulate respiration; usually measured as P_aCO_2.

carbon monoxide (CO) colourless, odourless, tasteless gas, formed by burning carbon or organic fuels with a scant supply of oxygen; inhalation causes central nervous system damage and asphyxiation.

carbonate carbonic acid salt.

carcinogenic causing carcinoma.

carcinoma malignant epithelial tumour that may develop in any part of the body; cancer.

cardia 1. cardiac opening. 2. the cardiac part of the stomach surrounding the oesophagogastric junction, distinguished by the presence of cardiac glands.

cardiac pertaining to the heart. *C. arrest* sudden, often unexpected stoppage of effective heart action requiring emergency cardiac care and cardiopulmonary resuscitation (CPR). *C. disease in pregnancy* in the UK today, most commonly resulting from congenital heart disease (previously due more to mitral stenosis after rheumatic fever or chorea). Pregnancy puts additional stress on the heart so that the condition often worsens; careful monitoring is essential; long-term antenatal admission to hospital may be necessary. Labour care aims to prevent problems of overexertion and cardiac overload although first stage is often short; forceps delivery or Caesarean may avoid the need for active second-stage pushing; third stage is the most dangerous for the mother because of increased blood volume from strong uterine contractions, possibly exacerbated by oxytocics: the obstetrician should be consulted about oxytocic administration for women with heart disease.

cardinal of first importance. *C. ligaments* two thickened bands of parametrium stretching from the uterine cervix to the lateral walls of the pelvis, which help to support the uterus; also known as transverse cervical or Mackenrodt's ligaments.

cardiogram graphic representation of the heart's action traced by the electrocardiograph.

cardiomyopathy, postpartum rare but potentially fatal complication of late pregnancy and the first 5 months after delivery in which myocardial inflammation and enlargement cause left ventricular heart failure and thromboembolic problems; management focuses on relieving congestive heart failure symptoms; full recovery may take several months and a few women require heart transplant.

cardiotocography (CTG) fetal heart activity (*cardio-*) and uterine contraction (*-toco-*) recording (*-graphy*) to assess fetal well-being in pregnancy or labour, via transducers placed on the maternal abdominal wall; the fetal heart rate may also be assessed via an electrode placed on the fetal scalp during labour. The recording is analysed for reduced baseline variability, decelerations and irregularities in the fetal heart rate in response to maternal uterine action and is one means of detecting fetal hypoxia.

cardiovascular relating to the heart and blood vessels.

caries decay or necrosis of bone. *Dental c.* decay of teeth.

carneous mole mass of blood clots surrounding a dead embryo and retained by the uterus. Also termed blood mole, fleshy mole, missed abortion. *See* TUBAL MOLE.

carotene deep yellow pigment converted to vitamin A by the liver.

carotid bodies small neurovascular structures in the bifurcation of the right and left carotid arteries containing chemoreceptors that monitor oxygen content in blood and help to regulate respiration.

carpal tunnel syndrome hand tingling and numbness resulting from pressure on the median nerve as it passes through the carpal tunnel in the wrist. Common in pregnancy as local oedema increases pressure; often worse at night, may be relieved by sleeping with the hands splinted. More severe cases may need physiotherapy, osteopathy or chiropractic; acupuncture and reflexology may also help; usually resolves spontaneously after delivery although very occasionally surgery is required to correct the problem.

carpopedal spasm muscular spasm of the hands and feet in TETANY.

carrier 1. person who carries pathogenic organisms in the body without symptoms of disease; organisms may be passed to others, e.g. haemolytic streptococci in the throat of a carrier could be transmitted to the genital tract of a recently delivered woman. 2. in genetics, an apparently normal individual who carries a RECESSIVE or SEX-LINKED GENE. *C. oil* an oil, e.g. grapeseed or sweet almond, in which essential oils used in aromatherapy are diluted and applied to the skin in massage as a means of preventing skin-to-skin friction.

cartilage specialised, fibrous connective tissue present in adults, forming most of the temporary skeleton in the embryo, providing a model in which most of the bones develop and constituting an important part of the organism's growth mechanism.

caruncle, caruncula small fleshy eminence, often abnormal. pl. *carunculae*. *Carunculae myrtiformes* small elevations of mucous membrane around the vaginal orifice; the remnants of the ruptured hymen.

case conference meeting of professionals involved in the care of a particular person (often a child), to agree patterns of action and monitor progress.

casein one of the proteins of milk; it is less digestible and present in larger quantities in cows' milk than in human milk.

caseinogen precursor of casein; converted into casein by rennin in the gastric juice of babies.

caseload midwifery system of midwifery care in which each midwife is responsible for a group of women, i.e. a caseload, resulting in better communication and continuity of care for the women and improved job satisfaction for the midwife.

case mix database computerised record system that combines all of the data received from patient administration and operational systems to provide comprehensive information about all treatment and services received by each patient during an episode of care; helps to develop expected care profiles for different groups, analyse and compare different treatment regimes and produce comparative costings for different treatments; may be used for medical audit.

cast structure moulded in a hollow organ and retaining the shape of the cavity of the organ when shed, e.g. a decidual cast shed from the uterus in tubal pregnancy or casts from the renal tubules found in the urine in kidney disease.

castration removal of the male testicles or the female ovaries.

catamenia menstruation.

cataract opacity of the crystalline lens or its capsule, which impairs vision. *C. cataract* sometimes occurs in newborn babies, either as a result of a familial condition or maternal RUBELLA in early pregnancy; also associated with GALACTOSAEMIA.

catecholamine sympathomimetic amines [dopamine, adrenaline (epinephrine) and noradrenaline (norepinephrine)], which play an important role in the body's physiological response to stress. Their release at the sympathetic nerve endings increases the rate and force of muscular contractions of the heart, thereby increasing cardiac output and constricting peripheral blood vessels, resulting in raised blood pressure; elevates blood glucose levels by hepatic and skeletal muscle glycogenesis; and promotes an increase in blood lipids by increasing the catabolism of fats.

catgut suture material made from sheep gut, used mainly for buried sutures as it is absorbed by the body.

catheter tube made of polythene, rubber, gum elastic or silver, perforated near its blind end; introduced into various hollow organs, vessels or canals for the purpose of CATHETERISATION.

catheterisation insertion of a catheter to introduce or withdraw fluid or to measure fluid pressure, e.g. bladder, cardiac or umbilical catheterisation.

cathode negative electrode.

cation ion carrying a positive electric charge, e.g. sodium (Na), copper (Cu).

cauda equina literally, horse's tail; the nerves into which the spinal cord divides at its termination in the lumbar region.

caudal block regional analgesia achieved by the introduction of the agent through the sacral hiatus. It is less reliable than entering the epidural space by the lumbar route. *See* EPIDURAL ANALGESIA.

caul occasional condition in which the amnion fails to rupture in labour and envelops the baby's head at birth; it should be ruptured as quickly as possible to establish a clear airway.

caulophyllum homeopathic remedy used to induce or accelerate labour in certain women, but which should not be used routinely or by the midwife without adequate training. *See also* HOMEOPATHY.

cautery hot instrument or chemical agent used to destroy tissue by burning it, sometimes used to treat cervical erosion.

cavity of the pelvis hollow within the pelvic walls, bounded by the pelvic brim (inlet) above and the outlet below.

cele suffix meaning 'a tumour', e.g. meningocele, a swelling consisting of a protrusion of meninges.

cell structural unit of which all multicellular organisms are made, consisting of a nucleus with central nucleolus, CHROMOSOMES with surrounding semifluid cytoplasm containing mitochondria, RIBOSOMES and other bodies, all contained within the cell membrane. All living cells arise from other cells,

either by division of one cell to make two, as in MITOSIS and MEIOSIS, or by fusion of two cells to make one, as in the union of the sperm and ovum to make the zygote in sexual reproduction. The cells of the body differentiate during development into many specialised types with specific tasks to perform and are organised into tissues and thence into organs.

cellulitis diffuse inflammatory process within solid tissues, characterised by oedema, redness, pain and functional disturbance, caused by infection with streptococci, staphylococci or other organisms. Usually occurring in the loose tissues beneath the skin, it may also occur in tissues beneath mucous membranes or around muscle bundles or surrounding organs. Pelvic cellulitis in tissues surrounding the uterus is called parametritis and may occur if infection has been introduced into the genital tract, as a complication of septic abortion or following labour.

cellulose carbohydrate; the fibrous outer covering of vegetable cells, which is not digestible in the alimentary tract of humans but which gives bulk and stimulates peristalsis.

Celsius internationally recognised unit of temperature (°C), previously called centigrade in the UK; water freezes at 0°C and boils at 100°C.

census enumeration of a population, first introduced in England and Wales in 1801 and repeated every 10 years (except 1941), which records name, address, sex, occupation, marital status and other social information.

centigrade *See* CELSIUS.

centile *See* PERCENTILE.

centimetre one-hundredth of a metre.

central nervous system brain and spinal cord.

central venous pressure (CVP) pressure of blood in the right atrium, which indicates the balance between cardiac output and venous return, measured via a catheter inserted through the median cubital vein to the superior vena cava; the distal end of the catheter is attached to a manometer, positioned at the bedside so that the zero point is at the level of the right atrium; each time the mother's position is changed the zero point on the manometer must be reset. Invaluable in situations in which the amount of blood lost cannot be accurately estimated, e.g. in concealed ABRUPTIO PLACENTAE, to ensure adequate fluid replacement without overloading the circulation. The normal range of fluid volume in the right atrium is from 15 to 110cm of saline when the zero point of the scale corresponds to the mid-axillary line.

centrifuge apparatus that rotates test tubes at great speed to precipitate bacteria, cells and other substances.

cephalhaematoma collection of blood beneath the periosteum of one of the cranial bones, which causes a fluctuant swelling to develop on the baby's head within 48 hours of birth; occasionally, the cranial bone beneath is fractured. A cephalhaematoma is distinguished from a CAPUT SUCCEDANEUM by the fact that it develops after birth and is limited to one bone; it takes several weeks to subside, but no treatment is necessary unless severe jaundice occurs.

Cephalhaematoma

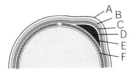

A, skin; **B,** subcutaneous tissue;
C, aponeurosis; **D,** periosteum;
E, blood under periosteum; **F,** bone.

cephalic version conversion to a head presentation. *See* VERSION.

cephalometry head measurement, used antenatally to measure the BIPARIETAL DIAMETER to assess fetal maturity and growth, most accurately by ULTRASOUND; after birth the baby's head is measured with a tape measure.

cephalopelvic relationship of the fetal head to the maternal pelvis. *C. disproportion* misfit between the fetal head and the maternal pelvis, assumed when the fetal head will not engage in the pelvis after 36 weeks of pregnancy; may be diagnosed in labour and may cause obstructed labour.

cephaloridine antibiotic derived from CEPHALOSPORIN, which, if given antenatally by the oral, intramuscular or intravenous route, will cross the placenta and enter the fetal circulation.

cephalosporin naturally occurring antibiotic, chemically similar to PENICILLIN.

cerclage encircling of a part with a ring or loop, as in correction of an incompetent cervix uteri or fixation of the adjacent ends of a fractured bone.

cerebellum hindbrain, below the cerebrum and behind the medulla oblongata.

cerebral pertaining to the cerebral hemispheres. *C. dysrhythmia* condition in which the brain shows an abnormal pattern of electrical waves on an electroencephalograph (EEG) tracing, occurring in epilepsy and eclamptic convulsions. *C. haemorrhage* bleeding from or into one of the cerebral hemispheres. *C. palsy* persistent motor disorder resulting from hypoxia *in utero*, asphyxia neonatorum and periods of apnoea and cyanosis, as in RESPIRATORY DISTRESS SYNDROME, HYPOGLYCAEMIA and other conditions.

cerebrospinal relating to the brain and spinal cord. *C. fluid* fluid in the ventricles of the brain, secreted by the choroid plexuses and circulating in the subarachnoid space and membranes surrounding the spinal cord. It protects the nerves in the brain and spinal cord from jar and injury. Excess cerebral fluid is found in HYDRO-CEPHALUS.

cerebrum largest part and centre of the higher functions of the brain, occupying the greater portion of the cranium and consisting of the right and left cerebral hemispheres.

cervical pertaining to the neck. 1. in obstetrics, pertaining to the cervix uteri or neck of the uterus. *C. canal* channel starting at the internal cervical os, communicating with the body of the uterus, and ending at the external os, opening into the vagina. *C. cerclage* see SHIRODKAR OPERATION. *C.cytology* examination of cervical cells to detect abnormal changes. *C. incompetence* failure of the cervix to hold the pregnancy in the uterus; a cause of second-trimester abortion, characterised by premature rupture of the membranes and painless expulsion of the fetus. *C. intraepithelial neoplasia (CIN)* classification of types of cervical dysplasia. CIN I is mild, reversible dysplasia; CIN II is moderate, reversible dysplasia; CIN III is severe, irreversible dysplasia and carcinoma *in situ*, requiring surgery to prevent the development of invasive carcinoma. 2. *C. vertebrae* small, joined neck bones.

cervicitis infection of the mucous membrane lining the cervix uteri. *Acute c.* occurs in GONORRHOEA. *Chronic c.* usually caused by low-grade infection following slight tearing of the CERVIX during delivery; the inflamed mucous membrane protrudes through the external os to the vaginal part of the cervix forming an erosion, which bleeds readily; treatment is by cauterisation to destroy infected tissues.

cervix constricted portion or neck. *C. uteri* neck of the uterus opening into the vagina; 2.5 cm long.

Chadwick's sign dark purplish discolouration and congestion of vaginal membrane caused by increased vascularity; a sign of pregnancy but

occurs in any condition in which there is pelvic congestion.

chancre the initial lesion of SYPHILIS, developing at the site of inoculation.

Changing Childbirth report (1993) Department of Health report that contained recommendations for improvements to provide women with more accessible, effective and efficient maternity care offering increased choice, control and continuity, with each woman cared for by a 'LEAD PROFESSIONAL'.

CHARGE syndrome syndrome including defects of the eyes, heart and ears, oesophageal atresia and growth retardation; may be associated with CHOANAL ATRESIA.

chemical change this differs from physical change in that a profound alteration in properties results, usually permanently and usually accompanied by the use of energy in a new substance, e.g. HYDROGEN (2 atoms) plus OXYGEN produces water.

chemical compound substance produced by chemical change that may then be broken up into its components only by chemical means, unlike a mixture, which can usually be separated mechanically.

chemoreceptor collection of cells sensitive to alterations in the chemicals contacting them, found in the carotid and aortic body; responsive to changes in the OXYGEN, CARBON DIOXIDE and HYDROGEN ion concentration in the blood. When OXYGEN concentration falls below normal in the arterial blood, chemoreceptors send impulses to stimulate the respiratory centre to increase alveolar ventilation and consequently OXYGEN intake by the lungs.

chemotherapy treatment of illness by chemical means, i.e. with medication. adj. *chemotherapeutic*.

chest thoracic cavity containing the lungs, heart, trachea, bronchi, oesophagus, large blood vessels and nerves.

chi-squared test statistical test to determine whether two or more groups of observations differ significantly from one another, i.e. more than would be expected by chance.

chickenpox varicella, an infectious childhood disease with an incubation period of 12–20 days and characterised by slight fever and eruption of transparent skin vesicles that dry up and may leave pits in the skin. Can be severe in neonates.

chignon large caput succedaneum seen on the head of a baby delivered by ventouse vacuum extraction. *See* VACUUM EXTRACTOR.

child abuse anything that individuals, institutions or processes do or do not do which directly or indirectly harms children or damages their prospects of a safe and healthy development into adulthood. If a child is seen to be in danger of suffering significant harm from physical, sexual, emotional or neglectful causes his or her name may be recorded in the Child Protection Register. If a midwife has reasonable cause to suspect the abuse of a child in a family in her care she must take the appropriate action to protect the child. *See also* CHILDREN ACT 1989.

child benefit weekly payment made to all primary carers of children under 16, or up to age 19 while still in full-time education, payable for each child, with higher rates for the first child and single parents.

child health clinic centre that healthy children attend regularly to be examined by a doctor and health visitor, to ensure normal progress and development.

child minder person approved by and registered with the local authority social services department to care for a small number of children aged from birth to 5 years during the day.

child protection procedures laid down in the Children Act 1989 that focus on the needs of the child; service providers should always consider the child's welfare and interests as paramount in any decision making; policies aim generally to support families to stay together where possible; replaces concept of parental rights with one of parental responsibility; midwives should have an understanding of child protection procedures as they may come into contact with families needing support and guidance. *C. p. register* record of children at risk of, or suspected of being at risk of, abuse; a key worker, usually a social worker, is appointed to ensure the Child Protection Plan is carried out; access to the register of named children is restricted to those with direct dealings with the children.

Child Support Agency government agency set up under the Child Support Act 1991 to operate a scheme for child maintenance in cases where the parents are living apart; responsible for assessing each case in which one parent has requested child maintenance, reviewing the situation at 2-yearly intervals and, if necessary, collecting the money from the absent parent.

childbirth process of giving birth to a baby, parturition. *Natural c.* approach whereby the mother and her partner are well prepared and remain in control of the labour, allowing it to progress naturally without medical intervention, drugs and other stimuli, if at all possible.

Children Act 1989 Act that brings together the comprehensive law relating to children, defining their rights, identifying parental responsibilities and detailing procedures to protect them. Child welfare is paramount in all court decisions, which should be made with minimum delay and, where possible, take into account the child's wishes. The court may issue a variety of orders, including a *contact order*, which requires the person with whom the child lives to permit access to another named person; a *residence order*, which settles arrangements over where a child lives; *care and supervision orders*, to place a child in local authority care; a *child assessment order*, to enable the child to remain in his or her normal residence whilst allowing access for assessment; and an *emergency protection order*, to remove a child from potential harm, usually to local authority care.

chiropody study and care of feet and the treatment of foot diseases, now known as podiatry.

chiropractic form of complementary medicine, similar to osteopathy, based on the principle that the musculoskeletal system is the body's main supporting framework, with all soft tissues attached either inside or outside this framework; trauma, injury, illness and environmental, dietary or genetic factors cause misalignment of the musculoskeletal system, thereby putting strain and tension on other parts of the body, triggering discomforts and disease. Treatment involves mobilisation and manipulation of joints to realign the spine and restore its relationship with the rest of the body. Chiropractic is effective in treating various pregnancy problems, e.g. backache, carpal tunnel syndrome and converting breech presentation to cephalic, and for treating colic in infants, hyperactivity in children, and menstrual and menopausal symptoms in non-pregnant women.

chiropractor practitioner of chiropractic.

Chlamydia trachomatis most common sexually transmitted bacterial infection, prevalent in those under 25 years or with multiple sexual partners; approximately 50% of men and 75% of women are asymptomatic or have non-specific urethritis; associated with subfertility, ectopic pregnancy, preterm labour and premature membrane rupture. Babies born to untreated mothers can contract severe conjunctivitis leading to blindness.

chloasma 'pregnancy mask' or skin pigmentation on the forehead, nose and cheeks.

chloral elixir hypnotic for babies containing 200 mg in 5 mL of solution. Dose: 30 mg/kg body weight for the first 2 weeks of life.

chloral hydrate hypnotic, sedative with mild pain-relieving properties, now rarely used.

chloramphenicol (Chloromyecetin) broad-spectrum antibiotic with specific activity against rickettsiae and many other bacteria. Side effects include serious, even fatal, blood dyscrasias; frequent blood tests are recommended during therapy.

chlordiazepoxide benzodiazepine antianxiety drug for short-term use; also used for acute alcohol withdrawal.

chlorhexidine (Hibitane) coal-tar derivative with wide antibacterial action, especially effective against coagulase-positive staphylococci; extensively used in antibiotic skin cleansers for surgical scrub, preoperative skin preparation and cleansing skin wounds.

chloride chlorine salt; an electrolyte that helps to maintain normal balance of the blood.

chlorothiazide diuretic and antihypertensive drug used to treat hypertension and oedema of congestive heart failure.

chlorphenamine (chlorpheniramine) maleate (Piriton) drug used to relieve allergy and for emergency treatment of anaphylactic reactions.

chlorpromazine (Largactil) antipsychotic agent and antiemetic phenothiazine drug; side effects include drowsiness and slight hypotension.

chlorpropamide antidiabetic drug, contraindicated in pregnancy; may cause neonatal hypoglycaemia.

choanal atresia membranous or bony obstruction of the posterior nares, which causes neonatal respiratory difficulty at or shortly after birth, leading to cyanosis.

cholecystitis inflammation of the gallbladder.

cholestasis of pregnancy *See* INTRAHEPATIC CHOLESTASIS.

chondroblast embryonic cell that forms cartilage.

chordee downward curvature of penis caused by congenital anomaly such as hypospadias.

chorditis inflammation of spermatic (or vocal) cords.

chorea St Vitus' dance, also called Sydenham's chorea. Disease related to rheumatism, probably bacterial, affecting the nervous system; characterised by irregular involuntary muscular movements. In pregnancy it is termed chorea gravidarum; occasionally seen in young primigravidae with a history of childhood rheumatism or chorea, in whom it puts additional strain on the already impaired heart.

chorioangioma collection of fetal blood vessels in WHARTON'S JELLY, forming a tumour on the placenta; little clinical significance but may be associated with POLYHYDRAMNIOS.

choriocarcinoma highly malignant NEOPLASM, occurring in about 3% of cases of HYDATIDIFORM MOLE; detected by raised serum or urinary chorionic gonadotrophin and by radioimmunoassay and treated with cytotoxic chemotherapy and, if necessary, hysterectomy.

chorioepithelioma former term for CHORIOCARCINOMA.

chorion outer of the two membranes enclosing the fetus *in utero*, derived from the TROPHOBLAST; opaque and friable, sometimes retained after delivery. *C. biopsy* removal of tissue from the gestational sac to identify chromosomal and other inherited disorders, which can be performed as early as 8 weeks' gestation and has the advantage over amniocentesis of facilitating termination before 12 weeks. *C. frondosum*

part of the chorion covered by villi in the early weeks of embryonic development before the placenta is formed. *C.laeve* non-villous, membranous part of the trophoblast, which develops into the chorion.

chorionic gonadotrophin *See* HUMAN CHORIONIC GONADOTROPHIN.

chorionic villi minute finger-like projections arising from the TROPHOBLAST and persisting in the chorion frondosum, having an outer SYNCYTIOTROPHOBLASTIC layer with multiple nuclei and without cell walls, and an inner CYTOTROPHOBLASTIC layer with cell walls and single nuclei within each cell. Fetal capillaries are embedded in mesoderm; oxygenated maternal blood spurts in cascades over the villi in the intervillous spaces, so that oxygen, nutrients, etc., may pass into the fetal circulation and CARBON DIOXIDE, etc., may pass out; after 24 weeks' gestation the cytotrophoblastic cell layer remains only in isolated areas.

chorionic villus sampling (CVS; placental biopsy) antenatal aseptic procedure used to obtain small samples of chorion frondosum via a needle or fine cannula inserted into the uterus transabdominally or transvaginally under ultrasound guidance; can be performed after 11 weeks' gestation but earlier than AMNIOCENTESIS although interpretation of CVS results can sometimes be difficult; used to determine fetal KARYOTYPE or obtain fetal DNA; there is a procedure-induced, operator-dependent risk of miscarriage of 1–2%.

chorionicity placental formation in MULTIPLE PREGNANCY; monochorionic twins are connected to a single placenta and have an increased risk of TWIN-TO-TWIN TRANSFUSION SYNDROME; dichorionic twins have two separate placentae, although they may fuse, and there is a lower risk of complications.

choroid plexus vascular fringe-like folds in the PIA MATER in the third, fourth and lateral ventricles of the brain; concerned with formation of cerebrospinal fluid.

Christmas disease hereditary haemorrhagic disease caused by deficiency of clotting factor IX; also called haemophilia B.

chromatin substance of the chromosomes, composed of DNA and basic proteins (histones); the material in the nucleus that stains with basic dyes. *Sex c.* Barr body; mass of condensed, inactive X chromosome found in cells of normal females.

chromatography technique for separating components of a substance dependent on differences in the absorbency of each component when passed through a medium such as paper; used for a wide variety of investigations, such as newborn blood-spot screening for SICKLE CELL DISEASE.

chromosome minute thread-like structures in the cell nucleus, composed of DEOXYRIBONUCLEIC ACID (DNA) and protein, carrying genes that transmit the inherited characteristics. Human cells carry 46 chromosomes, 22 pairs of autosomes and two sex chromosomes (XX or XY). *C. analysis* test to analyse fetal cells obtained by AMNIOCENTESIS or from a blood sample (lymphocytes); cells are cultured in the laboratory and cell division is arrested mid-stage by the drug colchicine; chromosomes are stained to produce a distinct pattern of light and dark bands along the chromosome, with each one being recognised by its size and banding pattern. An individual's chromosomal characteristics are referred to as the KARYOTYPE. *See also* GENE.

chronic prolonged or permanent, e.g. chronic disease; opposite of acute.

cilia fine hair-like processes that grow on the free border of certain epithelial cells. The lining of the fallopian tubes is ciliated epithelium; the cilia wave backwards and forwards, producing a current to propel the ovum from the ovarian end of the fallopian tube to the uterus. sing. *cilium.*

ciliated having cilia.

ciprofloxacin antimicrobial drug, active against Gram-negative organisms, particularly *Chlamydia*; use with caution during pregnancy and breastfeeding.

circulation movement in a circular course, as of the blood. *Fetal c.* circulation of blood in the fetus; the foramen ovale and ductus arteriosus bypass the lungs, and blood is carried to and from the placenta by the umbilical vessels and ductus venosus.

circumcision excision of the prepuce of the penis, which may be necessary if the urinary meatus of the prepuce is obstructed. Performed on healthy Jewish male children on the eighth day of life as a religious ceremony; PLASTIBELL is commonly used for circumcision in many hospitals. *Female c.* female genital mutilation, involving excision of the labia and clitoris and narrowing of the vaginal introitus, performed to ensure chastity and particularly common in areas such as the Sudan. Gynaecological complications include delay in labour, bladder-wall necrosis and urinary or vesicovaginal fistulae.

circumvallate literally, surrounded by a wall. *C. placenta* placenta with a distinct ridge on the fetal surface, caused by a peripheral double fold of chorion, liable to separate partially, causing antepartum haemorrhage.

clamp surgical instrument used to compress part of the body, e.g. to prevent or arrest haemorrhage. *Hollister c.* plastic device to occlude the umbilical cord vessels, applied at birth about 1–2 cm from the umbilicus for about 48 hours, then removed.

clavicle collar bone, articulating with the sternum and the acromion process of the scapula. *Fractured c.* an uncommon birth injury that may be due to traumatic breech delivery or shoulder dystocia, or uncommonly occurring spontaneously as a result of congenital OSTEOGENESIS IMPERFECTA. *See also* CLEIDOTOMY.

cleft lip congenital unilateral or bilateral defect resulting from the failure

Cleft lip

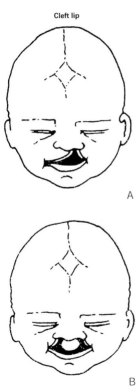

A

B

A, unilateral; **B,** bilateral.

of fusion of the median nasal and maxillary processes in the embryo; usually operable during the first few weeks or months of life.

cleft palate congenital defect in which there is a split or cleft in the palate, either centrally or on one side only, which interferes with sucking and speech and requires corrective surgery that is usually very successful. The most severe form is complete cleft of the palate accompanied by a bilateral CLEFT LIP.

cleidotomy rare procedure involving division of the fetal clavicles with scissors to facilitate delivery of obstructed shoulders, e.g. in a large ANENCEPHALIC fetus.

climacteric physiological changes occurring around the time of the MENOPAUSE.

clinic place where patients or clients receive advice and treatment.

clinical pertaining to or founded on actual observation and treatment of patients, as distinguished from theoretical or experimental. *C. trial* assessment of the effectiveness of modes of treatment by carefully following responses to therapy in defined patient groups. *Controlled c. trial* study in which one or more active treatments are compared with each other and with placebo. *Double-blind c. trial* comparison of different treatments (active and placebo) in which neither participants nor observers know who is receiving treatment until after the study is completed, an attempt to remove bias. *C. directorate* system of devolved management responsible for its own budgeting and use of resources, in which a clinical specialty such as obstetrics and gynaecology is headed by a director who is usually a medical practitioner and assisted by a senior midwife and a business manager. *C. governance* framework through which NHS organisations are accountable for continuous improvement of service quality and care standards by creating an environment in which excellence will flourish. *See also* NATIONAL INSTITUTE FOR HEALTH AND CLINICAL EXCELLENCE (NICE) *and* NATIONAL SERVICE FRAMEWORKS.

clinical nurse specialist nurse who has acquired advanced knowledge and skills in a specific area of clinical practice.

clinical risk index for babies professional scoring tool used to assess initial neonatal risks and for comparing performance of one neonatal intensive care unit with another.

clinical risk management systematic review of adverse events, usually related to delivery of patient care, in order to prevent further incidents.

clinical thermometer instrument for taking body temperature, orally, rectally, in the axilla.

clitoridectomy excision of the clitoris as in female CIRCUMCISION.

clitoris small sensitive erectile organ at the anterior junction of the labia minora; homologue of the penis.

clomethiazole edisilate (Heminevrin) hypnotic, sedative, anticonvulsant drug that depresses the central nervous system; used to treat insomnia, agitation, confusion, acute withdrawal symptoms in alcoholism and drug addiction, and for the control of sustained epileptic fits and eclampsia.

clomifene citrate (Clomid) GONADOTROPHIC drug used to stimulate ovulation.

clone cells that are genetically identical to each other and that are descended by asexual reproduction from the parent cell, to which they are also genetically identical.

clonic of the nature of a jerk; the convulsive stage of a fit.

Clostridium anaerobic Gram-positive spore-bearing BACILLUS, e.g. that of tetanus or gas gangrene.

clot blood cells that form a partially solidified mass in a matrix of fibrin; the solid part of blood after it escapes

from the blood vessels; may also occur in lymph.

clotrimazole (Canesten) antifungal agent administered vaginally as a pessary or cream to treat vaginal 'thrush'.

clotting formation of a jelly-like substance from blood shed at the site of an injury to a blood vessel. Occasionally clots form within blood vessels, causing arteriosclerosis, thrombosis or varicose veins. *C. time* time taken for shed blood to clot, usually 5 minutes. *See* COAGULATION.

cloxacillin semi-synthetic penicillin used to treat staphylococcal infections caused by penicillinase-producing organisms.

clubfoot *See* TALIPES.

coagulase substance produced by certain strains of staphylococci, which causes clotting in plasma; *coagulase-positive* staphylococci, e.g. *Staphylococcus aureus*, are much more dangerous, especially to neonates, than those that are coagulase negative, e.g. *S. albus*.

coagulation clot formation *C. disorder* condition occuring in severe placental abruption, intrauterine death, endotoxic shock and, rarely, amniotic fluid embolism, signified by reduced clotting factors, low fibrinogen and THROMBOCYTOPENIA; profuse bleeding occurs, blood fails to clot and fibrinogen is redirected, leading to DISSEMINATED INTRAVASCULAR COAGULATION (DIC). Investigations include cross-matching, full blood count, prothrombin time, clotting time, platelet counts and measurement of fibrinogen and fibrinogen degradation products; treatment is dependent on the test results.

coarctation of the aorta stricture of the aorta at, or just below, the ductus arteriosus; often diagnosed by absence of femoral pulses.

cocaine hydrochloride topical anaesthetic applied to mucous membranes, more commonly known as a recreational drug leading to psychological dependence in long-term users; absorbed through mucosal surfaces or smoked, as with the highly addictive 'crack'; powerful vasoconstrictor associated with spontaneous abortion, maternal hypertension, placental abruption, stillbirth and small for gestational age babies, possibly due to its appetite-suppressing effects, which lead to poor maternal weight gain. Arterial thrombosis is more common in pregnant cocaine abusers; maternal death results from cardiac arrhythmias, coronary ischaemia, intracranial aneurysms, cerebral haemorrhage or hypertensive convulsions, whereas fetal malformations include intestinal atresia, limb defects, genitourinary disorders and neurological problems.

coccus spherical micro-organism. *See* BACTERIA.

coccydynia persistent pain in the area of the COCCYX.

coccygeus one of two muscles arising from the ischial spines, inserted into the lateral borders of the sacrum and COCCYX, and forming part of the PELVIC FLOOR. Also called ischiococcygeus.

coccyx terminal bone of the spinal column, a fusion of four rudimentary vertebrae.

Cochrane database database of systematic reviews of published clinical research; international multidisciplinary collaboration of health professionals, consumers and researchers who review randomised controlled clinical trials related to pregnancy and childbirth; other medical specialties also have collaborative review groups to examine relevant research.

Code of Professional Conduct document produced by Nursing and Midwifery Council to inform nurses, midwives and health visitors of professional conduct standards required in their professional practice, and to inform the public, other professions and employers of professional conduct standards expected of a registered practitioner.

cohort group of people who possess a common characteristic, e.g. same sex or same profession, used in research to make generalisations derived from quantitative data.

coitus sexual intercourse, copulation. *C. interruptus* method of contraception where the penis is withdrawn from the vagina before ejaculation of semen.

colic severe spasmodic abdominal pain, common in infants up to 3 months old. The baby pulls up his legs, cries loudly, becomes red-faced and expels gas, either as flatus or burping. *Biliary c.* spasm from passage of a gallstone through the bile ducts. *Renal c.* spasm from passage of a stone along the ureter. Painful, ineffective, irregular uterine contractions are sometimes termed colicky.

coliform resembling *Escherichia coli*. *See* BACTERIA.

collapse state of prostration as a result of circulatory failure. *See also* SHOCK.

colloidal solution suspension in water or other fluid of molecules that do not readily pass through animal cell membranes, e.g. blood, plasma and plasma substitutes; valuable for treating shock because they are retained in the circulation.

colon section of the large intestine from the caecum to the rectum.

colostrum thin, yellow, milky fluid secreted from the breasts from 16 weeks of pregnancy and for 3–4 days after birth until lactation is initiated; high in protein and initially low in lactose, with fat content equivalent to breast milk; an important source of passive antibodies.

colour index measurement of the proportion of haemoglobin in red blood cells; normally 1, but <1 in iron-deficiency anaemia and >1 in megaloblastic anaemia.

colpo- pertaining to the vagina.

colpocele hernia of either bladder or rectum into vagina.

colphysterectomy removal of the uterus via the vagina.

colpoperineorrhaphy repair of the pelvic floor, vagina and perineal body, usually undertaken for PROLAPSE.

colporrhaphy repair of the vagina. *Anterior c.* for CYSTOCELE; *posterior c.* for RECTOCELE.

colposcope device for examining the vagina and cervix by means of a magnifying lens; used for the early detection of malignant changes.

colposcopy examination of vaginal and cervical tissue with a colposcope, usually performed after an abnormal cervical smear result to detect abnormal epithelium and benign tumours.

colpotomy incision of the vaginal wall. *Posterior c.* incision through the posterior vaginal fornix to the pouch of Douglas to drain a pelvic abscess.

columnar epithelium type of epithelium containing cylindrical cells.

coma deep unconsciousness from which it is not possible to rouse the patient, caused by cerebrovascular accident, diabetes mellitus, alcoholism, eclampsia or uraemia.

comatose in a coma.

combined test first-trimester Down's syndrome screening test performed via a NUCHAL TRANSLUCENCY (NT) ultrasound scan and by assessment of maternal blood for PREGNANCY-ASSOCIATED PLASMA PROTEIN-A (PAPP-A); results are combined with the maternal age-related Down's syndrome risk to give an overall result, giving higher SENSITIVITY and SPECIFICITY than that of NT or PAPP-A screening alone.

commensal organism that lives on another without harming it. *See also* LACTOBACILLUS ACIDOPHILUS.

Commission for Health Improvement (CHI) independent non-departmental government body for England and Wales with statutory powers, set up to improve quality of patient care by assisting the NHS to address unacceptable standards; replaced by Commission for Healthcare Audit and Inspection (CHAI), which now inspects both NHS and private institutions.

commissure connection. *Posterior c.* fold of skin connecting the labia minora posteriorly.

Committee on Safety of Medicines (CSM) UK organisation responsible for controlling the release of new drugs; also collects data on adverse reactions to drugs via the yellow card system, which enables the CSM to issue warnings about serious adverse effects.

Community Health Council organisation that represents consumer's interests at district level of the NHS; there is a paid secretary but other members are drawn from local organisations, working on a voluntary basis.

compatibility mixing together of two substances without chemical change or loss of power.

compensation in heart disease, ability of the weakened heart to still function adequately.

complement 1. that which adds to something or makes up a deficiency. 2. the thermolabile group of proteins in normal blood serum and plasma that, in combination with antibodies, causes the destruction of particular antigens (as bacteria and foreign blood corpuscles).

complementary making up a deficiency. *C. feed* artificial feed given to an infant to make up the deficient amount of a breastfeed, not now recommended for normal healthy babies. cf. SUPPLEMENTARY. *C. medicine* alternative medicine outside conventional health care but used in conjunction with orthodox medicine, including osteopathy, chiropractic, acupuncture, homeopathy, herbalism, massage, aromatherapy, reflexology, hypnotherapy, shiatsu and many more.

complete abortion bleeding from the genital tract before 24 weeks of pregnancy, resulting in miscarriage; products of conception are expelled, with no requirement for surgical evacuation of the uterus.

compound presentation rare complication of labour in which more than one part of the fetus presents, e.g. head and hand; head and foot; breech, hand and cord.

compression 1. pressing together, as in bimanual compression of the uterus to prevent haemorrhage. 2. in embryology, the shortening or omission of certain developmental stages.

computed tomography (CT) Radiological examination of internal organs using a computer to produce a series of images in cross-section that appear as 'slices' of the organ being examined; can show several different types of tissue in great detail, e.g. lung, bone, soft tissue, blood vessels, and can assist with diagnosis of certain infectious diseases, musculoskeletal disorders and cancers; occasionally, contrast dye is injected into the bloodstream to improve image quality. Also called computed axial tomography (CAT).

computed axial tomography (CAT) *See* COMPUTED TOMOGRAPHY.

computerised records many health records are now held on computer systems, required by law to be secure and to maintain confidentiality, usually achieved by limiting access; a manual record may also be kept. *See also* DATA PROTECTION ACT.

conception 1. formation of an idea. 2. fusion of spermatozoon and ovum to form a viable zygote, the onset of pregnancy.

condom contraceptive device, a sheath covering the penis, worn during sexual intercourse for both contraception and to prevent sexually acquired infections *Female c.* sheath inserted into the vagina.

condyloma wart-like growth near the external genitalia or anus, occasionally syphilitic in origin.

cone biopsy removal of a cone-shaped section from the cervix, performed to confirm diagnosis when a cervical smear test suggests presence of pre-cancerous cells.

confidential enquiry unique form of audit in which case notes are scrutinised by relevant professionals to identify substandard care and allow recommendations to be made for future practice, including the triennial Confidential Enquiry into Maternal Deaths (CEMD), the Confidential Enquiry into Stillbirths and Deaths in Infancy (CESDI) and the Confidential Enquiry into Perioperative Deaths.

congenital born with, term used to describe a malformation present at birth or an infection acquired *in utero*.

Congenital Disabilities (Civil Liabilities) Act 1976 Act, applicable in England, Wales and Northern Ireland, which entitles a child to recover damages if it is proven that he suffered as a result of a breach in duty of care, except where the breach occurred before conception with the knowledge of one or both parents. The same provisions are made in Scottish law. The accuracy and preservation of maternity records is therefore essential.

congenital dislocation of the hip (CDH) condition resulting from abnormal development of the acetabulum, femoral head or surrounding tissues, more common if there is a family history, in a breech presentation and in girls. About 1–2% of neonates have dislocated or dislocatable hips, usually found as part of the routine examinations performed by midwives and paediatricians in the first 24 hours of life and confirmed on ultrasound. Treatment is to stabilise the hip in abduction and flexion using a special harness; many dislocatable hips resolve spontaneously although a few children require surgery.

congenital heart defect structural defect of heart or great vessels, or both.

congenital infection infection acquired *in utero*, including rubella, cytomegalovirus, herpes simplex, HUMAN IMMUNODEFICIENCY VIRUS (HIV), toxoplasmosis.

congestion abnormal accumulation of blood in a part of the body.

congestive pertaining to or associated with congestion. *C. heart failure* a broad term denoting conditions in which the heart's pumping capability is impaired.

conjoined twins Siamese twins; rare congenital abnormality (1 in 200 000 births) whereby MONOZYGOTIC (identical) twins are fused together, usually involving the heads and trunks and occasionally the internal organs; may result from incomplete division of the embryonic cell mass or the embryos may become joined again after they have split; overall survival rate is 5–25%. *See also* TWINS.

conjugate 1. to join or yoke together, e.g. in the liver, bilirubin is combined with albumin by the activity of GLUCURONYL TRANSFERASE to render it water soluble so that it may be excreted via the gut. *See also* ICTERUS GRAVIS *and* JAUNDICE. 2. a conjugate diameter of the pelvis. *See also* PELVIS.

conjunctiva the mucous membrane lining the inner surface of the eyelids and covering the anterior aspect of the eye.

conjunctivitis inflammation of the conjunctiva. *See* OPHTHALMIA NEONATORUM.

connective tissue tissue that binds together or supports the structures of the body. Adipose tissue, areolar tissue, bone, cartilage, fat, blood and fibrous tissue are all connective tissues.

consanguinity blood relationship.

consent in law, voluntary agreement with an action proposed by another. Consent is an act of reason; the person giving consent must be of sufficient mental capacity and be in possession of all essential information to give valid consent. Written informed consent is generally required before many invasive clinical procedures, including amniocentesis and surgery.

constipation decrease in frequency of defecation, difficulty in defecating or a change in bowel habits from the norm; common in pregnancy as a result of smooth muscle relaxation because of the effects of progesterone. Excessive tea consumption, inadequate fluid intake, diet lacking fibre or prophylactic iron supplementation may exacerbate the condition. Postnatally, inhibition and a fear of damage to the already bruised area may contribute to poor bowel habits.

constriction ring localised annular spasm of the uterine muscle at any level but often near the junction of the upper and lower uterine segments. In the first and second stages of labour it may form round the neck of the fetus and in the third stage it forms an HOURGLASS CONSTRICTION of the uterus, causing a retained placenta. It may result from the use of oxytocic drugs in a uterus with uncoordinated function following early rupture of the membranes and especially if intrauterine manipulation is carried out. Relaxation may occur with inhalation of amyl nitrite but often deep anaesthesia is required.

consultant in public health medicine doctor responsible for public health functions, e.g. promoting health, preventing disease, fostering cooperation between the health and social services.

contagion communication of disease from one person to another by direct contact.

contingency screening method of antenatal Down's syndrome screening currently being developed; includes first-trimester BIOCHEMICAL SCREENING (hCG and PAPP-A); may be combined with NUCHAL TRANSLUCENCY SCAN. Women at high risk are then offered more precise diagnostic investigations;

those at low risk exit the screening programme; those with mid-range risks proceed to second-trimester biochemical screening to obtain results that combine first- and second-trimester values, improving DETECTION RATES and reducing the FALSE-POSITIVE RATE.

continuing professional development (CPD) further study after the attainment of basic qualifications. Under the Nursing and Midwifery Council's regulations, all midwives, nurses and health visitors are required to demonstrate periodic updating and refreshment throughout their professional lives, to enable them to provide contemporary, research-based care to patients and clients.

continuity of care term used to describe care given to one woman from booking until discharge to the health visitor in which good communication from one appointment to the next and between all professionals ensures that there are no omissions or duplications in the care of that mother. Continuity does not necessarily mean that only one professional is in contact with the mother: this would indeed be unrealistic. However, verbal and written communication between professionals should be comprehensive enough to avoid errors and to facilitate the mother's sense of security in the care she is receiving. Various schemes of care exist in an attempt to provide continuity of care. *See also* CASELOAD MIDWIFERY, CHANGING CHILDBIRTH REPORT, TEAM MIDWIFERY.

continuous inflating pressure (CIP) pressure of water used against a baby's spontaneous breathing in respiratory distress syndrome (RDS). Its purpose is to prevent HYPOXAEMIA, apnoeic attacks or rising levels of carbon dioxide in the blood (Pco_2).

continuous negative pressure (CNP) a rarely used method of treating a neonate with the RESPIRATORY DISTRESS SYNDROME. Sub-atmospheric pressure is applied to the baby's thorax in a body box.

continuous positive airway pressure (CPAP) a technique used to prevent total alveolar collapse on expiration in a baby with RESPIRATORY DISTRESS SYNDROME. Positive pressure of 2–5 cmH_2O is applied into the respiratory tract by the nasal or endotracheal route or by face mask. CPAP is used with patients who are breathing spontaneously. When the same principle is used in mechanical ventilation, it is called positive end-expiratory pressure (PEEP).

contraception the prevention of conception. *Barrier method c.* for women include occlusive caps, e.g. diaphragm, vault cap or vimule; should be used with spermicidal creams, foam or jelly for extra protection. Men use a condom or sheath; a female condom is available, although this is more to protect against HIV than for contraception. *Chemical c.* Oral contraceptive pills for women are either a combination of oestrogen and progesterone or progesterone alone; a male contraceptive pill is also being developed. Injectable progestogen is available for women requiring a method that is as reliable as possible. Intrauterine devices or coils can be inserted into the uterus and can remain *in situ* for several years. *'Natural' c.* includes the rhythm method or 'safe period', the temperature method, Billings' method and coitus interruptus or withdrawal. The most reliable method is sterilisation, of either the woman by laparoscopy or laparotomy, or the male by vasectomy.

contraceptive pertaining to contraception; any means used to prevent conception.

contracted pelvis pelvis in which any diameter of the brim, cavity or outlet is reduced to an extent that it interferes with labour progress.

contraction temporary shortening of muscle fibre, which returns to its original length during relaxation. Contractions of the uterus during pregnancy are painless and are termed Braxton Hicks contractions, after the obstetrician of that name. During labour they are usually painful and are accompanied by RETRACTION.

controlled cord traction method of delivering the placenta and membranes, in which, once the placenta is known to have separated, the midwife places the ulnar border of her left hand in the suprapubic region and pushes the contracted uterus upwards, while with her right hand she gains a firm hold on the cord and exerts gentle traction, following the curve of Carus. The membranes are eased out slowly and gently to avoid tearing them, which can lead to retained products. If an oxytocic drug is administered to facilitate separation of the placenta it is *not* necessary to await signs of separation and descent before attempting controlled cord traction; however, if the placenta has been allowed to separate physiologically it is *imperative* to await these signs to avoid risks to the mother of haemorrhage or even uterine inversion.

controlled drugs preparations subject to the Misuse of Drugs Act 1971, Misuse of Drugs (Notification of and Supply to Addicts) Regulations 1973 and the Misuse of Drugs Regulations 1985, which regulate the prescribing and dispensing of psychoactive drugs, including narcotics, hallucinogens, depressants and stimulants. Midwives using controlled drugs in a hospital or institutional setting must follow locally agreed procedures and policies. If pethidine is required for community use the midwife applies to the local supervisor of midwives for a signed supply order form to obtain the drug from an approved pharmacist; controlled drugs prescribed to an individual mother for home delivery legally belong to the woman. Unwanted controlled drugs must be surrendered to an authorised person, i.e. the pharmacist who provided the drug or a medical officer, but not the supervisor of midwives. Destruction of controlled drugs is carried out by the midwife in the presence of an authorised person, i.e. a supervisor of midwives, pharmaceutical officer, regional medical officer, police officer or inspector of the Home Office Drugs Branch.

controlled trial research method in which one group of subjects in a study do not receive the experimental treatment or investigation in an attempt to decrease the risk of error and increase the possibility that the study results accurately reflect reality.

convulsions violent involuntary contractions of voluntary muscle, due to eclampsia, epilepsy or hysteria in the mother; the commonest causes of neonatal convulsions are HYPOXIA, cerebral birth injury and HYPOGLYCAEMIA.

Cooley's anaemia uncommon, severe type of anaemia in Mediterranean races; thalassaemia.

Coombs' test blood test used to determine the presence of red cell antibodies to enable detection of HAEMOLYTIC DISEASE OF THE NEWBORN (HDN); if a mother is Rhesus negative cord blood is taken at birth to check ABO and Rhesus typing. *Direct C.t* or direct antiglobulin test (DAT) detects maternal antiglobulin antibodies coating the baby's red cells; if positive, HDN may develop; the baby's serum bilirubin levels should be checked. *Indirect C. t* or indirect antiglobulin test (IAT) is used to match blood products before transfusion.

copper cuprum, element, minute quantities of which are essential to health. Symbol Cu.

Copper-7 INTRAUTERINE CONTRACEPTIVE DEVICE containing copper wire embedded in the plastic shape.

co-proxamol *See* DEXTROPROPOXYPHENE HYDROCHLORIDE.

copulation sexual intercourse, coitus.

cord *See* UMBILICAL CORD.

cordocentesis percutaneous umbilical cord blood sampling (PUBS); fetal blood sampling; funipuncture; invasive antenatal investigation after 18 weeks' gestation to obtain a fetal blood sample, usually performed by entering the intrahepatic portal vein or by placental cord insertion to reduce haemorrhage. Risks include miscarriage, fetal haemorrhage and infection; fetal sedation by administering maternal opiates may reduce fetal blood movement during the procedure. Developments in chromosomal and genetic analysis from amniotic fluid and chorionic villus sampling mean that cordocentesis is less used now but it remains useful to check fetal blood indices and to perform *in utero* blood transfusions for haemolytic disease.

cornea transparent anterior part of the eyeball in front of the lens, covered by conjunctiva; severe infective conjunctivitis may cause ulceration, scarring and visual impairment. *See also* OPHTHALMIA NEONATORUM.

cornu literally, horn; junction of uterus and fallopian tube. pl. *cornua.*

coronal suture skull suture between the two frontal and the two parietal bones. *See* FETAL SKULL.

coronary encircling. *C. arteries* those that supply the heart. *C. thrombosis see* THROMBOSIS.

corpus body. *C. albicans* white scar left on the ovarian surface after retrogression of a corpus luteum. *C. luteum* literally, yellow body; structure, first greyish and later yellow, developing from the graafian follicle after ovulation and lasting 12 days before degenerating; if conception occurs it lasts about 14–16 weeks until the placenta is formed and fully functioning. *C. uteri* body of the uterus.

corpuscle small body or cell, e.g. the blood cell.

corrosive agent that destroys or eats into other substances.

cortex outer layers of an organ, e.g. the cortex of the cerebral hemispheres, kidney, suprarenal gland or ovary.

cortical necrosis irreparable damage to the renal cortex due to severe vasospasm of the arteries occurring after severe shock, especially ABRUPTIO PLACENTAE.

corticoids group of hormones secreted by the adrenal cortex.

corticosteroids steroid hormones produced by the ADRENAL cortex and their synthetic equivalents; divided into *glucocorticoids* (cortisol or hydrocortisone, cortisone, corticosterone), *mineralocorticoids* (aldosterone, desoxycorticosterone, corticosterone) and androgens. Also called adrenocortical hormones and adrenocorticosteroids.

cortisone STEROID hormone produced by the adrenal cortex; antiallergic and anti-inflammatory – used in allergic states, e.g. asthma, rheumatoid arthritis, severe skin conditions, ulcerative colitis. Hydrocortisone is similar; prednisone and prednisolone are synthetic forms of cortisone and hydrocortisone respectively.

coryza head cold, with headache, watery discharge from the eyes and nasal catarrh.

costal pertaining to the ribs.

cot death *See* SUDDEN INFANT DEATH SYNDROME (SIDS).

cotyledon placental division or lobe.

Council for Healthcare Regulatory Excellence UK statutory overarching body; promotes best practice and regulatory consistency in all healthcare professions, i.e. doctors, dentists, nurses, midwives, health visitors, opticians, osteopaths, pharmacists and other professions suuplementary to medicine.

counselling consultation and discussion process in which the counsellor listens and facilitates the client to solve problems, explore difficulties constructively and make appropriate decisions, so that the future may be approached more confidently and more constructively.

couvade psychosomatic condition in which the father experiences pregnancy symptoms.

Couvelaire uterus deep purplish-blue bruised appearance of the uterus in severe concealed abruptio placentae, caused by high uterine tension forcing blood between the myometrial fibres.

coxa hip joint. *C. valga* hip deformity with increased angle between the neck and the shaft of the femur. *C. vara* deformity with decreased angle between the neck and the shaft of the femur.

cracked nipple nipple damage occurring during breastfeeding as a result of the baby being incorrectly fixed on the breast, which causes pressure leading to soreness and bleeding; can be prevented by teaching the mother how to position the baby at the breast correctly. If the nipple is too sore to continue feeding, treatment involves mechanical milk expression to maintain lactation. Creams containing camomile or the application of moist camomile teabags may ease the discomfort and aid healing.

cramp painful spasmodic muscular contraction, usually in the calf; may be associated with vitamin B, calcium or salt deficiency and relieved by eating appropriate foods; ischaemia of leg muscles may cause night cramps, which may be eased by elevating the foot of the bed.

cranial relating to the cranium. *C. nerves* 12 pairs of nerves arising directly from the brain.

cranioclast instrument for crushing the fetal skull, rarely used now.

craniosacral therapy form of osteopathic treatment using very gentle manipulation of the cranium to release tensions within the skull, thought to cause various problems; successfully used to treat fractious babies after difficult forceps or vacuum extraction deliveries, and colic and hyperactivity in older infants.

craniostenosis premature closure of the cranial suture lines, requiring surgery to relieve raised intracranial pressure.

craniotomy perforation and extraction of the crushed fetal skull to allow vaginal delivery; now obsolete.

cranium the skull.

C-reactive protein (CRP) plasma protein produced by the liver in response to inflammation; used as a serum marker for inflammation; can give indication of underlying disease or effectiveness of treatment.

creatine non-protein substance synthesised in the body from amino acids (arginine, glycine, methionine); readily combines with phosphate and is stored as high-energy phosphate, necessary for muscle contraction.

creatinine nitrogenous compound, the end product of creatine metabolism, formed in muscle, passed into the blood and excreted in the urine. Raised serum creatinine levels indicate impaired kidney function or abnormal muscle wasting. A 24-hour urine collection and venous blood sampling to determine creatinine clearance allows the rate of creatinine excretion per minute to be calculated; may be undertaken in pregnant women with severe hypertension.

crèche DAY NURSERY.

Credé's expression technique to aid separation and expulsion of partially separated placenta in severe postpartum haemorrhage, involves massage to make uterus contract and squeezing of uterus behind and in front of the fundus to force the placenta into the vagina; intensely painful and shock-producing, rarely used.

cretinism congenital thyroid deficiency, causing arrested physical and mental development with dystrophy of bones and soft tissues, large head, short limbs, puffy eyes, thick protruding tongue, excessively dry skin, lack of coordination and mental handicap; treated with lifelong thyroid extract administration, which facilitates normal growth and mental development. The acquired or adult form is MYXOEDEMA.

cri du chat syndrome hereditary congenital syndrome characterised by hypertelorism, microcephaly, severe mental deficiency and a plaintive cat-like cry; results from the deletion of part of the short arm of chromosome 5.

cricoid ring shaped. *C. cartilage* ring-like cartilage forming the lower and back part of the larynx. *C. pressure* pressure applied to the cricoid cartilage during induction of general anaesthesia to occlude the oesophagus, preventing acid reflux from the stomach; pressure is maintained until the endotracheal tube is in position and the anaesthetist has checked that the seal provided by the cuff is effective.

criminal abortion termination of pregnancy performed outside the legal parameters of the 1967 Abortion Act; associated with high mortality and morbidity.

Criminal Records Bureau (CRB) Home Office Executive Agency, launched in 2002, which provides wider access to criminal record information through its disclosure service, enabling employers to identify individuals who may be unsuitable for work involving children or vulnerable adults. Midwives and others working in maternity care are required to undergo CRB checks before employment or training.

cross-matching vital procedure to ensure compatibility between donor and recipient blood in transfusion and organ transplantation; the donor's erythrocytes or leucocytes are placed in the recipient's serum and vice versa; absence of agglutination, haemolysis and cytotoxicity indicates that the donor and recipient are compatible.

crown–rump length (CRL) first-trimester ultrasound measurement of the fetal crown to rump length, used to assess fetal age accurately.

crowning moment during birth when the suboccipitobregmatic and biparietal diameters of the fetal head are distending the vulval ring, and the head no longer recedes between contractions.

cryosurgery operation using a refrigerated probe to remove abnormal tissue, e.g. cervical erosion.

cryptomenorrhoea subjective symptoms of menstruation without flow of blood.

culture 1. propagation of microorganisms or cells in a culture medium to obtain a sufficient sample for analysis, although increased availability of molecular techniques such as POLYMERASE CHAIN REACTION (PCR) has reduced the need to culture cells. 2. learned set of values, beliefs and attitudes common to a group of individuals; may relate to a society, organisation or profession; care should be taken not to discriminate or make assumptions about a person, based on perceptions of their culture or beliefs.

curette blunt or sharp metal loop used to remove unhealthy tissues by scraping or to obtain biopsy material. *Curettage* operation, using a curette, commonly performed to remove the uterine endometrium.

curve of Carus arc corresponding to the pelvic axis, the route taken by the fetus on its passage through the birth canal. *See diagram.*

Cushing's syndrome overactivity of the adrenal cortex resulting in excess glucocorticoids governing carbohydrate metabolism, leading to obesity, especially of the face and trunk, amenorrhoea, hirsutism (*see* HIRSUTE) and weakness.

cutaneous concerning the skin.

Section of bony female pelvis

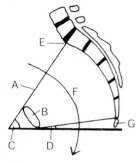

Curve of Carus and angles of inclination: **A,** plane of pelvic brim; **B,** symphysis pubis; **C,** angle of inclination of brim 55°; **D,** angle of outlet 5°; **E,** sacral promontory; **F,** curve of Carus; **G,** coccyx.

cyanocobalamin vitamin B12, found in liver, eggs and fish, essential for formation of erythrocytes and prevention of anaemia; administered intramuscularly for pernicious anaemia.

cyanosis blueness of the skin and mucous membranes because of a deficiency of oxygen.

cyclopropane gas used for general anaesthesia.

cyesis pregnancy. *Pseudocyesis* false pregnancy.

cyst tumour with a membranous capsule and containing fluid. *Chocolate c.* ovarian cyst associated with endometriosis. *Corpus luteum* or *luteal c.* cyst developing from the corpus luteum in HYDATIDIFORM MOLE. *Dermoid c.* cyst containing skin, hair, teeth, etc., caused by abnormal development of embryonic tissue. *Multilocular c.* ovarian cyst divided into compartments. *Papilliferous c.* ovarian cyst lined with papillae, which grow through the cyst wall into the peritoneal cavity, causing ascites. *Pseudomucinous c.* ovarian cyst containing mucin-like fluid. Gestational ovarian cysts should be diagnosed early and may be removed mid-trimester to avoid intrapartum complications and the risk of becoming malignant.

cystic fibrosis autosomal recessive inherited disease in which the mucus-secreting glands of the body secrete an unusually thick tenacious mucus, causing neonatal pancreatic fibrosis and MECONIUM ILEUS and, later, repeated chest infections. Diagnosis is by the serum immune-reactive trypsin (IRT) test; a sweat test, if carried out, shows raised sodium chloride and there may also be a raised ALBUMIN level in the meconium. One person in 25 is a CARRIER and, in Britain, one person in 2000 is affected. Also known as mucoviscidosis or fibrocystic disease of the pancreas.

cystic hygroma multilocated cystic collection of lymphatic fluid, commonly at the back of the neck, resulting from abnormal lymphatic development. Fetal cystic hygromas can be seen on ultrasound from 10–11 weeks' gestation and differentiated from enlarged NUCHAL TRANSLUCENCY because they are septated; associated with chromosomal abnormalities such as TURNER'S SYNDROME and EDWARD'S SYNDROME; CHORIONIC VILLUS SAMPLING or AMNIOCENTESIS is offered if seen on ultrasound. Fetal prognosis is usually poor, although cystic hygromas can occasionally disappear when the KARYOTYPE is normal.

cystitis inflammation of the bladder.

cysto- prefix relating to the bladder.

cystocele hernia of the bladder into the vagina, due to pelvic floor damage during childbirth. *See* COLPORRHAPHY.

Cystocele

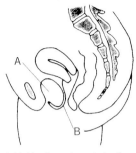

A, bladder; **B,** anterior vaginal wall.

cystoscope instrument for inspecting the interior of the bladder.

cystoscopy inspection of the interior of the bladder with a cystoscope.

cystotomy incision of the bladder, e.g. for the removal of calculi.

cyto- pertaining to cells.

cytogenetics branch of GENETICS involving the study of CHROMOSOMES.

cytology science of the structure and functions of cells to detect abnormalities. *Cervical c.* test to detect very early genital tract malignancy; routine in antenatal, postnatal and family planning clinics and for women over 35. *Vaginal c.* antenatal examination of desquamated cells from the vaginal wall for hormone changes suggesting placental insufficiency and fetal risk.

cytomegalic inclusion disease infection caused by cytomegalovirus, marked by nuclear inclusion bodies in large infected cells; may be congenital, with HEPATOSPLENOMEGALY, cirrhosis and microcephaly; acquired infection presents similarly to infectious mononucleosis.

cytomegalovirus (CMV) common infection that may cause severe fetal anomaly through damage to fetal cells, resulting in loss of function; incidence in primary infection is approximately 7%; adverse effects are more severe if infection occurs in the first trimester and may be indicated by early-onset INTRAUTERINE GROWTH RESTRICTION, bright (echogenic) bowel or cerebral VENTRICULOMEGALY. Up to 60% of women in developed countries have evidence of immunity from previous asymptomatic infection or mild infection presenting as general malaise, fever and lymphadenopathy.

cytoplasm all of the protoplasm of a cell, excluding the nucleus.

cytotrophoblast cellular layer of the trophoblast; Langhans' cell layer, less obvious after 19–20 weeks' gestation. *See also* CHORIONIC VILLI.

dactyl finger or toe.

dai *See* TRADITIONAL BIRTH ATTENDANT.

Danol danazol, anterior pituitary suppressant.

Data Protection Act 1984 Act giving people the right to know what information is held about them on computer, including health-related data, but does not apply to manual records; the 1990 Access to Health Records Act was passed to allow access to any computerised or manual health-related records made after 1991. Patients must apply to gain access to their records. The Data Protection (Subject Access Modification) (Health) Order 1987 restricted access to health information that might cause serious physical or mental harm to an individual or reveal the identity of another person.

database information that is collected, stored, reviewed and updated; used for evaluation and audit or as a research resource.

day nursery centre for daytime care of children up to age 5 years, provided by Department of Social Services or voluntary agencies. Priority is given to children from 'at risk' families and to those with special needs.

deafness lack or loss, complete or partial, of the sense of hearing. *Congenital d.* deafness present at birth, often due to antenatal infection, especially rubella.

death cessation of all physical and chemical processes occurring in all organs or cellular components. *Brain d.* in the UK, diagnosis of clinical brainstem death is governed by a set of guidelines ratified by the Medical Royal Colleges and their Faculties. *Cot d.* sudden infant death syndrome (SIDS). *D. certificate* certificate issued by registrar for deaths after receipt of a preliminary certificate completed and signed by an attending doctor, indicating the date and probable cause of death. Only after issue of this certificate, indicating that the death has been registered, can burial or cremation take place. *D. grant* payment made by Social Security from the Social Fund, which is payable to low-income families only and recoverable from the estate of the deceased. *D. rate* the number of deaths per stated number of persons (100 or 10 000 or 100 000) in a certain region in a certain time period.

decapitation severing of the head from the body; destructive operation now rarely used in obstructed labour.

decidua pregnant endometrium, thicker and more vascular than non-pregnant endometrium, into which the fertilised ovum embeds, facilitating transport of nutrition to the fertilised ovum; shed at the end of pregnancy. *D. basalis* part on which the ovum rests, covering the maternal placental surface. *D. capsularis* part covering the ovum as it projects into the uterine cavity. *D. vera* true uterine lining, not in contact with the ovum for the first 12 weeks of pregnancy. *See diagram.*

decidual cast expulsion of the decidua intact, in the shape of the uterine cavity, following death of the ovum in ectopic pregnancy. *See* ECTOPIC PREGNANCY.

decompensation inability of the heart to maintain adequate circulation marked by dyspnoea, venous engorgement, cyanosis and oedema.

Decidua

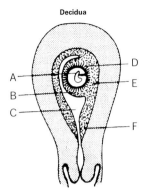

Sixth week of pregnancy.
A, Embryo; **B,** *D. capsularis*;
C, uterine cavity; **D,** chorionic villi;
E, *D. basalis*; **F,** *D. vera*.

deep transverse arrest obstruction of the fetal head during the second stage of labour, resulting from a first-stage occipitoposterior position in which the fetus has attempted to turn anteriorly (long rotation) with the head becoming caught between the ischial spines of the pelvic outlet, especially if they are prominent. KIELLAND'S FORCEPS delivery or manual rotation followed by WRIGLEY'S FORCEPS delivery is required to release the obstructed head. The baby may have excessive moulding leading to possible intracranial damage.

deep vein thrombosis (DVT) blood clot in a vessel, which can be life-threatening if it completely occludes the vessel, as in the coronary arteries causing heart attack or in the cerebral vessels causing cerebrovascular accident. The thrombosis may also move from its original site to another, causing problems elsewhere, e.g. pulmonary embolism. Newly delivered mothers are at risk of deep vein thrombosis because of changes in clotting factors that occur at term to prevent excess haemorrhage. Midwives should be alert to signs of thrombosis such as a red, tender, hot area on the calf.

defaecation evacuation of the bowels.

defibrillation termination of atrial or ventricular fibrillation, usually by electric shock.

deficiency disease caused by dietary or metabolic deficiency.

deflexion attitude of the fetus in which the head is not flexed, or only partially flexed, as may occur in occipitoposterior position.

degeneration structural change, which lowers the vitality of the tissue in which it takes place. *Fatty d.* fat is deposited in tissues. *Red d.* See NECROBIOSIS.

dehiscence bursting open or rupture, as in rupture of an abdominal wound after surgery; also, rupture of the graafian follicle at the point of ovulation.

dehydration excessive loss of body fluid or failure to take sufficient fluid to balance loss, often with ketoacidosis; occurs in severe vomiting, prolonged labour, excessive haemorrhage. Signs include dry inelastic skin, dry tongue and sunken eyes, acetone smell on the breath, scanty urine with ketones, electrolyte imbalance and abnormal blood reactions. Maternal dehydration with ketoacidosis can be life-threatening to the fetus; intravenous dextrose is administered, with saline if urinary chlorides are severely diminished. *D. fever* neonatal condition resulting from insufficient fluid intake, in which severe dehydration caused by diarrhoea, a depressed fontanelle, poor skin turgor and weight loss occur; the condition can be corrected orally if mild or intravenously if severe.

delay in labour unusual prolongation of labour; most common in the first stage – partogram shows if the rate of cervical dilatation is slower than expected (active-phase rate of 1 cm per hour in a primigravida or 1.5 cm per hour in a multipara); delay of 2 hours or more may require AUGMENTATION OF LABOUR. Second-stage delay is technically defined as more than 30–120 minutes in a nullipara and 10–60 minutes in a multipara but, in practice, as long as the fetal and maternal conditions remain satisfactory and gradual progressive descent of the presenting part is made, no action is taken. A physiological third stage of more than 2 hours, or an actively managed third stage of more than 30 minutes, in which there is delay in separation and expulsion of the placenta may require manual removal of the placenta and membranes.

deletion in genetics, loss of genetic material from a chromosome.

delirium mental disturbance of relatively short duration usually reflecting a toxic state, marked by illusions, hallucinations, delusions, excitement, restlessness and incoherence. May result from acute illness accompanied by excessively high fever.

delivery natural expulsion or extraction of the baby, placenta and fetal membranes at birth. *Abdominal d.* delivery of the baby through an incision made into the uterus via the abdominal wall (CAESAREAN SECTION). *Instrumental d.* delivery facilitated by the use of instruments, particularly forceps. *Spontaneous d.* delivery occurring without assistance of forceps or other mechanical aid. *Vaginal d.* complete expulsion of the baby, placenta and membranes via the birth canal, usually head first presenting by the vertex; breech delivery is also possible.

demand feeding feeding when the baby appears hungry and not according to a fixed timetable; also called 'on demand' feeding or baby-led feeding.

demography statistical science dealing with populations, including matters of health, disease, births and mortality.

denaturation test Singer's test; blood test to distinguish fetal from maternal blood.

denidation degeneration and expulsion during menstruation of certain epithelial elements, potentially the nidus of an embryo; the intended shedding of uterine lining when postcoital contraceptive pills are used.

Denis Browne splint special boot designed for correction of TALIPES.

denominator in obstetrics, a particular point on the presenting part of the fetus used to indicate its position in relation to a particular part of the mother's pelvis, e.g. the occiput in a vertex presentation, the sacrum in BREECH presentation or mentum (chin) in face presentation.

dental care See Appendix 12.

dental caries decay of teeth.

dentition teething. *Primary d.* eruption of temporary (milk) teeth, usually around age 6 or 7 months, continuing until the end of the second year. A full set consists of eight incisors, four canines, four premolars and four molars. *Secondary d.* appearance of the permanent teeth, commencing at 6 or 7 years and complete by 12–15 years, except for the posterior molars or 'wisdom teeth', which may appear between the ages of 17 and 25. There are 32 permanent teeth: eight incisors, four canines, eight premolars or bicuspids, and 12 molars.

deoxygenated deprived of oxygen. *D. blood* blood that has lost much of its oxygen in the tissues and is returning to the lungs for a fresh supply.

deoxyribonucleic acid (DNA) nucleic acid of complex molecular structure occurring in cell nuclei as the basic structure of GENES. DNA is present in all cells of every species and directs all activities of living cells, including its own replication and perpetuation in generation after generation of cells.

Department of Health (DH) the body responsible for administering the NHS.

Department of Social Security (DSS) central government department responsible for administering social security matters, including national insurance scheme, income support, child support, welfare benefits and social services.

Depo-Provera *See* MEDROXYPROGESTERONE ACETATE.

depression 1. lowering of the spirits; mood change experienced as sadness or melancholy. *Endogenous d.* occurs in manic-depressive psychosis, associated with slowing of thought and action and feelings of guilt. *Reactive d.* depression occurring as a result of some event that influences the person unfavourably. Either type may occur in the puerperium, usually starting in the first 2 weeks and developing gradually. Early recognition and treatment is essential to prevent increasing severity. Treatment involves support, psychotherapy and/or antidepressant drugs in mild cases, but psychiatric hospital admission, preferably in a mother and baby unit, antidepressants and, occasionally, electroconvulsive therapy may be required. 2. a dip, felt on palpation.

dermoid cyst tumour consisting of a fibrous wall lined with stratified epithelium and containing pulpy material in which epithelial elements such as hair are found.

descent downward movement, e.g. of the fetus during labour, through the brim, cavity and outlet of the pelvis. Descent is assessed by abdominal examination and may be measured in fifths. *See diagram.*

desquamation shedding of superficial epithelial cells from any part of the body.

destruction of controlled drugs a midwife must destroy any unwanted controlled drugs, obtained through a supply order procedure, in the presence of an 'authorised' person: a supervisor of midwives in England, Wales and Northern Ireland, a regional pharmaceutical officer in England, a pharmaceutical adviser for the Welsh Office, a chief administrative pharmaceutical officer of health boards in Scotland, a Northern Ireland Department of Health inspector appointed under the Misuse of Drugs Act 1971, regional medical officers in England, Scotland and Wales, an inspector of the Pharmaceutical Society of Great Britain, a police officer or an inspector of the Home Office Drugs Branch.

detection rate measure of a screening test's performance; the proportion of people found to be positive (or high risk) on a screening test; also known as sensitivity of a test.

detoxication process of neutralising toxic substances, a function of the liver.

detrusor general term for a body part, e.g. a muscle, that pushes downwards.

development process of growth and differentiation.

developmental pertaining to development. *D. anomaly* absence, deformity or excess of body parts as a result of faulty embryological development. *D. milestones* significant behaviours, used to mark the process of child development, e.g. sitting, walking, talking, etc. *D. tests* standard series of tests to assess children's development.

dexamethasone synthetic glucocorticoid used primarily as an anti-inflammatory agent in various conditions, including diseases and allergic states; also used in a screening test for diagnosis of CUSHING'S SYNDROME. May be given before preterm delivery to accelerate fetal lung maturity and reduce respiratory distress syndrome.

dextran polysaccharide preparation used as a plasma substitute to treat shock; it restores circulatory volume

Descent of the fetal head into the pelvis

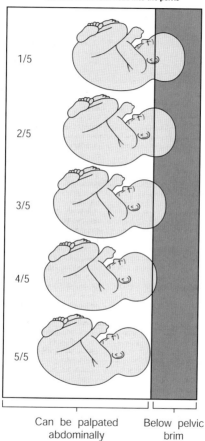

1/5

2/5

3/5

4/5

5/5

Can be palpated
abdominally

Below pelvic
brim

and does not leak out of blood vessels in the same way as physiological saline. It can be used when blood grouping is not possible and carries no risk of viral infections, unlike plasma.

dextropropoxyphene hydrochloride oral analgesic. Safety in pregnancy has not been established; may be addictive, especially if taken with alcohol.

dextrose glucose, monosaccharide; simplest form of carbohydrate.

diabetes insipidus rare disease in which there is a deficiency of antidiuretic hormone secretion from the posterior pituitary gland, characterised by polyuria, consequent thirst and dehydration; treated with vasopressin.

diabetes mellitus familial disease of deficient insulin secretion from the pancreatic islet cells or increased resistance to the action of insulin, possibly due to effects of anterior pituitary growth hormone; characterised by polyuria, weight loss, thirst and lassitude, leading to hyperglycaemia and ketosis, which may cause coma. Diabetes may be insulin dependent, in which the glucose tolerance test is abnormal and there are signs and symptoms of the disease, or non-insulin dependent, with an abnormal glucose tolerance test but no signs and symptoms. *Gestational d. m.* increased metabolic workload and insulin resistance of pregnancy, especially in women with a genetic predisposition or those with predisposing factors such as a previous baby weighing more than 4.5 kg, previous unexplained stillbirth or neonatal death, triggers a temporary diabetic state; these women are more prone to clinical diabetes later in life. Possible complications include maternal infections, hypertension, polyhydramnios, ketoacidosis, fetal abnormalities, death or hypoxia, cephalopelvic disproportion and birth trauma, and neonatal hypoglycaemia or respiratory distress

syndrome. Care is usually shared between the obstetrician and physician for close monitoring of maternofetal and diabetic conditions; the mother should be delivered in hospital, with careful observation of the blood sugar levels; Caesarean section may be necessary. Blood sugar monitoring continues postnatally when the mother's insulin requirements fall sharply; extra carbohydrate is required if the mother is breastfeeding.

diabetic pertaining to diabetes. *D. coma* loss of consciousness occurring as a result of severe ketosis.

diabetogenic inducing diabetes. In pregnancy susceptible women may become temporarily diabetic, but the condition may also recur in subsequent pregnancies and later life.

diacetic acid acetoacetic acid, colourless compound present in minute quantities in normal urine and in abnormal amounts in the urine of diabetic women and those who have excessive vomiting.

diagnosis determination of the nature of a disease. *Clinical d.* diagnosis made by studying actual signs and symptoms. *Differential d.* patient's symptoms are compared and contrasted with those of other diseases. *Tentative d.* provisional diagnosis judged by apparent facts and observations.

diagonal conjugate internal pelvic measurement between sacral promontory and lower border of the symphysis pubis, usually measuring 12.5 cm in a normal pelvis; the true conjugate is estimated as 1.3 cm less than this. In practice, the examining finger cannot normally reach the sacral promontory, unless the pelvis is unusually small, so the true conjugate is inferred as average because the promontory is out of reach. *See diagram.*

dialysis passage of salts, water and metabolites through a semipermeable membrane. *Renal d.* use of an artificial

**Measurement of the
diagonal conjugate**

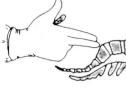

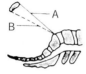

A, true conjugate; **B,** diagonal conjugate

kidney; the patient's blood is separated from the dialysing fluid by the membrane, retaining blood cells and plasma proteins and losing the toxic substances normally excreted by the kidney.

diameter straight line passing through the centre of a circle or sphere. *See* FETAL SKULL *and* PELVIS.

diamorphine hydrochloride heroin, powerful analgesic and drug of addiction.

diaphragm 1. muscular, dome-shaped partition separating the thorax from the abdomen, an important muscle of respiration; convex when relaxed and flattened as it contracts during inhalation, enlarging the chest cavity and allowing expansion of the lungs. In the second stage of labour the contraction of the diaphragm and abdominal muscles aids the expulsive force of the uterine contractions. 2. *Contraceptive d*. device of moulded rubber or other soft plastic material, fitted over the cervix uteri to prevent entrance of spermatozoa.

diaphragmatic hernia protrusion of an abdominal organ through the diaphragm into the thoracic cavity.

diaphysis shaft of a long bone.

diarrhoea frequent passage of loose stools, usually caused by infection; in the neonate there is rapid dehydration and disturbed electrolyte balance; if caused by infection it can be rapidly transmitted to others in a maternity unit, so the baby will need to be isolated. *See also* ESCHERICHIA COLI.

diastasis separation, e.g. of muscle as in diastasis recti or of cartilage as in symphysis pubis diastasis. *See* SYMPHYSIS PUBIS.

diastole resting stage of the cardiac cycle in which the cardiac muscle is relaxed following atrial and ventricular SYSTOLE.

diastolic pertaining to diastole. *D. murmur* abnormal sound produced during diastole occurring in valvular heart disease. *D. pressure* pressure of blood in the arteries during the resting stage of the cardiac cycle. *See* BLOOD PRESSURE.

diathermy high-frequency electrical currents used in physiotherapy and in surgical procedures to cauterise blood vessels to prevent excessive bleeding and to treat cervical erosions, neoplasms, warts and infected tissues; derived from the Greek words *dia* and *therma*, literally meaning 'heating through'. *See also* CRYOSURGERY.

diazepam oral, intramuscular or intravenous benzodiazepine tranquilliser, used as a preoperative anti-anxiety agent, skeletal muscle relaxant, anticonvulsant, e.g. in eclampsia and to treat alcohol withdrawal symptoms.

dicephalus fetus with two heads.

dichorial, dichorionic having two distinct chorions, as in dizygotic twins.

didactylism presence of only two digits on a hand or foot.

didelphia double uterus.

didymitis inflammation of the testicle; orchitis.

didymus 1. testis. 2. word termination designating a fetus with a duplication of parts or one consisting of conjoined symmetrical twins.

diembryonic production of two embryos from a single egg.

dienestrol synthetic OESTROGEN used in the treatment of atrophic vaginitis and kraurosis vulvae.

dietetics branch of medical science concerned with diet for maintenance of health and cure of disease.

diethylstilbestrol synthetic OESTROGEN.

dietician professional concerned with the promotion of good health through proper diet and with the therapeutic use of diet in the treatment of disease.

differential making a difference. *D. blood count* comparison of the numbers of different white cells present in the blood. *D. diagnosis see* DIAGNOSIS.

diffusion passage of substances in solution into an area of weaker concentration through a semipermeable membrane, e.g. OXYGEN, CARBON DIOXIDE, some minerals and urea diffuse across the placental CHORIONIC VILLI.

digestion process by which ingested food is changed and rendered suitable for absorption into the blood.

digit finger or toe.

digital pertaining to the finger (or toe). *D. examination* examination carried out with one or more fingers.

digitalis active principle of the foxglove plant. *D. purpurea* used in congestive heart failure and atrial fibrillation to slow and strengthen the heart beat.

digoxin drug obtained from the leaves of *Digitalis lanata*; used in the treatment of congestive heart failure.

dihydrocodeine tartrate (DF 118 Forte) oral and intramuscular analgesic; side effects include nausea, headaches, vertigo; avoid in asthmatics as it causes histamine release.

dilatation stretching of either an orifice or, occasionally, a hollow organ, either naturally, as in the cervix during labour, or artificially, as in the cervix before curettage of the uterine cavity.

dilator instrument used to effect dilatation, e.g. HEGAR'S DILATOR.

dimenhydrinate antiemetic preparation.

dimetria condition characterised by a double uterus.

dimorphism quality of existing in two distinct forms. *Sexual d.* 1. physical or behavioural differences associated with sex. 2. having some properties of both sexes, as in the early embryo and some hermaphrodites.

diodone contrast medium similar to iodoxyl, used in radiography.

diphtheria acute, specific infectious disease caused by *Corynebacterium diphtheriae* (Klebs–Löffler bacillus), which was highly dangerous before diphtheria immunisation was introduced. *See* Appendix 14.

diphtheroids non-pathogenic corynebacteria resembling the bacilli of diphtheria, common COMMENSALS of the throat, nose, ear, conjunctiva and skin.

diplococci cocci found always in pairs, which may be encapsulated, e.g. pneumococci, or intracellular, e.g. gonococci. *See* GONOCOCCUS.

diploid having two sets of CHROMOSOMES within the cells; in humans the diploid number is 46, i.e. 23 pairs.

diplosomatia condition in which complete twins are joined at some of their body parts.

direct antiglobulin test (DAT) test used to detect HAEMOLYTIC DISEASE OF THE NEWBORN. *See* COOMBS' TEST.

disability any restriction or lack (resulting from an impairment) of ability to perform an activity in the manner or within the range considered normal for a human being. *Developmental d.* substantial disability of indefinite duration, with onset before the age of

18 years, attributable to learning disability, autism, cerebral palsy, epilepsy or other neuropathy.

disaccharide carbohydrate formed of two simple sugar units, e.g. lactose in milk, sucrose and maltose; readily broken down into MONOSACCHARIDES.

disc circular or rounded flat plate. *Embryonic d.* flattish area in a cleaved ovum in which the first traces of the embryo are seen. *Intervertebral d.* layer of fibrocartilage between the bodies of adjoining vertebrae. *Prolapsed intervertebral d.* rupture of an intervertebral disc, commonly occurring in the lower back and occasionally the neck.

discharge flow of substances from the body. *Vaginal d. in pregnancy* hormonal changes increase the amount of discharge, which should be white, mucoid and non-irritating; there is a raised vaginal pH; profuse, offensive or irritating discharge should be investigated.

discoloration alteration in the colour of the skin or mucous membranes, e.g. Jacquemier's sign, the bluish discoloration of the cervix and vagina seen in early pregnancy.

discus proligerus compact mass of follicular cells surrounding the ovum before it is expelled from the graafian follicle.

disease any abnormal condition that causes local or general disturbance in body structure or function.

disinfect process to destroy microorganisms to a level that is not harmful to health.

dislocation displacement of a bone from its natural position; may be congenital, usually resulting from a faulty construction of the joint, e.g. the hip.

displacement movement to an unusual position, e.g. retroversion or PROLAPSE of the non-gravid uterus, which normally lies in the centre of the pelvic cavity, anteverted and anteflexed.

disproportion lack of harmony or lack of a proper relationship between one object and another. *Cephalopelvic d.* (CPD) disparity between the fetal head and the maternal pelvis, either because the head is too large or abnormally positioned, or because the pelvis too small or abnormally shaped; detected in the last 4 weeks of pregnancy by failure of the fetal head to engage, either spontaneously or on pressure, and confirmed on ultrasound. In severe CPD Caesarean section will be needed, but in mild CPD uterine contractions in labour help to mould the fetal head through the pelvis, often with increased flexion; in anticipation of this the mother may undergo TRIAL LABOUR.

disseminated intravascular coagulation (DIC) widespread formation of thromboses in the microcirculation, mainly in the capillaries; a secondary complication of conditions such as abruptio placentae, retained dead fetus, amniotic fluid embolism and various types of infections and bacteraemias, which introduce coagulation-promoting factors into the circulation. The intravascular clotting ultimately triggers haemorrhage as a result of the rapid consumption of fibrinogen, platelets, prothrombin and clotting factors V, VIII and X. Treatment consists of replacement of the relevant blood products. If the primary condition cannot be treated, intravenous heparin may inhibit the clotting process and raise the level of the depleted clotting factors.

distal situated away from the centre of the body or point of origin. Opposite of proximal.

Distalgesic *See* DEXTROPROPOXYPHENE HYDROCHLORIDE.

district general hospital hospital that provides a full range of specialist services in a catchment area.

diuresis increased secretion of urine.

diuretic drug that increases excretion of urine, e.g. furosemide (frusemide).

diurnal pertaining to or occurring during the daytime or period of light.

dizygotic pertaining to or derived from two separate zygotes (fertilised ova). *D. twins* twins originating from two ova and two spermatozoa, with separate placentae, chorions and amnions, and of the same or different sexes, more common than MONOZYGOTIC twins; also called binovular twins. *See also* MULTIPLE PREGNANCY.

Döderlein's bacillus non-pathogenic lactobacillus occurring normally in vaginal secretions; metabolism of glycogen within the vaginal squamous epithelium lining produces lactic acid and a pH of 4.5, which counteracts the alkalinity of cervical mucus and is hostile to pathogenic organisms.

dolichocephalic having a long head, where the anteroposterior diameter is increased.

domiciliary within or at home. *D. midwife* community-based midwife.

dominant inheritance mode of inheritance in which one parent passes on a characteristic to the offspring; one of the pair of GENES carries the characteristic and is dominant over the other gene, giving a 50% chance of the baby being affected, as in ACHONDROPLASIA. *See also* RECESSIVE inheritance.

'domino' booking maternity care plan in which a mother gives birth in a consultant unit, cared for by the community midwife and returning home any time after 6 hours following delivery; derived from *domi*ciliary midwife *in* and *out*.

donor one who gives, e.g. blood donor gives blood for transfusion, milk donor supplies excess milk for a human milk bank.

dopamine intermediate product in noradrenaline (norepinephrine) synthesis; neurotransmitter in the central nervous system. Synthetic dopamine is administered intravenously to correct haemodynamic imbalance in shock syndrome.

Doppler ultrasound procedure using a series of pulses to detect blood flow, e.g. in the fetal umbilical artery (to assess placental function), middle cerebral artery (to assess placental failure and fetal anaemia) and ductus venosus (to detect hypoxia); returning echoes from moving blood, which differ from those of surrounding stationary tissue, are reflected as sound waves and used to estimate speed and direction of blood flow; colour flow imaging helps to determine which vessels are being measured.

dorsal concerning the back. *D. position* mother lies on her back with head and shoulders slightly elevated.

double-blind trial test for the real effect of a new drug or treatment in clinical practice, in which neither the patients receiving nor the staff administering the treatment know which of two apparently identical treatments is the one being tested.

double uterus abnormal uterine development caused by failure of fusion of the müllerian ducts, producing two uterine bodies with or without duplication of the cervix and vagina, which may cause repeated miscarriages; very occasionally, two independent conceptions occur and implant into the two sections of the uterus; preterm labour is common.

douche 1. stream or jet of water or other fluid applied to some part of the body. *Vaginal d.* procedure in which up to 5 litres of warm saline is used to produce hydrostatic pressure to distend the vagina and thus cause INVERSION OF THE UTERUS to revert to its normal position. 2. apparatus used for a douche.

Douglas' pouch pouch of peritoneum between the upper third of the vagina in front and the anterior wall of the rectum behind.

doula from the Greek word meaning 'woman who serves other women'; in maternity care, one who provides emotional and practical support, most commonly during pregnancy and labour, but occasionally postnatally.

Down's syndrome chromosomal abnormality involving chromosome 21. Most commonly results from an extra chromosome, i.e. 47 chromosomes instead of 46 (*trisomy 21*), associated with increasing maternal age. Also caused by a translocation, usually between chromosomes 14 and 21; parents may have normal chromosomes or a similar translocated chromosome, in which case there is a 10% chance of a subsequent pregnancy being affected. Baby has slanting eyes, broad flat nose, brachycephaly, short neck with loose skin, HYPOTONIA, broad hands with a single palmar crease, third fontanelle, BRUSHFIELD'S SPOTS in the iris and other abnormalities, e.g. congenital heart disease as well as learning disabilities.

drainage tube tube inserted into a cavity, wound or infected area to allow the exit of excess fluids or purulent material.

dramatherapy therapeutic use of drama, in which clients are encouraged to act out their feelings to overcome problems; has been used successfully to treat infertility.

draught reflex *See* MILK FLOW MECHANISM.

drepanocyte sickle cell.

drepanocytosis occurrence of drepanocytes (sickle cells) in the blood.

dressing covering applied to a wound surface.

Drew–Smythe cannula S-shaped metal CATHETER used to puncture the hindwaters when the head is not engaged; rarely used now as it can cause placental separation.

droplet infection passage of pathogenic bacteria in minute droplets from the respiratory tract during talking, coughing, sneezing, etc.

drug 1. medicinal substance. 2. narcotic. 3. to administer a drug. *D. abuse* use of one or more drugs for recreational purposes. *D. addiction* state of periodic or chronic intoxication from repeated consumption of a drug; characterised by a psychological and a physical dependence on its effects, leading to a compulsion to continue using the drug, often in increasing doses, and to obtain it by any means; has detrimental effects on the individual and on society. *D. interaction* modification of the potency of one drug by another (or others) taken concurrently or sequentially, producing either harmful or therapeutic effects.

drugs in midwifery drugs categorised for use in pain relief in labour; induction and acceleration of labour; management of haemorrhage; resuscitation; and treatment of physiological and pathological disorders.

Dubowitz score method to assess gestational age in a low-birthweight infant.

Duchenne's muscular dystrophy childhood type of muscular dystrophy. 1. spinal muscular atrophy. 2. bulbar paralysis. 3. tabes dorsalis.

Ducrey's bacillus organism that causes soft chancre (*Haemophilus ducreyi*).

duct (ductus) tube or channel for conveying away the secretion of a gland.

ductus arteriosus fetal blood vessel bypassing the pulmonary circulation by connecting the pulmonary artery and descending aorta, and which normally closes at birth. The umbilical vein travels in the cord to the fetus and divides into two branches, one of which is the *ductus venosus*, and this joins the inferior vena cava.

Duffy blood group type of blood containing a rare antigen.

Dulco-lax *See* BISACODYL.

dunken *See* TRADITIONAL BIRTH ATTENDANT.

duodenum first part of small intestine, from pylorus to jejunum, 25–27 cm

(10–11 in) long. *Duodenal atresia* incomplete canalisation of the duodenum; causes projectile vomiting with bile when the baby starts feeding.

dura mater tough fibrous membrane lining the skull, forming the outermost covering of the brain and spinal cord. A double fold of inner dura mater, the falx cerebri, dips down between the cerebral hemispheres; a horizontal fold, the tentorium cerebelli, separates the cerebellum from the cerebral hemispheres above; both these membranes carry large venous sinuses that drain blood from the skull; they may be stretched and torn during labour, causing intracranial HAEMORRHAGE.

dural tap puncture of the dura mater, usually following regional anaesthesia, causing a leakage of cerebrospinal fluid and leading to persistent headache for up to a week; rest to avoid further loss of cerebrospinal fluid is required.

duration of pregnancy pregnancy averages 266 days from conception to delivery and 280 days (40 weeks) from the first day of the last menstrual period to delivery. If the woman knows the date of the first day of her last menstrual period, the estimated date of delivery (EDD) can be calculated by adding 9 months and 7 days for an average 28-day menstrual cycle; if the average cycle is x days less than 28, the EDD will be x days earlier; if the cycle is y days more than 28, the EDD will be y days later. The EDD is only a guide and women should be advised not to depend on the precise date. Normal labour may commence any time between 37 and 43 weeks of pregnancy but, in the case of pregnancy persisting for more than 10 days past the EDD, medical intervention may be advocated to expedite delivery; preterm labour is usually classified as occurring before 37 weeks' gestation.

Dutch cap contraceptive device. *See* DIAPHRAGM.

duty of care legal term denoting the responsibility to a patient or client of anyone who offers themselves as a skilled professional midwife, nurse or doctor, irrespective of any contractual agreement existing between the parties, based on a set of rules regarding the expected standard of care; these rules may be used to determine whether or not a professional has neglected their duty of care, based on the standards prevailing at the time of any legal case questioning the issue.

dydrogesterone orally effective, synthetic progestin used to diagnose and treat primary amenorrhoea and severe dysmenorrhoea, and in combination with oestrogen, for dysfunctional menorrhagia.

dys- prefix meaning 'difficult', 'disordered' or 'painful'.

dysentery notifiable intestinal infection characterised by severe diarrhoea with the passage of blood or mucus and pus; usually caused by a *Shigella* species or *Entamoeba histolytica*.

dyslexia impairment of ability to comprehend written language as a result of a central lesion. adj. *dyslexic*.

dysmature vague term commonly used to describe a baby who is small for gestational age.

dysmenorrhoea difficult or painful menstruation, characterised by cramplike lower abdominal pains, headache, irritability, mental depression, malaise and fatigue.

dyspareunia difficult or painful coitus.

dyspepsia indigestion.

dyspnoea difficult or laboured breathing.

dyspraxia impairment of movement resulting from immaturity in the brain's processing of information, associated with problems of perception, language and thought; affects up to 10% of the population and up to 2% severely; more common in males and may be familial.

69

dystocia difficult or abnormal labour.

dystrophia literally, difficult or abnormal growth. *Dystocia d. syndrome* rare obstetric sequence to which some short, heavily built, subfertile, hirsute women with android pelves may be prone; pre-eclampsia and occipito-posterior position of the fetus may occur.

dysuria difficult or painful micturition.

ecbolic oxytocic, i.e. causes uterine muscles to contract.

ecchymosis effusion of blood beneath the skin, causing discoloration; bruising.

echovirus group of viruses (enteroviruses) isolated from humans that produce many different human diseases, e.g. aseptic meningitis, diarrhoea and respiratory diseases.

eclampsia rare serious complication of PRE-ECLAMPSIA, characterised by epileptiform fits occurring towards term, during or shortly after labour. The midwife should call the doctor urgently, position the mother on her side, insert an airway if possible, administer oxygen until breathing resumes, check reflexes regularly and prevent the mother from harming herself. Intravenous magnesium sulphate or phenytoin to control fits may be given; ergometrine is contraindicated. The mother may start spontaneous labour; strong sedation may lead to misinterpretation of distress from contraction pain as onset of more fits. Repeated fits can cause cerebral haemorrhage, pulmonary oedema, renal or hepatic failure, or pneumonia from inhalation of debris. Risks to the fetus include hypoxia and death *in utero*, especially during apnoeic phases. Prompt recognition and early treatment of pre-eclampsia should prevent most cases of sudden fulminating pre-eclampsia, with impending eclampsia. adj. *eclamptic*.

econazole antifungal agent similar to clotrimazole or miconazole.

'ecstasy' methylenedioxymethamphetamine (MDMA) or 'E'; illicit drug, a synthetic hallucinogenic amphetamine for oral or rectal use. Concentration varies from 2–200 mg; tablets and capsules may contain other substances, e.g. caffeine, paracetamol or ketamine (anaesthetic). MDMA inhibits serotonin reasbsorption, reducing brain reserves, affecting mood and producing boundless energy in the early stages; prolonged use leads to loss of appetite, sweats, palpitations, insomnia, jaw stiffness, teeth grinding, frequency of micturition, cardiac arrhythmias, hepatotoxicity, and neurological and psychiatric damage. Hyperthermia is the most lethal effect, often accompanied by disseminated intravascular coagulation, metabolic acidosis, hyperkalaemia and acute renal failure.

ecto- prefix meaning 'outside'.

ectoblast ectoderm.

ectocervix part of the cervix protruding into the vagina.

ectoderm outer germinal layer of the developing embryo from which the skin, external sense organs, mucous membrane of the mouth and anus and nervous system are derived.

-ectomy suffix meaning 'cutting out', e.g. appendicectomy, hysterectomy.

ectopia abnormal position of any structure. *E. vesicae* uncommon congenital defect of the abdominal wall in which the interior of the bladder is exposed.

ectopic pregnancy embedding of a fertilised ovum, usually in the fallopian tube, but occasionally in the ovary, abdominal cavity or, rarely, in the cornu of the uterus (interstitial or angular pregnancy). Pregnancy usually terminates within 4–10 weeks because of separation of the gestational sac from the fallopian tube lining; peristaltic action of the tube moves it into the peritoneal cavity; slight vaginal bleeding occurs as the decidua is shed. Alternatively, tubal rupture occurs when the trophoblast has penetrated the fallopian tube more deeply, causing severe pain, intraperitoneal or intraligamentary haemorrhage and profound shock, requiring immediate blood transfusion and laparotomy to locate and ligate the bleeding vessels. The midwife's role involves management of the shock and haemorrhage until medical aid arrives, follow-up support and care. Very occasionally, abdominal pregnancy can progress almost to term with a live baby being delivered by laparotomy; the placenta, usually adherent to a major abdominal organ such as the liver, is left *in situ* to reabsorb slowly over a period of months.

Ectopic gestation

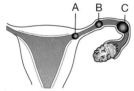

A, interstitial (angular); **B,** isthmic; **C,** ampullar.

ectro- prefix meaning 'miscarriage', 'congenital absence'.

ectrodactyly congenital absence of all or part of a digit.

ectromelia gross hypoplasia or aplasia of one or more long bones of one or more limbs. adj. *ectromelic*.

ectrosyndactyly condition in which some digits are absent; the remaining ones are webbed.

eczema allergic skin condition, often hereditary; infantile eczema may be precipitated by giving cows' milk feeds. If there is a family history of eczema, hay fever or asthma the mother should be encouraged to breastfeed her baby totally, as even one complementary feed can induce these conditions.

Edward's syndrome (trisomy 18) congenital disorder resulting from the presence of an additional chromosome 18; the second most common TRISOMY after DOWN'S SYNDROME (trisomy 21), occurring in approximately 1:3000 conceptions, the risk increasing with advancing maternal age. The baby shows evidence of varying levels of growth restriction with a small head, low-set ears, small jaw and mouth, clenched fist with overlapping fingers and may have defects in the heart or other organs; there will also be significant developmental delay. At least half die *in utero* and, of those born alive, approximately 50% die within 1 week and 90% within 5 months. Occasionally, the less severe MOSAIC trisomy 18 occurs in which not all cells have the extra chromosome 18.

effacement 'taking up' of the cervix in which the internal os dilates, opening out the cervical canal and leaving only a circular orifice, the external os; occurs in labour before cervical dilatation in nulliparae but simultaneously in multigravidae.

efferent carrying outward, i.e. from the centre to the periphery. *E. nerves* motor nerves that obey impulses from the nerve centres of the brain.

effleurage light, circular, stroking massage; abdominal effleurage in labour can reduce the perception of pain, as touch impulses reach the brain before pain impulses.

effusion escape of blood or serum into surrounding tissues or cavities.

egg 1. ovum, female gamete. 2. oocyte. 3. female reproductive cell at any stage before fertilisation and in derivatives after fertilisation, even after some development. *E. donor* woman who takes drugs to induce multiple ovulation after which the ova are removed by laparoscopy, fertilised *in vitro* and transferred to the uterus of a recipient.

Eisenmenger's syndrome large ventricular septal defect, overriding of the aorta and right ventricular hypertrophy, associated with a high maternal mortality.

ejaculation forcible, sudden expulsion, especially of semen from the male urethra, a reflex action occurring as a result of sexual stimulation.

elective planned. *E. Caesarean section* operative delivery planned when circumstances suggest it is the only safe way to deliver the baby, because of either the maternal or the fetal condition.

electrocardiogram (ECG) tracing of the heart's action shown by electrical waves, used in the diagnosis of heart disease.

electrode conductor through which electricity leaves its source to enter another medium. *Fetal scalp e.* electrode applied to the fetal scalp in labour to record the electrocardiogram (ECG).

electroencephalogram (EEG) tracing of electrical brain waves.

electrolyte substance that dissociates into electrically charged particles in solution (IONS), e.g. sodium bicarbonate, potassium chloride. *E. imbalance* disturbance of electrolyte levels diagnosed from blood tests, usually resulting from severe vomiting or renal failure.

electrophoresis technique in which movement of electrically charged particles under the influence of an applied electrical field enables substances, e.g. DEOXYRIBONUCLEIC ACID (DNA), to be separated into constituent parts; used for serum protein analysis and to analyse neonatal haemoglobin for sickle cell disease and other haemoglobinopathies.

eliminate to expel waste substances from the body, e.g. the kidneys eliminate urea, the bowel eliminates unabsorbed food products, the lungs eliminate carbon dioxide.

embolism blocking of a blood vessel by a solid or foreign substance introduced into the circulation; a large embolus causes immediate death whereas a smaller embolus causes collapse, chest pain, dyspnoea and cyanosis. Oestrogens appear to increase the risk of venous thrombosis so should not be used to suppress lactation. *Air e.* air bubbles enter the circulation, possibly during vaginal or intrauterine douching in pregnancy. *Amniotic fluid e.* amniotic fluid, and substances it may contain, enter the circulation, occasionally complicating labour. *Pulmonary e.* often a consequence of pelvic or leg vein thrombosis, and occasionally occurring after labour; part of the clot detaches and travels in the bloodstream until it is arrested in a branch of the pulmonary artery.

embolus foreign particle or substance circulating in the blood, e.g. a detached portion of thrombus, mass of bacteria, air bubble or amniotic fluid. pl. *emboli*.

embryo developing offspring of viviparous animals before birth; in humans the term embryo is used for the first 8 weeks after conception, the term fetus is used thereafter.

embryology science of the development of the embryo.

embryonic plate part of the inner cell mass of the blastocyst from which the embryo is formed.

embryotomy dissecting the fetus to facilitate delivery in cases of neglected obstructed labour where operating facilities are unavailable; extremely rare in modern obstetrics.

emergency condition requiring immediate attention. Midwives should not give treatment that they have not been trained to give or which is outside their sphere of practice, except in an emergency, in accordance with the NMC Midwives' Rules. *E. protection order* court order by which a child can be arbitrarily removed from his parents in the interests of his safety.

emetic substance used to induce vomiting, e.g. common salt in water, apomorphine.

emmenagogue any substance that may induce vaginal bleeding. adj. *emmenagogic.*

empowerment capacity to empower, to give power or authority; the philosophy that women should be empowered during pregnancy, labour and the puerperium to take control over their own care and to work in partnership with maternity care providers.

emulsion mixture of minute particles of a fatty or oily substance suspended in fluid.

encephalins *See* ENKEPHALINS.

encephalitis inflammation of the brain caused by viral infections, e.g. herpes simplex; bacterial infections, e.g. tuberculosis or syphilis; fungal infections, e.g. histoplasmosis; or protozoal infections, e.g. toxoplasmosis.

encephalocele hernia of the brain through a congenital or traumatic opening of the skull.

encephalopathy diffuse disease or damage of the brain. *Wernicke's e.* inflammatory haemorrhagic encephalopathy due to thiamine deficiency; a rare complication of hyperemesis gravidarum.

encopresis faecal incontinence, not due to organic defect or illness.

endemic pertaining to infectious disease that is always present in the locality.

endo- prefix meaning 'inside' or 'within'.

endocarditis inflammation of the endocardium or lining of the heart.

endocervicitis inflammation of the membrane lining the cervix uteri; CERVICITIS.

endocervix mucous membrane lining the cervical canal.

endocrine literally, secreting within; glands whose secretions (hormones) pass directly into the bloodstream.

endogenous originating inside the body, e.g. inside the birth canal in puerperal sepsis.

endometriosis tissue resembling and functioning similarly to the endometrium but outside the uterus; chocolate cyst of the ovary contains some endometrial material.

endometritis inflammation of the endometrium.

endometrium mucous membrane lining the body of the uterus.

endorphins opiate-like peptides produced naturally by the body at neural synapses at various points in the central nervous system pathway where they modulate the transmission of pain perceptions, raising the pain threshold and producing sedation and euphoria; the effects are blocked by naloxone, a narcotic antagonist.

endoscope instrument fitted with a light, used to inspect hollow organs and structures, e.g. CYSTOSCOPE and LAPAROSCOPE.

endotoxic shock rare condition associated with septicaemia caused by gram-negative organisms, especially *Escherichia coli, Clostridium welchii* and beta-haemolytic streptococci, which release endotoxins thought to cause widespread dilatation of arterioles in liver, lungs and other organs, so that diminished venous return causes profound shock; signs are similar to hypovolaemic shock but rigors may also occur. Urgent administration of appropriate antibiotics is required.

endotracheal within the trachea. *E. tube* airway catheter inserted into the trachea during intubation to assure patency of the upper airway and enable removal of secretions. *E. intubation* resuscitative process, sometimes accompanied by cardiac massage; also performed during general anaesthesia when a 'cuffed' tube is used, which protects the lungs because, when inflated, it prevents any regurgitated gastric fluid from passing the 'cuffed' area and entering the lungs.

enema injection of fluid into the rectum.

energy (calorie) requirement every bodily process requires energy, which is derived from food that is reduced by digestion to usable 'fuel', which the body 'burns'; the amount of energy required varies from one person to another: a pregnant woman requires 2500 cal (625 kJ) per day. Excess energy is stored as fat, providing a supplementary energy source if the diet is inadequate.

engagement entry of the presenting fetal part into the true pelvis. In a cephalic presentation the head is engaged when the BIPARIETAL DIAMETER has passed the plane of the pelvic brim, usually at about 36 weeks' gestation in a primigravida but possibly not until after the onset of labour in a multipara.

engorgement of the breasts painful accumulation of secretion in the breasts, often accompanied by oedema and lymphatic and venous stasis at the onset of lactation, which can be avoided by early on-demand breastfeeding with the baby correctly positioned at the breast. A firm supporting brassiere or breast binder may be helpful but care should be taken not to create pressure on the oedematous tissue. Dark green cabbage leaves applied over the breasts exert an osmotic pressure to relieve the engorgement. The leaves are wiped (not washed to prevent onset of osmosis) and cooled in the refrigerator, then applied over the breasts; when they become wet they are replaced with dry leaves; the process is repeated until relief is obtained.

enkephalins two naturally occurring pentapeptides isolated from the brain, with potent opiate-like effects, probably serving as neurotransmitters; classified as ENDORPHINS.

ensiform cartilage lowest part of the sternum, the xiphisternum, used as a marker when undertaking antenatal abdominal examination to estimate gestation.

enteritis intestinal infection. *See* DYSENTERY.

entoderm cells in the inner cell mass that line the yolk sac and later develop into the epithelium of the fetal alimentary tract, trachea, bronchi, bladder and urethra.

Entonox a mixture of NITROUS OXIDE and OXYGEN (50% of each), premixed in a blue cylinder with a white collar, approved by the Nursing and Midwifery Council (NMC) for use by midwives as a means of administering analgesia in labour; the mother controls the amount of gas received by inhaling as required, either through a face mask or a mouth piece.

enuresis involuntary micturition; bedwetting, as a result of psychological, neurological or pathological causes.

environmental health concept that the health of any individual can be affected by his or her environment, e.g. pollution and poor housing.

environmental health officer local authority employee responsible for improving and regulating the environment and enforcing statutory regulations related to, for example, housing, food hygiene, refuse collection, infestation, air pollutants and noise.

enzyme biological catalyst; substance present in small amounts that produces a chemical reaction, e.g. milk sugar (lactose) is broken down by the enzyme lactase in the small intestine to form GLUCOSE and GALACTOSE.

eosin red stain used in the identification of cells and bacteria.

eosinophil white blood cell in which the granules can be stained red with eosin.

Epanutin *See* PHENYTOIN SODIUM.

ephedrine adrenergic alkaloid used as a bronchodilator, antiallergen, central nervous system stimulant, mydriatic agent and pressor agent.

epicanthus vertical fold of skin either side of the nose, sometimes covering the inner canthus (junction of eyelids), prominent in certain races and babies with Down's syndrome.

epidemic situation in which any disease has attacked a large number of people at one time.

epidemiology study of the distribution of factors determining health and disease in human populations, to enable the prevention and control of disease.

epidermis non-vascular outer layer or cuticle of the skin.

epidermolysis bullosa severe, usually fatal, autosomally RECESSIVE skin disorder characterised by a profusion of fluid-filled blisters resembling PEMPHIGUS NEONATORUM.

epididymis elongated, cord-like structure along the posterior border of the testis, whose coiled duct provides for the storage, transport and maturation of spermatozoa.

epidural analgesia injection of local analgesic, e.g. BUPIVACAINE HYDROCHLORIDE, into the epidural space to block the spinal nerves. Injection is by one of two routes: caudal, through the sacrococcygeal membrane covering the sacral hiatus, or lumbar, through the intervertebral space and ligamentum flavum. Used in prolonged labour; occipitoposterior position; breech presentation; forceps delivery; to reduce hypertension in pre-eclampsia or eclampsia; multiple or preterm delivery; Caesarean section; maternal cardiac or respiratory disease; or as a result of client preference. Dangers include sudden hypotension

leading to fetal hypoxia; spinal or dural tap; toxic reactions to the drug; neurological sequelae from injury or haematoma; higher risk of instrumental delivery because of poor head flexion as a result of the relaxed pelvic floor; infection. An intravenous cannula is inserted to provide a means of immediate treatment in the event of a problem and the mother should be positioned carefully to avoid hypotension. The midwife monitors maternal blood pressure and fetal heart rate frequently, especially after the first dose of bupivacaine, which is given by the anaesthetist who inserts the epidural cannula, and after each 'top up', which midwives may be trained to administer. *See also* MOBILE EPIDURAL *and* SPINAL ANAESTHESIA.

epigastrium upper and middle abdominal region within the sternal angle. adj. *epigastric*. Epigastric pain in pre-eclamptic women may indicate the onset of ECLAMPSIA and is due to hepatic oedema and/or haemorrhage.

epiglottis lid-like cartilaginous structure overhanging the entrance to the larynx.

epilepsy paroxysmal transient nervous system disturbance resulting from abnormal electrical activity of the brain; anticonvulsive drugs are required to prevent maternal seizures, which lead to intrauterine hypoxia, but they may have a teratogenic effect on the fetus, causing lip, palate and heart defects.

epileptiform resembling an epileptic fit, as in eclampsia.

epiphysis end of a long bone with the shaft separated by cartilage in children; ossification of the fetal epiphyses provides a guide to fetal maturity. pl. *epiphyses*.

episiorrhaphy repair of an EPISIOTOMY.

episiotomy mediolateral or median (midline) incision in the thinned-out perineal body to enlarge the vaginal orifice during delivery, carried out under local anaesthetic, usually lidocaine (lignocaine) 0.5% 10 mL or 1% 5 mL. Performed to expedite delivery in cases of fetal distress; before forceps delivery or ventouse extraction; to reduce risk of intracranial damage in preterm or breech delivery. Appropriately trained and competent midwives are permitted by the Nursing and Midwifery Council to infiltrate the perineum, perform an episiotomy and repair perineal trauma.

Episiotomy

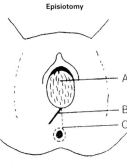

A, fetal head; **B,** mediolateral incision; **C,** midline incision.

epispadias abnormal urethral opening on the dorsal surface of the penis.

epistaxis nose bleed.

epithelial tissue *See* EPITHELIUM.

epithelium layer of cells covering all outer surfaces and lining all inner surfaces, including cavities, glands and vessels.

epsilon-aminocaproic acid antifibrinolytic drug used to prevent the breakdown of FIBRIN by PLASMIN, used in cases of severe abruptio placentae.

Epstein's pearls small white epithelial spots at the junction of the hard and soft palate.

Equal Opportunities Commission *ad hoc* body set up in 1975 to help enforce the Sex Discrimination Act 1975 and the Equal Pay Act 1970.

Erb's paralysis upper arm paralysis caused by injury to the upper trunk of the brachial plexus nerves as they leave the spinal cord in the cervical region; several muscles are paralysed so that the arm hangs medially rotated with the elbow extended and wrist and fingers flexed. It results from traction on the fetal neck, e.g. during the birth of the head in breech delivery or in SHOULDER PRESENTATION before vertex delivery.

erectile having the power to become erect. *E. tissue* vascular tissue that becomes congested and swollen under stimulus, causing erection of the part, e.g. the nipple of the female breast, the male penis.

ergometrine active alkaloid principle of ergot; oxytocic drug effective in preventing or controlling postpartum haemorrhage and commonly used in conjunction with oxytocin as Syntometrine. Acts within 45 seconds when given intravenously and within 7 minutes if administered intramuscularly, and gives a sustained uterine contraction. Oral ergometrine is used to treat secondary postpartum haemorrhage resulting from retained products of conception.

ergonomics scientific study of humans in relation to their work and the effective use of human energy.

ergot drug obtained from a fungus that grows on rye; causes strong sustained contraction of muscle, especially the uterus.

erosion of the cervix during pregnancy red zone around the columnar epithelium near the external cervical os as a result of hormonal changes, which cause softening and increased HYGROSCOPIC qualities of the collagen connective tissue; usually resolves spontaneously after delivery.

erythema redness of the skin.

erythroblast immature, nucleated red blood cell.

erythroblastosis fetalis haemolytic disease of the newborn in which ERYTHROBLASTS are found in the neonatal circulation.

erythrocyte red blood cell; minute biconcave disc containing haemoglobin, which acts as a carrier of oxygen. *E. sedimentation rate* rate at which red blood cells settle at the bottom of a tube of blood, normally no more than 10 mm per hour, but increased in normal pregnancy and in infection to an average of 78 mm per hour.

erythromycin antibiotic similar to penicillin.

erythropoiesis formation of red blood cells.

Esbach's albuminometer graduated glass tube for estimating the approximate amount of albumin in urine.

Escherichia coli Gram-negative bacillus normally inhabiting the intestine, which may cause urinary tract infections and epidemic diarrhoeal diseases, especially in babies and children; may cause endotoxic shock if it enters the circulation. *See also* GRAM STAIN.

essential hypertension persistently high blood pressure of unknown cause, but often hereditary; diagnosed antenatally if first trimester blood pressure is over 140/90 mmHg; condition may worsen, remain static or improve in pregnancy. Antihypertensive drugs decrease renal and placental blood flow so are used with caution. Dangers include pre-eclampsia, ECLAMPSIA, abruptio placentae, subarachnoid haemorrhage, cardiac or renal failure, placental insufficiency, small for gestational age baby or stillbirth.

essential oils highly concentrated plant substances used in aromatherapy for their therapeutic properties resulting from the chemical constituents; they should always be diluted in a carrier oil and rarely taken by mouth. Many essential oils are contraindicated in pregnancy, labour and during breast-feeding.

estimated date of delivery *See* EXPECTED DATE OF DELIVERY.

ethambutol tuberculostatic agent.

ethics rules or principles that govern correct conduct, and personal and social values. Midwives must adhere to the NMC Code of Professional Conduct for the Nurse, Midwife and Health Visitor 2000, which provides guidance and advice for standards of practice and conduct that are essential for the ethical discharge of the practitioner's responsibility; the Midwives' Code of Practice provides guidance specifically related to the role of the midwife.

ethinyloestradiol contraceptive pills containing oestrogen and progesterone; usual dose 30 mg, commenced 3–4 weeks postpartum but contraindicated during breastfeeding.

ethnic pertaining to a social group that shares cultural bonds or physical (racial) characteristics. *E. minority* social grouping of people who share cultural or racial factors but who constitute a minority within the greater culture or society.

ethnography study of the culture of a single race; data are collected through observation, usually during a period of residence with the group being studied.

ethnomethodology sociological theory concentrating on case studies using participant or non-participant observation.

ethyl chloride local anaesthetic applied topically to intact skin.

etiology *See* AETIOLOGY.

eugenics study of measures that may be taken to improve future generations.

euphoria feeling of well-being, not always justified by the circumstances.

Eustachian tube narrow tube connecting the tympanum (middle ear) with the nasopharynx.

eutocia normal labour or childbirth.

evacuation emptying. *E. of retained products of conception (ERPC)* surgical emptying of the uterus to remove blood clots and placental tissue, to prevent or control severe uterine postpartum haemorrhage.

evaluation fourth stage in a process approach to care, in which the effectiveness of care is judged.

eversion turning inside out; to turn outward.

evidence-based practice systematic appraisal of clinical situations; use of contemporary research findings as a justification for clinical decision making.

evisceration destructive operation to remove abdominal and thoracic organs of a dead fetus when a tumour or gross ascites has delayed vaginal delivery; rarely used now.

evolution natural development; the process of unfolding or opening out. *Spontaneous e.* rare spontaneous delivery of a fetus in the transverse lie in which the shoulder escapes first, followed by the thorax, pelvis and limbs, and finally the head. cf. spontaneous EXPULSION.

ex- prefix meaning 'out of', 'outside', 'away from'.

exacerbation increase in the gravity or seriousness of disease symptoms.

exchange transfusion method of TRANS-FUSION in which a sample of blood is withdrawn from the patient and replaced by the same volume of donor blood, used in neonates to treat severe hyper-bilirubinaemia and anaemia, usually resulting from Rhesus incompatibility; sometimes called replacement transfusion.

excreta waste matter excreted from the body: faeces, urine, sweat, sputum, etc.

exercise in pregnancy women should be encouraged to continue gentle exercise to which they are accustomed, for as long as they feel comfortable; yoga, aerobics, pilates or Aquanatal exercises are popular antenatal activities. *See also* POSTNATAL EXERCISES.

exfoliation falling off in scales or layers. adj. *exfoliative. Lamellar e. of newborn* congenital hereditary disorder in which the baby is completely covered with parchment-like membrane that peels off within 24 hours, after which there may be complete healing or the scales may reform and the process is repeated. In the severe form, the baby (harlequin fetus) is completely covered with thick, horny, armour-like scales and is usually stillborn or dies shortly after birth; also termed ichthyosis congenita, ichthyosis fetalis or lamellar ichthyosis.

exocrine 1. secreting externally via a duct. 2. denoting such a gland or its secretion.

exogenous of external origin.

exomphalos rare herniation via the umbilicus of abdominal contents covered with peritoneum; in unanticipated cases, the midwife should cover the area with a sterile non-adhesive dressing and cotton wool, to avoid damage from infection, and call medical aid.

exotoxin potent toxin formed and excreted by bacterial cells into the surrounding medium, most commonly due to *Clostridium*; diphtheria, botulism and tetanus are all caused by bacterial toxins.

expected date of delivery (EDD) calculated by counting forwards 9 months and adding 7 days from the first day of the last normal menstrual period or counting back 3 months and adding 7 days. Adjustments are made for a regular long cycle by adding the number of days that the cycle is in excess of 28 or, in a regular short cycle, by subtracting the number of days that the cycle is less than 28.

expression pressing out. 1. pressure on the uterus to facilitate the expulsion of the placenta. *See* CREDÉ'S EXPRESSION. 2. mechanical or digital pressure on the areola to compress the lacteal sinuses so that milk is removed from the breast.

expulsion forcible driving out, e.g. of the fetus from the uterus. *Spontaneous e.* the manner in which a very small macerated fetus can be forced through the pelvis with the shoulder presenting so that the head and trunk are born together.

exsanguinate to deprive of blood, as after a severe haemorrhage.

extension drawing out, lengthening, opposite of flexion; e.g. in normal labour the occiput escapes under the pubic arcula, forced downwards by uterine contractions and forwards by the pelvic floor muscles, and the head extends, pivoting under the symphysis pubis.

external os opening from the cervical canal into the vagina.

external version manoeuvre designed to convert a malpresentation to one that is more likely to result in a vaginal delivery, e.g. breech presentation to cephalic, or transverse or oblique lie to longitudinal lie, in either a cephalic or breech presentation. Complications include true cord knots, placental abruption, fetal distress.

extra- prefix meaning 'outside'.

extracellular fluid fluid outside the cells.

extracorporeal membrane oxygenation (ECMO) neonatal ventilation method involving oxygenation of the blood supply outside the body, using technology similar to cardiac bypass support, allowing the lungs to rest and recover; baby must be at least 34 weeks' gestation and weigh over 1.8 kg.

extrauterine pregnancy embedding of the fertilised ovum outside the uterine cavity, e.g. in the abdominal cavity, ovary or, most commonly, the fallopian tube. *See* ECTOPIC PREGNANCY.

extravasation discharge or leaking of fluid from its normal channel into surrounding tissue, e.g. escape of blood or lymph from a vessel.

extrinsic of external origin. *E. factor* haematopoietic vitamin that combines with intrinsic factor for absorption and is needed for erythrocyte maturation; also called VITAMIN B12, CYANOCOBALAMIN.

extubation removal of a tube used in intubation.

exudation outward flow of a liquid or semi-liquid substance, e.g. of sebum from the sebaceous glands.

face area from mentum or chin to the supraorbital ridges; composed of 14 fused bones.

face presentation cephalic presentation with fetal spine and head extended and the face lowest in the pelvis; occurs in about 1:500–600 deliveries. May result from occipitoposterior position with insufficient flexion, possibly due to android pelvis, causing the biparietal diameter to be caught in the sacrocotyloid diameter, extending the head. Anencephaly is a less common cause now that ultrasound scans diagnose this early in pregnancy. The denominator is the mentum: labour may be uncomplicated with spontaneous delivery in a mentoanterior position, especially in a multipara with a small baby; spontaneous delivery is unlikely in a mentoposterior position unless the chin rotates anteriorly – there is a risk of persistent mentoposterior position with obstructed labour, in which case Caesarean section is necessary. The baby's face will be bruised and oedematous at delivery.

Face presentation

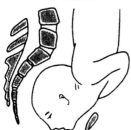

face-to-pubes persistent occipitoposterior position, in which the attitude of the head is military, neither flexed nor extended, and the sinciput, meeting the pelvic floor first, has rotated forwards bringing the occiput to the hollow of the sacrum; first- and second-stage delay is common. Maternal squatting may enlarge the pelvic outlet sufficiently to facilitate vaginal delivery but severe stretching and laceration of the pelvic floor often occurs. Forceps delivery is sometimes necessary. *See* PERSISTENT OCCIPITO-POSTERIOR.

Face-to-pubes delivery

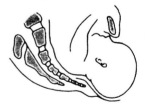

facial paralysis paralysis of the facial muscles, usually one side only, as a result of seventh cranial (facial) nerve injury, sometimes after forceps delivery; usually resolves spontaneously within a few days.

factor agent or element contributing to production of a particular result. *Anti-haemophilic f. (AHF)* factor VIII, one of the CLOTTING factors. *Anti-haemorrhagic f.* vitamin K. *Clotting f.*, *coagulation f.* factor (of which there are 12 or more) essential for normal blood clotting, whose absence, deficiency or excess may lead to an abnormal clotting mechanism. *Extrinsic f. see* EXTRINSIC. *Intrinsic f.* glycoprotein secreted by the parietal cells of the gastric glands, necessary for absorption of VITAMIN B12; deficiency causes pernicious anaemia. *F. V Leiden mutation (fVL)* inherited blood coagulation disorder that increases risk of thrombosis and strokes in the presence of other risk factors, e.g. obesity, surgery; associated with poor placentation, fetal loss and pre-eclampsia; screened for during a THROMBOPHILIA SCREEEN. *Releasing f.* factor produced in one structure that triggers the release of hormones from another structure. *Rhesus f.* genetically determined antigens present on the surface of erythrocytes; *see* RHESUS FACTOR.

faeces food residue and other waste products excreted from the bowels.

Fahrenheit scale of temperature measurement (°F); registers freezing point of water at 32°F, normal temperature of the human body at 98.4°F, boiling point of water at 212°F. For comparison with Celsius, *see* Appendix 8.

faint temporary loss of consciousness due to generalised cerebral ischaemia; syncope.

falciform sickle-shaped.

fallopian tubes uterine tubes, oviducts; two narrow canals, each 10 cm long, leading from the uterine cornua to the ovaries.

Fallot's tetralogy combination of four congenital cardiac defects: pulmonary stenosis, ventricular septal defects, right ventricular hypertrophy, dextroposition of the aorta in which it overrides the interventricular septum and receives venous as well as arterial blood.

false labour painful uterine contractions simulating labour, but without cervical dilatation, possibly due to increasing muscle contractility but without normal uterine FUNDAL DOMINANCE.

false pelvis region between the brim of the true pelvis and the crests of the ilia.

false-positive rate measure of a screening test's performance; the proportion of people who have a positive screening result but do not have the condition.

falx sickle, or a sickle-shaped structure.

falx cerebri sickle-shaped fold of dura mater separating the two cerebral hemispheres of the brain.

familial occurring in families, as in inherited conditions, e.g. haemophilia and acholuric jaundice.

family group of people residing together, usually related by blood or marriage. *Extended f.* nuclear family and their close relatives, e.g. children's grandparents, aunts and uncles. *Nuclear f.* couple and their children by birth or adoption living together and isolated from their extended family. *Single-parent f.* lone parent and offspring living as a family unit.

family planning arrangement, spacing and limitation of children in a family, depending on parental preferences and social circumstances. *See* CONTRACEPTION.

fascia sheet or band of fibrous connective tissue, either arranged loosely around organs and blood vessels or in dense strong sheets, often between muscles forming their attachments. *Pelvic f.* fascia of the pelvic cavity, with a parietal layer lining the walls and covering the pelvic floor and a visceral layer surrounding and supporting the pelvic organs; the part around the uterus is called the parametrium.

fat 1. adipose or fatty body tissue. 2. neutral fat; triglyceride (or triacylglycerol), a compound of fatty acids and glycerol.

fat soluble capable of being dissolved in fats, e.g. vitamins.

favism acute haemolytic anaemia caused by ingestion of fava beans. *See* GLUCOSE-6-PHOSPHATE DEHYDROGENASE.

febrile feverish; pyrexial.

fecundation fertilisation.

fecundity ability to produce offspring.

female genital mutilation female circumcision involving excision of labia majora, labia minora and clitoris and sometimes partial closure of the introitus; prevalent in areas such as the Sudan. Complications include problems with micturition and intercourse preconceptionally; excision and separation of the tissues may be required in labour or Caesarean section may be necessary.

feminisation 1. normal development of female sexual characteristics. 2. development of female sexual characteristics in the male. *Testicular f.* condition in which the individual is phenotypically female but lacks nuclear sex chromatin and is genetically male (has one X and one Y chromosome).

femoral pertaining to the femur. *F. artery* principal artery of the thigh, a continuation of the external iliac artery. *F. vein* main vein of the thigh, a continuation of the popliteal vein, passing up the leg through the groin and continuing as the external iliac vein.

femur thigh bone, from the hip to the knee, articulating with the innominate bone at the acetabulum.

fenestrated possessing a window-like opening or *fenestra*, as in the blades of midwifery forceps. *F. placenta* or *placenta fenestrata; see* PLACENTA.

fentanyl intravenous or intramuscular analgesic for intra- and postoperative pain.

Fentazin *See* PERPHENAZINE.

ferment to induce chemical changes as a result of enzymes with specific actions.

fern test cervical cytology to determine the amount of oestrogen in cervical mucus; oestrogen in the dried cervical mucus has a fern-like appearance on low-power microscopy.

ferritin iron–apoferritin complex; one of the forms in which iron is stored in the body.

ferrous containing iron in its plus two oxidation state. *F. fumarate* anhydrous salt, a combination of ferrous iron and fumaric acid; used as a haematinic. *F. gluconate* haematinic, less irritating to the gastrointestinal tract than other haematinics, generally used as a substitute when ferrous sulphate cannot be tolerated. *F. sulphate* most widely used haematinic to treat iron deficiency anaemia, less irritating than equivalent amounts of ferric salts and more effective.

fertile capable of producing offspring. *F. period* 1. 9 days surrounding ovulation when fertilisation of the ovum is theoretically possible; including the day of ovulation, it is normally classified as 5 days before and 3 days after ovulation; assessed over several months by recording the basal temperature. 2. period of a woman's life during which she may be able to achieve pregnancy, usually between the ages of 15 and 45.

fertility ability to produce young. *See also* SUBFERTILITY *and* INFERTILITY.

fertilisation impregnation, conception; union of the spermatozoon and the ovum to create a new human being, with traits such as sex and biological determinants specified by the genes and chromosomes present. *In vitro f.* artificial fertilisation of the ovum under laboratory conditions. *In vivo f.* artificial fertilisation within the reproductive tract.

fetal pertaining to the fetus. *F. abnormality see* MALFORMATION. *F. alcohol syndrome* condition resulting from heavy maternal consumption of alcohol, characterised by delivery of a small for gestational age baby with abnormalities of facial features and mental retardation. *F. death see* INTRAUTERINE DEATH. *F. haemoglobin* haemoglobin F, which differs from adult haemoglobin as it has a greater affinity for and higher capacity for oxygen; it forms 85% of the haemoglobin of a full-term baby at birth. *F. heart sounds* fetal heart beat, auscultated and counted via the abdominal wall, uterus and amniotic fluid, which may be continuously recorded with a fetal heart monitor. *F. maturity* assessment of the developmental stage of the fetus, usually by ultrasound, including measurement of the long bones of the femurs and size of the head. *F. blood sampling see* CORDOCENTESIS. *F. distress* clinical manifestation of fetal hypoxia. Maternal medical causes include disturbance of respiration, e.g. eclampsia or epilepsy; inadequate circulation, e.g. cardiac failure, severe anaemia, hyper- or hypotension; diabetes mellitus; infection. Uterine causes include hypertonicity or excessive retraction in obstructed labour; partial placental separation; placental insufficiency. Fetal causes include intracranial birth trauma; severe Rhesus incompatibility with gross anaemia; congenital abnormality; intrauterine infections; multiple pregnancy; malpresentation and malposition; cord prolapse; true knots; traction on the cord. Diagnosis is made from abnormal fetal heart rate and regularity, meconium-stained amniotic fluid, excessive fetal movements; delivery is expedited either by instrumental delivery or Caesarean section. *See also* CARDIOTOCOGRAPHY.

fetal skull fetal bony head structure; the *vault* contains the brain and is composed of two frontal bones divided by a frontal suture, two parietal bones divided by the sagittal suture and separated from the frontal bones by the coronal suture, and one occipital bone separated from the parietal bones by the lambdoidal suture. The membranous junction of three or more sutures forms the anterior fontanelle or BREGMA and the

posterior fontanelle or LAMBDA. Sutures and fontanelles felt on vaginal examination enable the midwife to determine the position of the fetal head in a cephalic presentation; *see* figure and Appendix 4. The *base* of the skull is composed of two temporal bones, one ethmoid bone and one sphenoid bone and part of the occipital bone, and contains an opening called the foramen magnum through which the spinal cord passes. The *face* is composed of 14 fused bones. *Diameters* of the skull are assessed to estimate progress in labour, and are taken longitudinally or transversely; circumferences may also be assessed. Within the skull are the brain and intracranial membranes, the FALX CEREBRI and the TENTORIUM CEREBELLI, carrying the venous sinuses by which blood is drained from the head: the SUPERIOR and INFERIOR LONGITUDINAL SINUSES, the STRAIGHT SINUS, the

Vault of the fetal skull

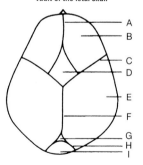

A, frontal suture; **B,** frontal bone; **C,** coronal suture; **D,** anterior fontanelle or bregma; **E,** parietal bone; **F,** sagittal suture; G, posterior fontanelle or lambda; **H,** lambdoid suture; **I,** occipital bone.

**Longitudinal diameters
(with diameters (cm))**

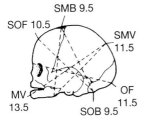

SOF, suboccipitofrontal; SMB, submentobregmatic; MV, mentovertical; SOB, suboccipitobregmatic; OF, occipitofrontal; SMV, submentovertical.

TRANSVERSE SINUS and the GREAT VEIN OF GALEN. If delivery or MOULDING are excessive the membranes and sinuses may be torn, causing intracranial haemorrhage.

fetocide injection to dispose of a fetus affected by serious abnormality in a twin pregnancy, to enable the other to grow and develop normally.

fetoscopy visualisation of the fetus by inserting an endoscope through the maternal abdominal wall into the uterus, now replaced by ULTRASONOGRAPHY.

fetus human embryo from 8 weeks of pregnancy until birth. *F. papyraceus* one of a set of twins that dies *in utero* in early pregnancy and becomes flattened against the uterine wall, usually expelled with the placenta, resembling a piece of parchment.

fever pyrexia, high body temperature; illness characterised by pyrexia.

fibre thread-like structure; muscle cell. *Dietary f.* ingested foodstuffs that cannot be broken down by intestinal enzymes and juices, passing through the small intestine and colon undigested, e.g. vegetables, cereals, fruits; assist in preventing constipation.

fibrin insoluble protein formed by the action of thrombin upon fibrinogen; necessary for blood clotting: it forms a network of minute long strands in which blood cells get caught.

fibrinogen protein formed in the liver that circulates in blood plasma; activated by THROMBIN when tissue injury occurs and forms FIBRIN, which arrests haemorrhage by clotting. Preparations containing human fibrinogen, e.g. fresh frozen plasma and cryoprecipitate, are used to restore blood fibrinogen levels after extensive surgery or to treat diseases or haemorrhagic conditions complicated by AFIBRINOGENAEMIA; pure fibrinogen is rarely used to avoid transmitting hepatitis.

fibrinolysin 1. PLASMIN. 2. a proteolytic enzyme formed from profibrinolysin (plasminogen) by the action of physical agents or by specific bacterial kinases; used to promote dissolution of thrombi.

fibrinolysis dissolution of fibrin by enzymatic action. adj. *fibrinolytic.*

fibrocystic disease *See* CYSTIC FIBROSIS.

fibroid 1. composed of fibrous tissue. 2. benign uterine tumour; submucosal, interstitial or subserous, or occasionally intracervical, commonly seen in primigravidae over 30. Problems in pregnancy are rare although, occasionally, red degeneration or miscarriage occurs; labour difficulties are unlikely but fibroids near the placental site may interfere with uterine contractions, causing postpartum haemorrhage. Fibroids usually decrease in size spontaneously in the puerperium.

fibromyoma fibroid.

fibroplasia formation of fibrous tissue as in wound healing. *Retrolental f.* retinal vascular proliferation and tortuosity with the presence of fibrous tissue behind the lens, leading to retinal detachment and arrested eye growth, often as a consequence of the use of excessively high oxygen concentrations in the care of preterm infants.

fibrosis formation of fibrous tissue; fibroid degeneration. adj. *fibrotic*. *Cystic f.* hereditary disorder with widespread dysfunction of exocrine glands, chronic pulmonary disease, pancreatic deficiency, high levels of electrolytes in sweat and, sometimes, biliary cirrhosis. *See also* CYSTIC FIBROSIS.

fibula lateral and smaller of the two bones of the leg.

filter porous substance permitting passage of fluids and materials in solution whilst retaining solids, e.g. cellulose acetate filter to remove bacteria and sterilise a solution, as in EPIDURAL ANALGESIA.

filtrate fluid that has passed through a filter.

fimbria finger-like fringe, as in the extremity of the fallopian tube. pl. *fimbriae*. adj. *fimbriated*.

first-degree perineal laceration *See* PERINEAL LACERATION.

first stage of labour from onset of painful regular uterine contractions and dilatation of the cervix until full dilatation of the cervix.

fission cleavage or splitting; reproduction by division of a cell into two equal parts. *Nuclear f.* splitting of the nucleus of an atom.

fissure cleft; either normal, as in a cerebral fissure, or due to disease, e.g. anal fissure.

fistula abnormal passage between two cavities or between a cavity and the surface of the body. *Rectovaginal f.* opening between vagina and rectum, usually due to severe and/or neglected laceration of the perineal body. *Vesicovaginal f.* opening between bladder and vagina, sometimes due to prolonged pressure in neglected obstructed labour.

fit seizure; convulsion, as in eclampsia or epilepsy.

flaccid limp; without tone, as in the muscles of a baby with severe asphyxia.

flagellum whip-like protoplasmic filament by which some bacteria move, e.g. *Trichomonas vaginalis*, a flagellated protozoon. pl. *flagella*.

Flagyl *See* METRONIDAZOLE.

flank side of the abdomen, between the ribs and the iliac crest.

flat pelvis pelvis in which the anteroposterior diameter of the brim is much shorter than the transverse diameter; the two described are platypelloid or rachitic. *See* PELVIS.

flatulence presence of gas or air in the stomach or intestine, causing discomfort or sometimes severe pain.

flatus gas in the bowel.

fleshy mole CARNEOUS MOLE; mass of clotted blood surrounding a dead embryo retained in the uterus.

flexion bending; normal attitude of the fetus *in utero*. *See* ANTEFLEXION *and* RETROFLEXION.

'flooding' severe uterine bleeding; lay term for MENORRHAGIA or METRORRHAGIA.

flora *Intestinal f.* bacteria normally residing within the lumen of the intestine.

flucloxacillin antibiotic active against most staphylococci and streptococci, including the majority of penicillinase-producing staphylococci, given orally, intramuscularly or intravenously.

fluid liquid or gas. *Amniotic f.* fluid within the amnion that bathes the developing fetus and protects it from mechanical injury. *Body f.* fluid within the body, composed of water, electrolytes and non-electrolytes that are continuously in motion. *Intracellular f.* fluid within the cell, constituting about two-thirds of the total body fluid. *Extracellular f.* fluid outside the cell, constituting about one-third of the total body fluid. *Cerebrospinal f.* fluid within the ventricles of the brain, subarachnoid space, and central canal of the spinal cord. *F. balance* normal volume of body water and its solutes (electrolytes and non-electrolytes), with normal distribution of fluids within the intracellular and extracellular compartments; total volume of body fluids is normally about 60% of the body weight. *F. balance chart* observation and recording of fluid intake and output for women susceptible to or suffering from disturbances in the balance of body fluids, as in severe pre-eclampsia.

fluorescence *in situ* hybridisation (FISH) diagnostic chromosome test used to identify TRISOMY and sex chromosome ANEUPLOIDY (but does not analyse the whole KARYOTYPE), performed after CHORIONIC VILLUS SAMPLING or AMNIOCENTESIS on uncultured cells to obtain rapid results (within 24–48 hours). Technique relies on coloured DEOXYRIBONUCLEIC ACID (DNA) probes, which attach to specific chromosome regions through hybridisation. Fluorescent spots appear and the number of spots in each cell can then be counted. Two spots indicate normal DIPLOID chromosomes; three spots indicate TRISOMY. *See also* QUANTITATIVE FLUORESCENCE POLYMERASE CHAIN REACTION (QF-PCR).

fluorescent treponemal antibody-absorbed test (FTA-abs) specific treponemal antibody test to confirm diagnosis of syphilis when the initial VENEREAL DISEASE RESEARCH LABORATORY (VDRL) test is positive; sensitive to early stages of infection.

folate large group of compounds derived from FOLIC ACID, necessary for various biochemical reactions in the body, especially DNA synthesis. Serum and erythrocyte folate levels are used to assess body stores; low levels are found in megaloblastic anaemia secondary to folate deficiency.

folic acid constituent of vitamin B complex, necessary for development of normal red blood cells; found in green vegetables, liver and yeast; also produced synthetically. Preconceptional deficiency may contribute to fetal neural tube defects: all women planning to conceive are encouraged to take folic acid supplements. Antenatal deficiency, resulting from inability of the body to absorb or utilise vitamin B, causes megaloblastic anaemia, as rapidly dividing fetal cells compete for folic acid to form cell nuclei.

follicle very small sac or gland. *graafian f.* small vesicle containing an ovum, formed in the ovary; one follicle matures during each menstrual cycle. *See* GONADOTROPHIC.

follicle-stimulating hormone (FSH) hormone released from the anterior pituitary gland, stimulating one or more GRAAFIAN FOLLICLES to mature during each menstrual cycle.

fomites substances or objects that transmit infectious organisms by contamination.

fontanelle membranous space where two or more sutures meet between the cranial bones of the skull. *Anterior f.* bregma. *Posterior f.* lambda. *See* FETAL SKULL.

footling presentation breech presentation in which one or both feet present before the buttocks. *See also* BREECH PRESENTATION.

foramen opening or hole, especially in a bone. *F. magnum* occipital bone opening through which the medulla oblongata becomes continuous with the spinal cord. *Obturator f.* large hole in the os innominatum of the pelvis. *F. ovale* opening between the two atria of the fetal heart.

forceps surgical instrument with two blades used for lifting or compressing an object, e.g. *dressing f.*, *dissecting f.* *Artery f.* compress bleeding points during an operation. *Midwifery f.* used in second-stage labour to deliver the baby's head if it is safer for the mother or baby, e.g. KIELLAND'S, NEVILLE BARNES and WRIGLEY'S FORCEPS. *Vulsellum f.* with claw-like ends. *See* Appendix 3.

foreskin prepuce; skin covering the glans penis.

forewaters amniotic fluid in the part of the bag of membranes lying below the presenting part of the fetus. *See also* HINDWATERS.

formaldehyde powerful disinfectant gas that produces formalin when in solution; used for preservation of specimens.

formalin *See* FORMALDEHYDE.

formula 1. prescription or recipe, especially for an infant's feed. 2. group of symbols making a certain statement, as in chemical symbols.

fornix arch; there are four fornices in the vault of the vagina, in front of (*anterior f.*), behind (*posterior f.*) and at the sides (*lateral f.*) of the cervix. pl. *fornices*.

Fortral *See* PENTAZOCINE HYDROCHLORIDE.

fossa pit or hollow, e.g. the iliac fossa, depression on the inner surface of the iliac bone.

foster children children in the care of FOSTER PARENTS.

foster parents responsible adults who, under the Children Act, are paid to care for children unrelated to them.

Fothergill's operation operation for uterovaginal prolapse; also called Manchester operation.

Foundation for Study of Infant Deaths (FSID) registered charity, providing support for parents whose baby's death has apparently been a 'cot death'; sponsors research into the syndrome.

fourchette fold of skin between the posterior extremities of the labia minora.

fracture break, usually of bone; occurs occasionally in difficult deliveries, e.g. depressed fracture of the skull, or in breech delivery, e.g. fracture of the clavicle, humerus or femur.

fraenum, frenum, frenulum small ligament that checks the movement of an organ, e.g. the *f. linguae* membranous connection between the floor of the mouth and lower surface of the tongue. *See* TONGUE TIE.

fragilitas ossium OSTEOGENESIS IMPERFECTA; fragile brittle bones.

Frankenhauser's plexus ganglion near the uterine cervix from which sympathetic and parasympathetic nerves supply the vagina, uterus and other pelvic viscera.

friable easily torn, broken or crumbled, e.g. placental chorion is friable and may be torn and partially retained in the uterus after delivery.

Friars' balsam compound tincture of benzoin; decongestant when inhaled as a vapour.

frigidity coldness; sexual unresponsiveness to physical stimulation in women, usually because of psychological causes.

frontal pertaining to the forehead. *F. bones* two bones forming the forehead in the fetus. *F. suture* membranous channel between the two frontal bones. *F. headache* serious symptom of severe PRE-ECLAMPSIA or impending ECLAMPSIA caused by cerebral oedema.

fulminating bursting forth, violently explosive; applied to conditions appearing suddenly and severely, e.g. pre-eclampsia and eclampsia.

fundal pertaining to the fundus, e.g. of the uterus. *F. dominance* normal uterine contractions originate from a pacemaker in the fundus, the wave of contraction gradually weakening as it passes over the upper and lower segments of the uterus. *F. pressure* rarely used method in which the contracted FUNDUS UTERI is used as a piston to expel the placenta and complete the third stage of labour.

fundus base of an organ or the part furthest removed from the opening. *F. uteri* top of the uterus, the part furthest from the cervix.

fungus group of eukaryotic organisms (mushrooms, yeasts, moulds, etc.); thrush is a fungal condition.

funic pertaining to the umbilical cord. *F. souffle* soft whispering sound from the umbilical cord, synchronising with fetal heart sounds.

funipuncture *See* CORDOCENTESIS.

funis umbilical cord.

funnel pelvis pelvis that narrows from above downwards, e.g. ANDROID PELVIS, in which the outlet is smaller than the brim.

Furadantin *See* NITROFURANTOIN.

furosemide (frusemide) diuretic that blocks reabsorption of sodium and chloride in the ascending loop of Henle; used in pregnancy for treatment of pulmonary oedema and occasionally for oliguria and acute renal failure; dose is 20–40 mg intravenously or intramuscularly; may inhibit lactation.

g

gag 1. instrument for holding open the jaws. 2. to retch, or strive to vomit. *G.reflex* elevation of the soft palate and retching, elicited by touching the back of the tongue or the wall of the pharynx; pharyngeal reflex.

Gairdner headbox perspex box placed over the baby's head into which additional oxygen is provided to increase the oxygen concentration of inspired air.

gait walk or carriage; abnormal gait in a pregnant woman may indicate pelvic deformity.

galact-, galacto- word element meaning 'milk'.

galactischia suppression of milk secretion.

galactogogue agent that is said to increase the secretion of milk.

galactorrhoea excessive flow of breast milk.

galactosaemia genetically determined biochemical disorder in which lack of an enzyme necessary for metabolism of galactose leads to high levels of galactose in the blood and tissues, causing failure to thrive, hepatomegaly and jaundice, and ultimately, mental retardation and death if untreated; exclusion of all galactose- or lactose-containing foods from the diet will control the condition.

galactose MONOSACCHARIDE resulting from the digestion of LACTOSE, converted to glucose by the liver.

galactose-1-phosphate uridyltransferase enzyme that converts galactose to glucose; deficiency causes galactosaemia.

galea aponeurotica tendon of the occipitofrontalis muscle, which forms a layer of the scalp.

Galen, vein of *See* GREAT VEIN OF GALEN.

gall bladder sac on the under part of the liver, holding and concentrating bile secreted by the liver. *G. b. changes in pregnancy* dilatation of the gall bladder in pregnancy slows the rate of emptying, causing thickened bile and an increased chance of OBSTETRIC CHOLESTASIS, whereas incomplete emptying may also lead to gallstones, which are relatively common in asymptomatic women.

gamete male or female reproductive cell.

gamete intrafallopian transfer (GIFT) infertility treatment involving retrieval of oocytes from the ovary at laparoscopy and placing them sequentially with sperm into the fallopian tubes; suitable for women with unexplained infertility and those with at least one patent, healthy fallopian tube when the male sperm parameters are near normal. *See also* ZYGOTE INTRAFALLOPIAN TRANSFER.

gamgee tissue absorbent wool covered with gauze, used for dressing wounds, etc.

gamma globulin class of plasma proteins composed almost entirely of IgG, an IMMUNOGLOBULIN protein containing most antibody activity and providing almost all known antibodies circulating in the blood. Commerical preparations are derived from blood serum and used to prevent, modify and treat various infectious diseases, providing passive immunity, usually for about 6 weeks against infections to which most of the population has antibodies. Gamma globulin with high anti-Rhesus antibody activity is given to Rhesus-negative mothers within 72 hours of delivery to prevent natural formation of antibody; other types can raise the body's resistance to measles, mumps and poliomyelitis.

ganglion nerve centre from which nerve fibres proceed.

gangrene death of tissue, usually applied to a large area or definite organ. *Dry g.* due to failure of arterial blood supply, e.g. process by which the umbilical cord dries and separates from the umbilicus about 5–7 days after birth. *Moist g.* caused by putrefactive changes, e.g. umbilical cord infection when it remains moist, becomes offensive and separation is delayed. *See also* GAS GANGRENE.

Gardnerella See BACTERIAL VAGINOSIS.

gargoylism type of MUCOPOLYSACCHARIDOSIS.

gas vaporous matter in its least dense form, neither solid nor liquid, where molecules are in constant movement; air is a mixture of several gases: oxygen, nitrogen, traces of carbon dioxide, argon and helium.

'gas and oxygen' analgesia *See* INHALATION ANALGESIA *and* ENTONOX.

gas gangrene infection of damaged tissues by the anaerobic organism *Clostridium welchii*, occurring occasionally after criminal abortion and, very rarely, after labour.

gastric pertaining to the stomach.

gastritis inflammation of the stomach lining.

gastro- prefix meaning 'relating to the stomach'.

gastroenteritis inflammation of the lining of the stomach and intestine; acute condition of diarrhoea and vomiting producing rapid and severe dehydration, particularly dangerous in babies; immediate isolation from other babies is vital; oral or intravenous fluids are given to combat dehydration, correct electrolyte balance and treat the infection.

gastrointestinal pertaining to the stomach and intestines. *G. tract* alimentary tract.

gastrojejunostomy surgical anastomosis of the stomach to the jejunum, performed to bypass obstruction in babies born with duodenal atresia.

gastro-oesophageal reflux in pregnancy common physiological disorder caused by relaxation of the cardiac sphincter at the stomach entrance leading to regurgitation of acid stomach contents; common with large fetus or multiple pregnancy; may accompany gestational sickness; postural adaptations may exacerbate or reduce the problem; antacids may be given to relieve oesophageal burning.

gastroschisis congenital fissure of the abdominal wall.

gastrostomy creation of an opening into the stomach to allow administration of food and liquids when stricture of the oesophagus or other conditions make swallowing impossible.

gate control theory of pain theory proposed by Melzack and Wall in 1965 of a neural mechanism in the dorsal horns of the spinal cord that acts like a gate, increasing or decreasing nerve impulse flow from peripheral fibres to the central nervous system; the position of the gate determines how much information is transmitted to the brain and the amount of pain perceived. Anxiety and anticipation cause the gate to open, increasing pain levels; other factors may cause the gate to close, reducing pain perception. TRANSCUTANEOUS ELECTRICAL NERVE STIMULATION (TENS) applied to nerve fibres in the skin impairs transmission of painful stimuli from the peripheral to central nervous systems, closing the gate, and, in conjunction with endorphin release from the brain, effectively reduces pain, e.g. in labour.

gauze large-mesh, thin cotton material, used for dressings.

Geiger counter instrument used to detect radioactive substances.

gemellology scientific study of twins and twinning.

gemeprost pessaries that soften and dilate the cervix, used to facilitate first-trimester transcervical procedures (1 mg is administered 3 hours before surgery) and for second-trimester termination of pregnancy (1 mg is given every 3 hours up to a maximum of five doses, then, if necessary, a second course is commenced 24 hours later).

gender category to which an individual is assigned on the basis of sex.

gene single unit of hereditary factors located in a defined position on a CHROMOSOME; composed of DEOXYRIBONUCLEIC ACID (DNA), consisting of a complex double chain of molecules carrying individual genetic codes and controlling day-to-day functions and reproduction of all body cells, e.g. synthesis of structural proteins and enzymes that regulate various chemical reactions taking place in a cell. Genes are capable of replication by mitosis; each daughter cell carries an exact replica of the genes of the parent cell and can carry hereditary traits through successive generations without change. Occasionally, abnormal or mutant genes occur, e.g. as in PHENYLKETONURIA, a condition in which there are two abnormal RECESSIVE genes.

general anaesthesia only occasionally used in obstetrics because of the increased use of REGIONAL ANAESTHESIA; remains a significant cause of maternal death, notably due to MENDELSON'S SYNDROME, which can be prevented by antacid therapy and the application of CRICOID PRESSURE.

General Medical Council (GMC) regulating body of all UK doctors; medical equivalent of the Nursing and Midwifery Council.

generic 1. pertaining to a genus. 2. general, non-proprietary; e.g. drug name not protected by a trademark.

genetic counselling consultation at which a geneticist explains the chances of recurrence of hereditary diseases, advising couples on any risk to future children.

genetics study of heredity.

genital relating to the organs of reproduction.

genitalia organs of reproduction.

genitourinary pertaining to the genital and urinary organs.

genome entire genetic complement of a cell or organism; the human genome is thought to have approximately 30 000 genes.

genotype classification of the genetic makeup of an individual. *See* GENE.

gentamicin antibiotic complex, effective against many gram-negative bacteria, especially *Pseudomonas*, and certain gram-positive bacteria, especially *Staphylococcus aureus*; used to treat septicaemia and neonatal sepsis, particularly of the central nervous system; should be avoided in pregnancy because of the risk of fetal eighth cranial nerve damage.

gentian violet antibacterial, antifungal, antihelminthic dye; applied topically for mould and gram-positive bacterial infections of the skin and mucous membranes and administered orally in pinworm and liver fluke infections.

genu knee.

genupectoral position knee–chest position, i.e. face downwards, resting on knees and chest. *See* POSITION.

genus classificatory group of animals or plants comprising one or more species.

German measles *See* RUBELLA.

germicide agent that destroys microorganisms.

gestagen hormones with progestational activity.

gestalt whole perceptual configuration. *G. therapy* psychotherapeutic approach that encourages individuals to cease intellectualising difficulties and to focus on feelings and emotions, gaining emotional insight and balance.

gestation pregnancy. *G. period* in humans approximately 40 weeks from the first day of the last normal menstrual period. *Ectopic g.* pregnancy outside the uterus. *G. sac* placenta and membranes containing the amniotic fluid and fetus during pregnancy.

gestational pertaining to gestation. *G. hypertension* raised blood pressure during pregnancy, which may progress to pre-eclampsia or eclampsia. *G. diabetes* former term for impaired glucose tolerance during pregnancy, which reverts to normal after delivery; these women are more likely to develop overt clinical diabetes mellitus in later life.

gigantism abnormal overgrowth of whole or part of the body, due to overactivity of the anterior pituitary growth hormone.

Gigli's operation pubiotomy. *See* SYMPHYSIOTOMY.

Gigli's saw fine wire instrument for sawing through bone.

gingivitis inflammation and bleeding of the gums.

girdle belt. *Pelvic g.* bony ring of the pelvis formed by the two innominate bones and the sacrum.

glabella area on the frontal bone above the nose and between the eyebrows.

gland collection of cells that secrete or excrete materials not related to their own metabolic needs. *Endocrine g's* secrete hormones into the bloodstream, e.g. thyroid gland secretes thyroxine.

glans acorn-shaped body, e.g. rounded end of the penis and the clitoris.

globin protein constituent of haemoglobin; also, any of a group of proteins similar to typical globin.

globulins class of plasma proteins, further subdivided into alpha (α), beta (β) and gamma (γ) globulins. *See also* GAMMA GLOBULIN *and* IMMUNOGLOBULIN.

glomerulus tuft of capillaries invaginated in the kidney tubule at its commencement in the renal cortex.

glossal pertaining to the tongue.

glottis vocal apparatus of the larynx, consisting of the true vocal cords and the opening between them.

glucagon the polypeptide hormone secreted by the alpha cells of the islets of Langerhans in response to hypoglycaemia or to stimulation by growth hormone; increases blood glucose concentration by stimulating glycogenolysis in the liver; administered to reverse hypoglycaemic coma, especially caused by hyperinsulinism.

glucocorticoid any corticoid substance that increases gluconeogenesis, raising the concentration of liver glycogen and blood sugar, i.e. cortisol (hydrocortisone), cortisone and corticosterone.

glucose dextrose found in fruits and honey; monosaccharide to which carbohydrates are reduced by digestion, producing energy for the body's cells and controlled by insulin. Surplus glucose is stored as glycogen in the liver and muscle, readily available when needed. Normal fasting glucose levels in the blood range between 70 and 90 mg per 100 mL (3.9–5.6 mmol/L); excessively high levels of glucose (hyperglycaemia) may indicate DIABETES MELLITUS, HYPERTHYROIDISM and hyperpituitarism; a GLUCOSE TOLERANCE TEST assesses the body's ability to metabolise glucose. Glucose is present in the urine of women with untreated diabetes mellitus.

glucose-6-phosphate dehydrogenase (G6PD) important enzyme in red blood cells. G6PD deficiency is an inherited X-linked RECESSIVE trait common in black races and Mediterranean people; absence leads to attacks of HAEMOLYSIS and severe or fatal anaemia following the intake of fava beans (favism), for example.

glucose tolerance test (GTT) test to diagnose gestational DIABETES MELLITUS, in which the mother's blood glucose levels are monitored before and after ingesting 75 g glucose; a fasting blood glucose level between 5.5 and 7.0 mmol/L and a glucose level between 7.8 and 11.1 mmol/L 2 hours after glucose ingestion suggests impaired glucose tolerance; levels higher than these values indicate gestational diabetes. Indications for the test include previous gestational diabetes, previous MACROSOMIA, close relative with diabetes (type 1 or type 2), POLYHYDRAMNIOS or maternal obesity (body mass index >35 kg/m²).

glucuronyl transferase liver enzyme; converts fat-soluble toxic bilirubin to the water-soluble non-toxic type.

glutaraldehyde antiseptic used to treat viral warts.

gluteal pertaining to the buttocks.

glycerol suppositories rectally administered medication to stimulate rectal activity.

glycogen carbohydrate polysaccharide stored in the liver and muscles.

glycosuria glucose in the urine. In pregnancy this may be related to carbohydrate ingestion and the inability to store it; a lowered renal threshold for sugar; DIABETES MELLITUS.

glycosylated haemoglobin See HbA$_{1c}$.

gnathic pertaining to the jaw or cheeks.

goblet cell goblet-shaped cell in the cubical epithelium of the fallopian tubes, producing a glycogen secretion to nourish the ovum.

goitre thyroid gland enlargement seen as a marked swelling in front of the neck, sometimes causing pressure on the trachea.

gonad organ producing ova or spermatozoa; in the female the ovary and in the male the testis.

gonadotrophic stimulating the gonads. _G. hormones_ those of the anterior pituitary lobe or placenta.

gonadotrophin any hormone that stimulates the gonads, e.g. follicle-stimulating hormone and luteinising hormone produced by the anterior pituitary. _Chorionic g._ gonad-stimulating hormone produced by the cytotrophoblast cells of the chorionic tissue, which later forms the placenta; female urine is tested for the presence of human chorionic gonadotrophin (hCG) to confirm pregnancy.

gonococcal pertaining to or caused by gonococci. _G. ophthalmia_ acute conjunctivitis due to gonococcal infection, which, in newborn babies, may lead to corneal ulceration; it was previously the commonest cause of blindness in babies and young children. _See_ OPHTHALMIA NEONATORUM.

gonococcus _Neisseria gonorrhoeae_; gram-negative intracellular diplococcus, the causative agent of gonorrhoea.

gonorrhoea sexually transmitted disease resulting from gonococcal infection; infects mucous membranes of the cervix, urethra and Bartholin's glands and may spread to cause salpingitis or septicaemia; any vaginal infection in pregnancy should be investigated and treated early. Incubation period is 1–16 days; may cause purulent vaginal or urethral discharge and burning pain on micturition but is usually symptomless; diagnosis is confirmed by smear and cultures; infection is treated with penicillin.

Goodell's sign softening of the cervix uteri and vagina; sign of pregnancy.

graafian follicle oestrogenic hormone-secreting cystic structure developing in the ovarian cortex during the menstrual cycle, with an outer covering or theca folliculi and a lining of granulosa cells surrounding the ovum within the follicle. When ripe the follicle ruptures, discharging the ovum (ovulation), and develops into a CORPUS LUTEUM.

Graafian follicle

A, follicular fluid; **B**, granulosa cells; **C**, ovum.

gram (g) unit of weight of the metric system.

Gram stain bacteriology stain; microorganisms that retain it are said to be Gram-positive; those that lose it are Gram-negative.

grand mal major epileptic seizure with loss of consciousness and convulsive movements, as distinguished from PETIT MAL, a minor seizure.

grande multigravida woman in her fourth or subsequent pregnancy, but who has not necessarily delivered live babies in previous pregnancies.

grande multipara woman of high parity, who has delivered four or more babies; increasing parity presents an increased risk of problems in pregnancy, labour and the puerperium.

granulation process of wound healing; granulations appear as small red projections on the surface of the wound, bringing a rich blood supply to the healing surface.

granulosa cells oestradiol-secreting cells lining the graafian follicle.

granulosa lutein cells granulosa cells after ovulation, which secrete oestradiol and progesterone.

gravid pregnant.

gravida pregnant woman. See PRIMIGRAVIDA and MULTIGRAVIDA.

gravity weight. *Specific g.* weight compared with that of an equal volume of water; specific gravity of water is 1.000 g/mL; specific gravity of normal urine is 1.010–1.020 g/mL, which is increased if solids are dissolved in it, e.g. sugar, and decreased when inadequate urea is excreted, e.g. in chronic nephritis.

great vein of Galen large cerebral vein passing from the midbrain and entering the junction of the inferior longitudinal and straight sinuses; extreme, abnormal or rapid fetal skull moulding during delivery may cause the cerebral membranes and the cerebral veins to be torn, resulting in intracranial haemorrhage.

grey-scale display ultrasonic method of showing different tissue textures, in which the amplitudes of the echo sound waves are shown on the screen as different shades of grey, and dense structures, e.g. bone, are white and fluids, e.g. amniotic fluid, are black. Many ultrasound machines can now view blood flow in colour.

grey syndrome potentially fatal condition seen in preterm babies caused by a reaction to chloramphenicol, characterised by an ashen grey cyanosis, vomiting, abdominal distension, hypothermia and shock.

grief sorrow, usually caused by death; the normal grieving process takes 2 or 3 years, following a pattern of numbness and denial, anger, guilt, bargaining and depression, and finally acceptance and readjustment.

groin junction of the front of the thigh with the trunk.

group B streptococcus (GBS) bacterial COMMENSAL found in rectum or vagina of 20–25% of pregnant women; many babies are colonised with GBS at birth and have no ill effects, but 1:16 000 babies develop infection in the first week of life and it is a leading cause of neonatal bacterial sepsis, pneumonia and meningitis, with 1:10 affected babies dying. Maternal risk factors include preterm delivery, prolonged membrane rupture and chorioamnionitis. Prophylactic intrapartum antibiotics may reduce the severity of neonatal effects; neonatal risk factors include previous baby with early-onset GBS infection, GBS identified in maternal swabs or maternal urine, maternal pyrexia in labour >38°C, preterm labour and prolonged rupture of membranes >18 hours.

group practice team of health-care professionals working together, e.g. general practitioners, NHS or independent midwives.

growth hormone substance stimulating growth; anterior PITUITARY GLAND secretion directly influencing protein, carbohydrate and lipid metabolism, and controlling the rate of skeletal and visceral growth; increased growth hormone production occurs in babies of poorly controlled diabetic mothers.

guardian *ad litem* someone from the local authority social services department appointed by a court to look after the interests of a child before a full adoption order is granted; the prospective adoptive parents have continuous possession of the child and, to ensure that the home will be satisfactory, they are visited and interviewed by the guardian *ad litem*, who makes a detailed report to the court.

gum gingiva enlarged, spongy, fluid-retaining gums caused by pregnancy oestrogen.

gumma syphilitic lesion found in the third or tertiary stage of syphilis in any part of the body.

Guthrie test blood-spot test for PHENYLKETONURIA, part of the NEWBORN BLOOD-SPOT SCREENING programme, which also screens for CYSTIC FIBROSIS, HYPOTHYRIDISM and SICKLE CELL DISEASE.

gynae- prefix meaning 'woman'.

gynaecoid woman-like, with feminine characteristics. *G. pelvis* typically female pelvis.

gynaecologist doctor specialising in women's health, particularly conditions of the reproductive tract.

gynaecology branch of medicine concerned with diseases of the female genital tract.

gynandroid hermaphrodite or a female pseudohermaphrodite.

gynandromorphism presence of chromosomes of both sexes in different tissues of the body, producing a mosaic of male and female sexual characteristics. adj. *gynandromorphous*.

habitual abortion three or more miscarriages, treated with hormone therapy, cervical CERCLAGE or antibiotics, depending on cause. *See also* ABORTION.

HbA₁c (glycosylated haemoglobin) most widely used measure of diabetic glycaemic control; elevated blood glucose causes glucose to bind with haemoglobin, producing glycosylated haemoglobin; in well-controlled diabetes the level should be below 7%. Test is performed monthly in cases of maternal diabetes.

haem insoluble, non-protein, iron protoporphyrin constituent of haemoglobin, other respiratory pigments and many cells; responsible for the oxygen-carrying properties of the haemoglobin molecule.

haema-, haemo-, haemato- prefixes denoting or relating to blood.

haemagglutination agglutination of erythrocytes.

haemagglutinin antibody that causes agglutination of erythrocytes.

haemangioma tumour made up of blood vessels clustered together; sometimes present at birth in various parts of the body, appearing as a network of small, blood-filled capillaries near the surface of the skin, forming a flat red or purple birthmark (a 'strawberry' or 'raspberry' mark); most disappear in childhood although the 'port-wine' stain type tends to persist.

haematemesis vomiting of blood; in newborn babies it may indicate HAEMORRHAGIC DISEASE or be due to swallowed maternal blood; fetal and maternal blood may be distinguished by SINGER'S TEST.

haematinic 1. improving the quality of blood. 2. agent that improves the quality of the blood, increasing the haemoglobin level and number of erythrocytes, e.g. iron preparations, liver extract and B complex vitamins.

haematocele collection of blood in a cavity. *Pelvic h.* collection of blood in the pouch of Douglas, usually due to tubal abortion or rupture.

haematocolpos accumulation of blood in the vagina.

haematocrit *See* PACKED CELL VOLUME.

haematology science dealing with the nature, functions and diseases of blood.

haematoma localised collection of extravasated blood in an organ, space or tissue; may occur in the vagina, vulva or perineum as a result of trauma during labour. Trauma to the fetus in labour may cause cephalhaematoma, due to rupture of small blood vessels between the skull and pericranium; it develops a few hours after birth and does not cross suture lines.

haematometra accumulation of blood in the uterus.

haematopoiesis formation and development of blood cells, usually in bone marrow but also in the spleen, liver and lymph nodes (extramedullary haematopoiesis).

haematoporphyrin iron-free derivative of haem, a product of the decomposition of haemoglobin.

haematosalpinx accumulation of blood in the fallopian tube.

haematuria blood in the urine, due to injury, infection or disease of any of the urinary organs.

97

haemoconcentration loss of fluid from the blood into the tissues, as in shock or dehydration.

haemodialysis procedure to remove toxic waste from the blood in cases of acute or chronic renal failure.

haemodilution increase of plasma in the blood in proportion to the cells; occurs normally in pregnancy as the blood volume increases (*see* HYDRAEMIA), or in haemorrhage, when fluid is drawn from the tissues into the blood to maintain the volume of circulating blood.

haemoglobin pigment contained in red blood cells enabling them to transport oxygen; compound of the ferrous iron-containing pigment haem combined with the protein globin. Each haemoglobin molecule contains four atoms of ferrous iron, one in each haem group, and can unite with four molecules of oxygen. Oxygenated haemoglobin (oxyhaemoglobin) is bright red in colour; haemoglobin unbound to oxygen (deoxyhaemoglobin) is darker. *In utero* fetal haemoglobin (HbF), which is formed in the liver and spleen, has an increased affinity for oxygen; when erythropoiesis shifts to the bone marrow in the first year of life, the adult haemoglobins HbA and HbA$_2$ start to be produced.

haemoglobinopathies inherited haemoglobin disorders in which the baby has an abnormal quantity (thalassaemia syndromes) or quality (e.g. SICKLE CELL DISEASE) of the globin chains of haemoglobin.

haemolysin ANTIBODY with COMPLEMENT that releases haemoglobin from red blood cells.

haemolysis liberation of haemoglobin from red blood cells; in excess it causes ANAEMIA and JAUNDICE; some microbes, e.g. beta-haemolytic streptococcus, form haemolysins specifically to destroy red blood corpuscles. In a transfusion reaction or in HAEMOLYTIC DISEASE OF THE NEWBORN, incompatibility causes the red blood cells to clump together; the agglutinated cells eventually disintegrate, releasing haemoglobin into the plasma; kidney damage may result as the haemoglobin crystallises and obstructs the renal tubules producing renal shutdown and uraemia. Other haemolysins include snake venoms, and certain vegetable and chemical poisons.

haemolytic pertaining to, characterised by or producing HAEMOLYSIS. *H. disease of the newborn* blood dyscrasia of newborn babies characterised by haemolysis of erythrocytes usually as a result of incompatibility between the baby's and mother's blood. In Rhesus incompatibility the fetus has Rhesus-positive blood and the mother has Rhesus-negative blood; the mother builds up antibodies against the fetal cells, which pass through the placenta to the fetal circulation, destroying the fetal erythrocytes very rapidly. To compensate for this rapid destruction of red blood cells there is increased bone marrow production and early release of immature red blood cells (erythroblasts). Also called erythroblastosis fetalis.

haemophilia inherited disease of delayed blood clotting, carried by the mother as a sex-linked recessive gene but occurring only in males; over 80% have haemophilia A, with deficiency of clotting factor VIII; 15% have haemophilia B (Christmas disease), with deficiency of factor IX. Treatment aims to raise deficient clotting factor level and maintain it to stop local bleeding.

Haemophilus influenzae serotype B (Hib) bacterial infection carried in the nasopharynx of approximately 75% of children, spread by coughing and sneezing, especially in day nurseries; causes bacteraemia, bacterial meningitis, otitis media, sinusitis, epiglottitis, pneumonia, cellulitis, joint and muscle pains and osteomyelitis. Treatment is by administration of cephalosporins or sulphur drugs; erythromycin is ineffective. Children are offered routine immunisation at 3, 4 and 12 months of age.

haemopoiesis *See* HAEMATOPOIESIS.

haemoptysis coughing up blood from the lungs, distinguishable from vomited blood by its bright colour and frothy character.

haemorrhage escape of blood from its vessels either externally or within the body. *Antepartum h.* bleeding before delivery, usually classified as any bleeding in pregnancy after 24 weeks' gestation; causes are *accidental h.* or abruption of a normally situated placenta; PLACENTA PRAEVIA bleeding from an abnormally situated placenta; or incidental causes. *Cerebral h.* bleeding due to rupture of a cerebral blood vessel, associated with hypertensive conditions, e.g. eclampsia, essential hypertension. *Concealed h.* bleeding in which the amount of blood loss revealed is much less than the actual amount; clinical signs are not in keeping with the measured blood loss. *Intracranial h.* bleeding occurring in the baby as a result of difficult delivery causing a tear at the junction of the TENTORIUM CEREBELLI and FALX CEREBRI and the blood vessels they contain. *Intraventricular h.* bleeding occurring between the ventricles in the brain in small and preterm babies. *Petechial h.* subcutaneous haemorrhage occurring in minute spots, sometimes seen in the newborn when the cord has been tightly around the neck or following a difficult delivery. *See also* POSTPARTUM HAEMORRHAGE.

haemorrhagic characterised by haemorrhage. *H. disease of the newborn* condition occurring in the first week of life; haemorrhage is usually from the gut, showing as haematemesis or melaena, or can be from the umbilicus, from puncture sites or internally, showing as haematuria; associated with very low levels of blood prothrombin and treated by administering vitamin K (1 mL phytomenadione intramuscularly) and blood transfusion; must be clearly differentiated from haemolytic disease of the newborn.

haemorrhoids piles; varicose veins of the lower rectum and canal (internal), or around the anal orifice (external). In pregnancy they often enlarge and become painful because of relaxation of smooth muscle by PROGESTERONE; constipation, increased vascularity and congestion increase the dilatation of the veins causing discomfort, which can be relieved by applying local analgesic ointment or suppositories. Vaginal delivery aggravates the condition by direct pressure from the fetal head increasing venous congestion and stasis. They usually resolve spontaneously postnatally as hormone levels fall, and medical or surgical treatment is not usually necessary.

haemostasis arrest of bleeding.

haemostatic astringent drug (styptics) or other agent capable of arresting bleeding.

hair analysis test used in preconception care to assess nutritional status and detect concentrations of up to 18 metals; high levels of some metals, e.g. lead, may be associated with congenital abnormalities; deficiencies, e.g. of zinc, can be treated with dietary advice and/or supplements.

hallucination false perception or psychosis, triggering false beliefs of seeing, smelling, hearing, tasting or feeling objects or people; may be *organic*, as a result of bacterial toxins, drugs or thyrotoxicosis, *psychogenic* or *functional*, with no apparent changes in the central nervous system; stress, e.g. childbirth, can precipitate the condition if there is an inherited susceptibility. *See also* PUERPERAL PSYCHOSIS.

halothane colourless, non-flammable, volatile liquid used for general ANAES-THESIA; rarely used for obstetric anaesthesia as postpartum haemorrhage may result because of relaxation of the uterus.

hamamelis witch hazel, an astringent for haemorrhoids or oedema of the vulva.

hand presentation in labour with an uncorrected oblique lie, shoulder presentation and arm prolapse, or in COMPOUND PRESENTATION, the fetal hand may present; on vaginal examination a hand can be distinguished from a foot by the ability of the thumb to abduct, the absence of a prominent heel and the digits being longer than toes.

haploid half the number of chromosomes characteristically found in somatic (diploid) cells of an organism.

hard chancre contagious syphilitic ulcer of the first stage; may be seen on the labium.

hare lip *See* CLEFT LIP.

Hartmann's solution solution of sodium chloride, sodium lactate, and calcium and potassium phosphate used intravenously as a systemic alkaliser and as a fluid and electrolyte replenisher.

hashish extract of the hemp plant, *Cannabis sativa*, smoked or chewed for euphoric effect; marijuana. Not recommended in pregnancy as long-term use may adversely affect mother or fetus.

headache pain in the head; in early pregnancy dilatation of the cerebral blood vessels resulting from progesterone action causes physiological headaches, but those occurring after 20 weeks' gestation may be a late sign of pre-eclampsia; if there are other prodromal signs of eclampsia, e.g. raised diastolic blood pressure, nausea, visual disturbances or epigastric pain, immediate action should be taken to prevent or control imminent fits. *Spinal h.* occasional complication

of epidural anaesthesia when the dura mater is inadvertently punctured causing loss of cerebrospinal fluid; may persist for about a week.

headbox Perspex box placed over the baby's head into which additional oxygen can be administered.

head circumference measurement of head circumference, usually the sub-occipitobregmatic diameter (33 cm) or occipitofrontal diameter (35 cm).

head fitting attempt to fit a non-engaged fetal head into the maternal pelvic brim at term or in labour, to exclude CEPHALOPELVIC DISPROPORTION; if it does not fit, ultrasound or X-ray pelvimetry provide more accurate, detailed information to assess if vaginal delivery is possible.

Heaf test form of tuberculin testing.

healing restoration of structure and function of injured or diseased tissues, with healing processes including blood clotting, inflammation and repair.

health 'a state of complete physical, mental and social well-being, not merely the absence of disease or infirmity' (World Health Organization definition).

health centre strategically-placed building in the community providing a full range of primary health care, commonly focused around the general practitioner's services and sometimes providing facilities for minor surgery.

health education various methods of education aiming to prevent disease; midwives and health visitors are responsible for promoting good health, especially with mothers and young babies.

Health and Safety at Work Act 1974 comprehensive legislation dealing with the welfare, health and safety of all employers and employees, except domestic workers in a private house.

health visitor (HV) registered nurse who has completed a 1-year full-time course in social and preventive medicine; responsible for health education of and disease prevention in mothers and children under 5; some specialise in care of the elderly, disabled or other special groups; the midwife liaises with the health visitor when care of the mother and baby is transferred to the health visitor between 10 and 28 days after delivery.

hearing test neonatal screening test, part of the National Newborn Hearing Screening Programme; enables early diagnosis of hearing loss, which occurs in 1–2 in 1000 babies, and early treatment, so that communication and social skills can be developed at a normal rate. The OTOACOUSTIC EMISSIONS (OAE) test and the AUTOMATED AUDITORY BRAINSTEM RESPONSE (AABR) test are now performed in place of the less reliable distraction test at 7 months of age.

heart organ that pumps blood into the arteries for transfer to every part of the body; cardiac output is increased in pregnancy because of the increase in blood volume, body weight, metabolism and size of the uterus. *H. disease in pregnancy* there are four grades of heart disease, which may deteriorate by at least one grade during pregnancy; previously, mitral stenosis due to childhood rheumatic fever or chorea was the main type of heart disease in pregnancy but, now, girls born with congenital heart disease survive into adult life and may become pregnant; care is shared between obstetrician and cardiologist, and delivery should be in a consultant maternity unit. *H. defects* disorders, some of which may be congenital, e.g. FALLOT'S TETRALOGY, PATENT DUCTUS ARTERIOSUS. *H. failure* inability of the heart to pump sufficient blood to assure a normal flow through the circulation. *H. murmur* any sound in the heart region other than normal heart sounds.

heartburn burning sensation in the chest, caused by regurgitation of stomach contents into the lower oesophagus. In pregnancy it results from relaxation of the cardiac sphincter of the stomach; may be a particular problem at night but can be relieved by sleeping propped up on pillows; antacid medications give transient relief; osteopathy, acupuncture or homeopathy may be effective treatments.

heat shield Perspex shield placed over a low-birthweight and/or sick baby in an incubator to prevent radiant and convective heat loss.

Hegar's dilators series of graduated dilators used to dilate the cervix uteri.

Hegar's sign little-used test for pregnancy, elicited between the sixth and tenth weeks of gestation when the embryo only occupies the upper part of the uterus; lower part above the cervix is greatly softened and on bimanual examination almost allows the fingers to meet.

Hegar's sign

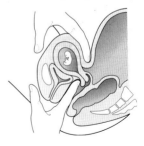

Hellin's law formula used to calculate the incidence of spontaneously-occurring multiple pregnancies in the UK: twins, 1:89 pregnancies; triplets, 1:89^2

or 1:7921 pregnancies; quadruplets, 1:89³ or 1:704969 pregnancies.

HELLP syndrome severe coagulation complication of pregnancy-induced hypertension (pre-eclampsia) occurring between 32 and 34 weeks' gestation in approximately 0.17–0.85 of all live births, characterised by haemolysis, elevated liver proteins and low platelets; a variation of pre-eclampsia/eclampsia syndrome. Associated with significant maternal mortality and morbidity resulting from DISSEMINATED INTRAVACULAR COAGULATION, acute renal failure, pulmonary oedema and subcapsular liver haematoma or hepatic rupture, and perinatal death due to intrauterine growth retardation and birth asphyxia. Symptoms include malaise, epigastric or right upper quadrant pain, nausea and vomiting, as well as non-specific symptoms suggestive of viral syndrome, but blood pressure may be relatively normal; diagnosis is confirmed by blood and platelet counts, liver function tests and coagulation studies. Intensive care is required to stabilise the mother's condition, expedite delivery and prevent further complications; liver transplant may be required in those with severe hepatic problems.

hemiplegia paralysis of one side of the body.

hemisphere half a sphere; one of the two halves of the cerebrum.

heparin anticoagulant formed in the liver and circulating in the blood. Administered subcutaneously or intravenously to treat thrombosis by preventing the conversion of prothrombin into thrombin; rapidly excreted. Protamine sulphate is used to counteract overdosage but, if used in excess, may also act as an anticoagulant.

hepatic pertaining to the liver.

hepatitis inflammation of the liver, usually caused by blood-borne viral infection. H. A virus causes mild disease, not normally problematic in pregnancy;

H. B virus is very infectious, spread through sexual intercourse, blood transfusion or sharing of contaminated equipment for intravenous injection, and universal antenatal screening is recommended. The disease may be asymptomatic or cause fatigue, nausea, vomiting and pain in the right upper quadrant over the liver, leading to chronic liver disease over time; mothers with positive screening results should be referred to a hepatologist, as serious long-term morbidity is possible. Vaginal delivery is acceptable, but fetal scalp electrodes should not be used in labour; the neonate should receive prompt vaccination. H. C screening is not routine in pregnancy, but should be offered to high-risk mothers (e.g. intravenous drug abusers who share contaminated needles, hepatitis B-/HIV-positive mothers); antenatal and intrapartum management is as for hepatitis B but no neonatal vaccine is available; there is no contraindication to breastfeeding.

hepatomegaly enlargement of the liver.

hepatosplenomegaly enlargement of the liver and spleen.

herbal medicine phytotherapy; complementary or alternative medicine in which plants are used for their therapeutic properties; many herbal remedies are contraindicated in pregnancy and labour and many more interfere with pharmacological preparations; the mother should seek expert help and avoid routine use of any herbal medicines in pregnancy.

hereditary transmissible or transmitted from parent to offspring; genetically determined.

heredity INHERITANCE from parents and ancestors by offspring of physical and mental characteristics, which are transmitted in genes according to laws described by Gregor Mendel.

hermaphrodite having the characteristics of both sexes; partial development of both male and female sex organs may occur; true hermaphrodites are rare, whereas PSEUDOHERMAPHRODITES are relatively more common.

hernia protrusion of peritoneum and other abdominal structures through a defect in the wall of the cavity. *Diaphragmatic h.* protrusion into the thorax of any of the abdominal contents, e.g. stomach, gut, resulting from serious congenital malformation; emergency surgery is required. *Femoral h.* protrusion, usually of a loop of bowel, through the femoral canal, more common in females. *Hiatus h.* protrusion of part of the stomach through the diaphragm into the thorax, which may be responsible for severe heartburn in pregnancy. *Inguinal h.* protrusion of bowel through the inguinal canal into the groin or scrotum; much commoner in males and may be present at birth. *Umbilical h.* protrusion of bowel through the gap in the recti at the umbilicus, common in babies of African descent; almost always heals spontaneously.

heroin morphine-based narcotic used therapeutically as an analgesic; also abused illicitly for its euphoriant effects; can cause physical dependence.

herpes inflammatory skin eruption characterised by small vesicles. *H. gestationis* skin eruption of unknown origin occurring occasionally in early or middle pregnancy, causing considerable irritation. *H. simplex* or *labialis* 'cold' sore on the face or lip, associated with head colds and fevers. *Genital h.* lesions on the cervix, vulva and surrounding skin in women and on the penis in men, usually caused by type 2 virus. To prevent neonatal herpes, Caesarean section is recommended for women presenting with clinical genital tract herpes within 2 weeks of delivery. *Congenital h. simplex* very serious neonatal condition with generalised vesicular rash, causing encephalitis and death. *H. zoster* shingles; extremely painful condition caused by the chickenpox virus in which the eruption follows the course of a cutaneous nerve.

heterogeneous dissimilar, made up of different characteristics.

heterosexual 1. pertaining to, characteristics of, or directed towards the opposite sex. 2. person with erotic interests directed towards the opposite sex.

heterozygous carrying dissimilar genes, e.g. a man whose blood is Rhesus positive, but who may transmit either Rhesus-positive or Rhesus-negative genes to his children. cf. HOMOZYGOUS.

heuristic encouraging or promoting investigation; conducive to discovery.

hexachlorophene antiseptic widely used in midwifery.

hiatus space or gap. *H. hernia. See* HERNIA.

Hibitane *See* CHLORHEXIDINE.

high-frequency oscillation ventilation (HFOV) ventilation method used for extreme prematurity, sometimes combined with nitrous oxide; pressure is used to allow optimum lung expansion; oscillation (bounce) is added to aid gas distribution.

higher education institution university providing degree and diploma programmes, e.g. in midwifery and nursing.

highly active antiretroviral therapy (HAART) *See* ANTIRETROVIRAL THERAPY.

hilot *See* TRADITIONAL BIRTH ATTENDANT.

hindwaters amniotic fluid surrounding the fetus, separated from the forewaters below the presenting part.

Hirschsprung's disease congenital absence of the parasympathetic nerve ganglia in the anorectum or proximal rectum, leading to absence of peristalsis, enlargement of the colon, constipation and obstruction; requires surgical correction. Also called aganglionic megacolon or congenital megacolon.

hirsute hairy.

histamine chemical substance produced when tissue is injured; thought to be a factor in anaphylactic shock, which is characterised by dilatation and increased permeability of capillaries; antihistamine drugs counteract effects.

histogram graph in which values found in a statistical study are represented by lines or symbols placed horizontally or vertically to indicate frequency of distribution.

histology visualisation of the minute structure, composition and function of tissues and organs.

history taking detailed synopsis of the woman's personal and family medical, surgical and obstetric history, current pregnancy and lifestyle, recorded by the midwife at the first antenatal appointment and forming the basis on which care is planned for the current pregnancy, labour and after childbirth.

Hodge pessary pessary used to maintain the position of the uterus following correction of a retroversion. *See* PESSARY.

Hogben test pregnancy test using a *Xenopus* toad; rarely used.

holism philosophy viewing an individual as a functioning whole rather than a composite of several systems.

holistic pertaining to totality or whole; in health care, the client's physical, emotional, psychological, social and spiritual needs are recognised as interdependent; she is treated as a complete person, rather than focusing only on the presenting condition.

Homans' sign pain in the calf when the foot is dorsiflexed and the leg extended; sign of deep vein thrombosis.

home birth *Planned h. b.* women can choose to deliver their babies at home and receive care from the community midwife and general practitioner, or sometimes from an INDEPENDENT MIDWIFE; the midwife is legally obliged to provide appropriate care for any woman within her area of practice, even if the mother's wish for a home birth is against professional advice. *Unplanned h. b.* occurs when a baby who is intended to be born in hospital is born unexpectedly or prematurely at home, or when the pregnancy is concealed.

home help service social services department providing domestic and housekeeping assistance to those in need, on either a short-term or long-term basis; payment is according to means.

homeostasis tendency of biological systems to maintain stability while continually adjusting to conditions that are optimal for survival, e.g. maintenance of body temperature. The two basic homeostatic regulators are negative feedback control, e.g. hormonal secretions from ENDOCRINE glands, which are typically regulated by the closed-loop feedback control system, and on–off switches, in which a response either does or does not occur, e.g. responses of the nervous system.

homeopathy complementary, energy-based medicine in which conditions are treated with minute doses of substances that, in large quantities, would actually cause the symptoms they are intending to treat (often referred to as 'treating like with like'); the remedy chosen must be matched exactly to the symptom picture of the individual. Homeopathy is not a pharmacological therapy, unlike HERBAL MEDICINE, so it will not interact with drugs. *See also* ARNICA.

homogeneous having the same nature or being of the same composition throughout.

homologous having the same structure or pattern.

homosexual 1. pertaining to the same sex. 2. individual who is sexually attracted to someone of the same sex.

homosexuality attraction for and desire to establish a sexual relationship with a member of the same sex.

homozygous having a pair of genes that are the same, e.g. a homozygous Rhesus-positive man can only transmit Rhesus-positive genes and all his children will be Rhesus positive even if the mother is Rhesus negative. cf. HETEROZYGOUS.

hookworm parasitic roundworm that enters the human body through the skin and migrates to the intestines, where it attaches itself to the intestinal wall and sucks blood from it for nourishment, causing blood loss and anaemia; found mainly in temperate regions where conditions are very insanitary, and in the tropics and subtropics; shoes should be worn out of doors as hookworm usually enters the body through the soles of the feet.

horizon specific anatomical stage of embryonic development, of which 23 have been defined, beginning with the unicellular fertilised egg and ending 7–9 weeks later with the beginning of the fetal stage.

hormone chemical substance secreted into the bloodstream by an endocrine gland and exerting an effect on some other part of the body.

hospital delivery mode of delivery advised for any woman whose medical condition is unfavourable, or whose previous or current obstetric history suggests potential problems in the forthcoming labour; the mother is legally entitled to reject any advice to have her baby in hospital and to request a HOME BIRTH.

hourglass constriction CONSTRICTION RING in the uterus, occurring in the third stage of labour; an uncommon cause of retained placenta; relieved by the inhalation of amyl nitrite or by anaesthesia.

human chorionic gonadotrophin (hCG) pregnancy hormone produced initially by the embryo and later by the

Hourglass constriction

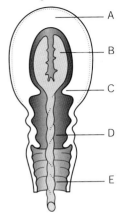

A, upper uterine segment; **B,** placenta; **C,** hourglass constriction; **D,** lower uterine segment; **E,** vagina.

TROPHOBLAST to prevent corpus luteum disintegration and maintain progesterone production to sustain the pregnancy; may also influence immune tolerance of pregnancy. Present in maternal blood and urine and forms the basis of early pregnancy testing; hCG measurement may be total (whole molecule), intact (beta part of the molecule) or free beta (one part of the beta molecule), the latter being commonly used in conjunction with other hormones in maternal serum screening for Down's syndrome. Levels are raised in multiple pregnancy, chorion carcinoma and Down's syndrome.

Human Fertilisation and Embryology Act 1990 amended version of the 1967 Abortion Act. Termination of pregnancy must be performed before 24 weeks of pregnancy by a registered medical practitioner, with agreement from a second doctor that the woman or her family would suffer physical, mental or social trauma if the pregnancy were to continue or if the baby is at risk of gross physical or mental abnormality. Termination may be performed at any time if there is serious risk to the mother's life if the pregnancy continues.

human immunodeficiency virus (HIV) blood-borne retrovirus, transmitted through sexual intercourse, blood transfusion, sharing of contaminated equipment for intravenous injection and vertical transmission from mother to baby; primarily infects immune cells, e.g. CD4 T cells, macrophages and dendritic cells, eventually destroying them and adversely affecting the immune system, leading to ACQUIRED IMMUNE DEFICIENCY SYNDROME (AIDS). Routine antenatal screening is offered, as prophylactic measures, e.g. antiretroviral drugs, avoiding breastfeeding and avoiding vaginal delivery unless the viral load is very low, can greatly reduce the incidence of vertical transmission. HIV-positive mothers receive specialist care shared between obstetrician and genitourinary physician. HIV is pandemic in the developing world, with an estimated 2 million HIV-positive women becoming pregnant every year.

human placental lactogen (hPL) placental hormone that aids growth and development of the breast, thought to resemble growth hormone and to affect carbohydrate metabolism.

humerus bone of the upper arm.

humid moist.

humidity degree of moisture in the atmosphere.

Huntington's disease chorea; rare hereditary disease appearing in adulthood between the ages of 30 and 45 years; characterised by mental deterioration, speech disturbance and quick involuntary movements caused by degenerative changes in the cerebral cortex and basal ganglia; total incapacitation and death ensue.

Hutchinson's teeth typical notching of the borders of the upper incisor teeth occurring in congenital syphilis.

hyaline resembling glass. *H. membrane* protein material in the alveoli of babies with hyaline membrane disease, also called respiratory distress syndrome (RDS); the baby has increasing difficulty in breathing from birth, with expiratory grunting and rib and sternal recession; preterm babies and those of diabetic mothers are particularly at risk; caused by lack of SURFACTANT in the lungs, demonstrated at post-mortem examination.

hyaluronidase enzyme that can hasten the absorption of drugs into body tissues. Found in the testes and present in semen; permeability of connective tissue is increased by its action and it disperses the cells of the corona radiata around the newly released ovum, thereby facilitating entry of the spermatozoon and consequently conception.

hydatidiform mole vesicular mole; benign neoplasm of the TROPHOBLAST, often the precursor of CHORIOCARCINOMA, appearing as a collection of hydropic vesicles. Incidence is 1 in 2000 pregnancies. Signs and symptoms of early pregnancy, notably nausea and vomiting, are often severe but no embryonic development occurs; the uterus must be evacuated surgically and the woman tested at intervals to ensure there is no regrowth of vesicles, which could progress to choriocarcinoma; she is usually advised to refrain from conceiving for 2 years.

hydraemia modification of the blood in which there is an excess of plasma in relation to the cells; occurs physiologically in pregnancy.

hydralazine antihypertensive drug administered orally or intravenously; contraindicated in early pregnancy and in women with tachycardia.

hydramnion, hydramnios excessive accumulation of amniotic fluid. *See* POLYHYDRAMNIOS *and* OLIGOHYDRAMNIOS.

hydro- prefix signifying water or hydrogen.

hydrocele swelling caused by accumulation of fluid, especially in the tunica vaginalis surrounding the testicles; common in the newborn and usually disappears spontaneously.

hydrocephalus 'water on the brain'; congenital malformation in which an increased amount of cerebrospinal fluid distends the ventricles of the brain. Often incompatible with life, though in milder cases the baby may survive and can be treated by an operation in which cerebrospinal fluid is diverted from the ventricles into the bloodstream. Can be diagnosed antenatally through an investigation of failure of the head to engage or persistent breech presentation or through observation of an unusually large fetal head; the most accurate method of diagnosis is serial cephalometry by ULTRASOUND.

hydrochloric acid strong acid secreted into the gastric juice; chemical symbol, HCl. Very acidic gastric juice (pH less than 2.0) aspirated into the lungs; is the main cause of bronchospasm in MENDELSON'S SYNDROME.

hydrocortisone hormone secreted by the adrenal cortex.

hydrogen gas that combines with OXYGEN to form water (H_2O); symbol H.

hydrogen ion concentration proportion of HYDROGEN ions in the blood; determines blood pH.

hydrogen ions HYDROGEN atoms carrying a positive electrical charge; cations.

hydromeningocele protrusion of the meninges containing fluid through a defect in the skull or vertebral column.

hydromyelomeningocele defect of the spine marked by a protrusion of the membranes and tissue of the spinal cord, forming a fluid-filled sac.

hydronephrosis collection of urine in the pelves of the kidney, resulting in atrophy of the kidney structure due to the constant pressure of the fluid until, finally, the whole organ becomes one large cyst. The condition may be congenital, caused by malformation of the kidney or ureter, or acquired, resulting from obstruction of the ureter by a tumour or stone, or back pressure from stricture of the urethra.

hydrops fetalis severe oedema of the fetus caused by blood incompatibility, usually resulting in either STILLBIRTH or neonatal death.

hydrosalpinx distension of the fallopian tube by an aqueous fluid.

hygiene science of health. *Communal h.* maintenance of the health of the community by provision of a pure water supply, efficient sanitation, good housing, etc. *Personal h.* cleanliness and care of the body and clothing.

hygroscopic readily absorbing moisture.

hymen fold of skin, partly occluding the vaginal introitus in a virgin; ruptured during sexual intercourse, leaving small tags of skin called *carunculae myrtiformes. Imperforate h.* membrane that completely occludes the vaginal orifice.

hyoscine (scopolamine) drug with antisalivary and amnesic properties.

hyper- prefix meaning 'excessive' or 'above normal'.

hyperbilirubinaemia excess of bilirubin in the circulating blood.

hypercalcaemia abnormally high concentration of calcium in the blood. *Idiopathic h.* neonatal condition associated with vitamin D intoxication, characterised by elevated serum calcium levels, increased skeletal density, mental deterioration and nephrocalcinosis.

hypercapnia abnormal increase in carbon dioxide in the blood.

hyperdactyly presence of supernumerary digits on the hand or foot.

hyperemesis excessive vomiting. *H. gravidarum* uncommon serious complication of pregnancy, characterised by severe and persistent vomiting, the aetiology of which is not fully understood.

hyperglycaemia excess of glucose in the blood (normal adult value is 3.3–5.3 mmol/L; 60–95 mg/100 mL). Persistent hyperglycaemia is a sign of DIABETES MELLITUS.

hyperkalaemia abnormally high concentration of potassium in the blood.

hypernatraemia abnormally high concentration of sodium in the blood, usually diagnosed when the plasma sodium is above 150 mmol/L; usually due to water depletion and extracellular fluid loss, or to excess salt intake. Occurs if a baby has excessive salt in milk feeds or becomes dehydrated; convulsions occur and can lead to brain damage. The condition can be prevented by giving low-sodium feeds, 25–50% normal strength, to a baby suffering from diarrhoea.

hyperphenylalaninaemia excess phenylalanine in the blood, as in phenylketonuria.

hyperplasia growth by multiplication of cells, occurs in the uterus during pregnancy.

hyperprolactinaemia increased levels of prolactin in the blood; associated with infertility and may lead to galactorrhoea (excessive or spontaneous milk flow); it has been reported to cause impotence in men.

hyperptyalism abnormally increased secretion of saliva.

hyperpyrexia excessively high body temperature, i.e. over 40°C (104°F).

hypertension abnormally high blood pressure, occurring in several diseases, e.g. acute or chronic nephritis, coarctation of the aorta. *Essential h.* raised blood pressure of unknown aetiology in an individual who is otherwise healthy; a common disease in the adult population, which, if not treated and controlled, may lead to damage of the blood vessels in the heart, brain and kidneys. In pregnancy, a reading of 140/90 mmHg, or a rise of more than 15–20 mmHg above the level recorded in the first trimester, is regarded as the upper limit of normal. *Pregnancy-induced h.* pre-eclampsia and eclampsia, of unknown cause; may be complicated by proteinuria and may lead to eclampsia with epileptiform fits and a high risk of maternal or fetal mortality.

hyperthyroidism thyrotoxicosis; excessive thyroid gland activity resulting in a raised basal metabolic rate and exophthalmos.

hypertonic 1. relating to hypertonia or excessive tone or tension, as in a blood vessel or muscle. *H. action of the uterus* abnormal uterine action in which the muscle tone is excessive; contractions are extremely painful, the intermissions brief with inadequate relaxation, labour is prolonged and exhausting to the mother and the fetus becomes hypoxic. The mother should be under epidural care and may benefit from EPIDURAL ANALGESIA and intravenous oxytocin but, if there is no progress, a Caesarean section may be needed. cf. HYPOTONIC. 2. applied to solutions that are stronger than physiological saline, e.g. hypertonic saline.

hypertrophy growth resulting from increase in the size of cells. *See also* HYPERPLASIA.

hyperventilation overbreathing, in which an excessive amount of carbon dioxide is removed from the blood; transient respiratory alkalosis commonly results; occasionally occurs when a woman is overbreathing in labour. Symptoms include faintness, palpitations or pounding of the heart, fullness of the throat and tetany, with muscular spasms of the hands and feet. Reassurance and a return to normal breathing is usually sufficient to rectify the situation.

hyperviscosity excessive viscosity of the blood, e.g. in polycythaemia when the number of red blood cells is increased; venesection to remove excess red cells may be necessary.

hypervolaemia abnormal increase in the volume of circulating fluid (plasma) in the body.

hypnosis state of apparent deep sleep in which a person acts only under the influence of some external suggestion.

hypnotherapy complementary medicine in which hypnosis is used to affect behavioural changes in the client through induction of a trance-like state so that the person is more relaxed and open to suggestion and, if pertinent, long-forgotten memories may be brought back to the conscious mind. Conditions with a psychological component can therefore be treated, such as problematic habitual behaviour, enuresis or severe anxiety states. It may assist in altering the woman's perception of pain and discomfort in labour, and has even been used as an alternative to general anaesthesia for Caesarean section.

hypnotic agent that produces sleep.

hypo- prefix meaning 'lacking in' or 'below normal'.

hypocalcaemia low level of calcium in the blood. *Neonatal h.* can occur within 48 hours of delivery or between the fifth and eighth days of life; convulsions may occur, especially in babies fed on unmodified cows' milk formula as the high phosphorus content of the formula contributes to the condition; a very rare complication of EXCHANGE TRANSFUSION.

hypocapnia diminished CARBON DIOXIDE level in the blood.

hypochondria morbid preoccupation or anxiety with one's health.

hypochondrium region of the ABDOMEN.

hypochromic deficient in pigmentation or colouring, as with red blood cells deficient in iron.

hypodactyly less than the usual number of digits on the hand or foot.

hypodermic beneath the skin, e.g. injections into the subcutaneous tissues. *H. syringe* plastic or glass syringe, used for hypodermic injections.

hypofibrinogenaemia deficiency of fibrinogen in the blood; rare but serious cause of postpartum haemorrhage, often associated with disseminated intravascular coagulation, severe abruptio placentae, amniotic fluid embolism and intrauterine death.

hypogastric arteries branches of the internal iliac arteries, which in the fetus pass out into the umbilical cord to carry deoxygenated blood to the placenta.

hypogastrium *See* ABDOMEN.

hypoglycaemia abnormally low blood sugar; may develop in a diabetic woman receiving insulin if insufficient carbohydrate is ingested. *Neonatal h.* occurs when the blood glucose level is less than 1.7 mmol/L in the baby at term and less than 1.2 mmol/L in low-birthweight babies; may occur very soon after delivery in a baby of a diabetic (or gestational diabetic) mother when too much insulin is produced (hyperinsulinaemia) for extrauterine needs, or within 24–48 hours of delivery in a SMALL FOR GESTATIONAL AGE BABY or any baby after severe ASPHYXIA, due to lack of GLYCOGEN in the liver. Fits or APNOEA may occur, leading to brain damage. In babies at risk, symptomatic hypoglycaemia may be prevented by early feeding and hourly screening with Dextrostix during the first few days of life.

hypomagnesaemia abnormally low magnesium content of the blood, manifested chiefly by neuromuscular hyperirritability.

hypomenorrhoea menstruation at intervals longer than 1 month.

hyponatraemia deficiency of sodium in the blood; salt depletion; present when the sodium concentration is less than 135 mmol/L. Symptoms include muscular weakness and twitching, progressing to convulsions if unrelieved.

hypopituitarism SHEEHAN'S SYNDROME; deficiency of secretion from the anterior lobe of the pituitary gland. May follow severe postpartum haemorrhage, with failure of lactation and subsequent amenorrhoea and sterility.

hypoplasia underdevelopment of a part or organ. adj. *hypoplastic*.

hypoprothrombinaemia lack of prothrombin in the blood causing bleeding. *See* HAEMORRHAGIC DISEASE OF THE NEWBORN.

hypospadias malformation in which the urinary meatus opens on the undersurface of the penis.

hypostatic pertaining to decreased movement. *H. pneumonia* may develop if an ill or elderly patient, or one with eclampsia, lies supine for long periods.

hypotension blood pressure below the normal range. *Postural b.* temporary fall in blood pressure on standing, resulting in dizziness and, occasionally, fainting; common in pregnancy.

hypotensive pertaining to low blood pressure. *H. drugs* drugs that lower the blood pressure, e.g. hydralazine and bupivacaine, as used in epidural anaesthesia.

hypothalamus part of the brain lying near the third ventricle; controls activity of the pituitary gland, the sympathetic and parasympathetic nervous systems, food intake and temperature regulation, and possibly has other functions.

hypothermia fall in body temperature to subnormal levels. *Neonatal h.* the neonate may lose heat rapidly because of the body's large surface area, especially if not dried well at delivery; worse in preterm infants who lack brown fat to help them maintain their temperature. Extreme chilling causes the baby to use up energy and oxygen

Mild hypospadias

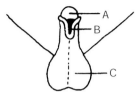

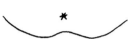

Severe hypospadias

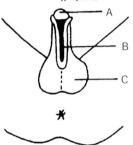

A, glans penis; **B,** urethral orifice; **C,** scrotum.

and, if the temperature falls below 35°C, neonatal cold injury develops, which may lead to death.

hypothesis theory presented as a basis for argument or discussion.

hypothyroidism condition resulting from deficiency of thyroid secretion: called cretinism in babies and myxoedema in adults.

hypotonia deficient muscle tone, often applied to the abdominal and uterine muscles.

hypotonic lacking tone. *H. uterine action* weak, ineffective contractions with prolongation of labour unless intravenous oxytocin is used, when the contractions usually become normal. cf. HYPERTONIC. *H. solution* solution that is more dilute than physiological saline.

hypovolaemia abnormally low circulating blood volume.

hypovolaemic pertaining to hypovolaemia. *H. shock* haemorrhagic shock; occurs following antepartum or postpartum haemorrhage. Emergency treatment is required to maintain an airway, administer OXYGEN and replace fluids intravenously; volume of fluid required is estimated by the use of a central venous pressure line. The midwife should assist with emergency treatment, maintain contemporaneous records, keep the woman as calm and undisturbed as possible and avoid her overheating.

hypoxaemia low OXYGEN tension in arterial blood; low $P\text{CO}_2$.

hypoxia diminished OXYGEN tension in the body tissues. *See also* ANOXIA.

hysterectomy removal of the uterus. *Abdominal h.* removal via an abdominal incision. *Pan-h.* old term for removal of the uterus and adnexa. *Subtotal h.* removal of the body of the uterus only. *Total h.* removal of the body of the uterus and cervix. *Vaginal h.* removal *per vaginam*. *Wertheim's h.* in addition to the uterus, fallopian tubes and ovaries, the parametrium, upper vagina and all the local lymphatic glands are excised: a successful method of treatment of carcinoma of the cervix.

hysteria psychoneurosis, with widely varied symptoms but no organic disease.

hystero-oophorectomy excision of the uterus and one or both ovaries.

hystero-salpingectomy excision of the uterus and one or both of the uterine tubes.

hystero-salpingography radiography of the uterus and uterine tubes after instillation of a contrast medium.

hysterotomy operation carried out between 12 and 24 weeks' gestation consisting of making an incision into the abdominal wall and uterus to remove an ovum or evacuate contents of the uterus.

iatrogenic caused by treatment.

ichthammol ammoniated coal tar product, used in ointment form for certain skin diseases.

ichthyosis rare congenital skin abnormality characterised by scaliness and desquamation of the skin of the whole body.

icterus jaundice; yellow staining of the skin and mucous membranes due to excess bile pigments in the blood and tissues. *I. neonatorum* jaundice of the newborn. *I.gravis neonatorum* severe jaundice of the newborn, usually caused by Rhesus ISOIMMUNISATION.

identical exactly alike. *I. twins* twins of the same sex developed from a single fertilised ovum; MONOZYGOTIC TWINS.

ideology science of development of ideas; body of ideas characteristic of an individual or social unit.

idiopathic of unknown cause.

idoxuridine analogue that prevents replication of DNA viruses; used topically in herpes simplex keratitis.

ileocaecal valve valve at the junction of the ileum and the caecum.

ileum last part of the small intestine, terminating at the caecum.

ileus paralysis of the wall of the gut; functional obstruction preventing peristaltic action. A complication of Caesarean section and other abdominal operations. *Meconium i. see* CYSTIC FIBROSIS.

iliac pertaining to the ilium. *I. crest* crest of the hip bone. *I. fossa* large shallow depression forming much of the inner surface of the ilium above the pelvic brim.

iliopectineal pertaining to the ilium and pubes. *I. line* ridge crossing the innominate bone from the sacroiliac joint to the *I. eminence*, a small protrusion marking the fusion of the ilium and os pubis.

ilium upper broad part of the innominate bone.

imaging production of diagnostic images, e.g. radiography, ultrasonography, scintigraphy.

immature not mature, insufficiently developed.

immune protected against infectious diseases, foreign tissue, foreign nontoxic substances and other ANTIGENS. *I.-reactive trypsin (IRT) test* blood test to diagnose cystic fibrosis.

immunity resistance of the body to infectious diseases, foreign tissues, foreign non-toxic substances and other ANTIGENS. *Humoral i.* occurs in body fluids and is concerned with antibody and complement activities; dependent on B lymphocytes, which mature into plasma cells primarily responsible for forming antibodies *Cell-mediated or cellular i.* involves various activities designed to destroy or contain cells recognised by the body as alien and harmful; dependent on T lymphocytes, which are primarily concerned with delayed immune responses, e.g. rejection of transplanted organs, defence against some slowly developing bacterial diseases, allergic reactions and certain autoimmune diseases. *Acquired i.* immunity produced specifically in response to an ANTIGEN; involves a change in the behaviour of cells and production of antibody as a primary response; after a short while the body becomes sensitised; the secondary response is produced more quickly and is more marked. *Active i.* natural, i.e. from infectious diseases, or artificial, i.e. from injection of living or dead organisms or their products in the form of toxins and toxoids. *Passive i.* natural, e.g. maternal immunoglobulin G (IgG) via the placenta, which protects the infant from various infectious diseases for a few months (although undesirable antibodies such as anti-D immunoglobulin may also be transmitted to the fetus), or acquired, e.g. the temporary immunity that follows the injection of antibodies of human (GAMMA GLOBULIN) or, more rarely, animal origin. *Natural or innate i.* non-specific; provided by intact cellular barriers of epithelium and humoral substances, e.g. COMPLEMENT and LYSOZYME; affected by genetic factors, age, race and hormone levels.

immunisation rendering immune. *I. programme see* Appendix 14.

immunoglobulin antibody; variety of chemical compound found mainly in GAMMA GLOBULIN; major component of the humoral immune response system, synthesised by lymphocytes and plasma cells and found in serum and other body fluids and tissues. There are five classes of immunoglobulin (Ig): IgA – two types with antiviral properties, of which secretory IgA is present in non-vascular fluids, e.g. colostrum and breast milk; IgD, found in trace quantities in serum; IgE, the reaginic antibody, increased in those with allergy; IgG, the most abundant and the major antibody in the secondary humoral response of immunity, the only immunoglobulin to cross the placenta; IgM, principally concerned with primary antibody response.

immunological pregnancy test standard method to diagnose pregnancy in which increased serum or urinary HUMAN CHORIONIC GONADOTROPHIN (hCG) levels are detected using immunological techniques, e.g. latex particle agglutination or, more commonly, an anti-hCG antibody 'sandwich' assay. In this assay hCG binds to a conjugate, the mixture migrates down a test strip and when it comes into contact with a line of anti-hCG antibodies a colour change occurs, indicating a positive result.

impacted driven into, wedged, lodged in a narrow strait, e.g. impacted shoulder presentation.

imperforate having no opening. *I. anus* congenital malformation requiring surgery.

impetigo skin blisters or raw patches, especially on trunk and buttocks of the baby, usually caused by STAPHYLOCOCCI or, occasionally, streptococci; the severe form, PEMPHIGUS NEONATORUM, is highly contagious.

implant introduction into the body tissues of drugs or tissue.

implantation act of planting or setting in, e.g. of a fertilised ovum in the endometrium. *I. bleeding* nidation or decidual bleeding; vaginal bleeding at the time and from the site of embedding of the blastocyst; coincides closely with the first missed menstrual period and may cause erroneous calculation of the expected date of delivery.

implementation third stage of the process approach to midwifery care; preceded by ASSESSMENT and planning and followed by EVALUATION.

impotence absence of sexual power; the man is unable to achieve or maintain a penile erection of sufficient rigidity to perform sexual intercourse successfully. adj. *impotent.*

impregnate 1. to saturate or instil. 2. to render pregnant.

imprinting species-specific, rapid learning during a critical period of early life in which social attachment and identification are established.

inborn errors of metabolism rare inherited disorders occurring in about 1:5000 births, mainly due to enzyme deficiencies, usually autosomal recessive; includes PHENYLKETONURIA and GALACTOSAEMIA.

incarcerated imprisoned, held fast. *Retroverted i. gravid uterus* retroverted pregnant uterus that does not antevert spontaneously; by 14 weeks' gestation it is so large that it becomes trapped under the sacral promontory and cannot rise out of the pelvis; may lead to acute retention of urine, abortion or, very rarely, SACCULATION OF THE UTERUS.

Incarceration of a retroverted gravid uterus

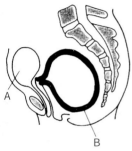

A, bladder; **B,** gravid uterus.

incest sexual activity between persons so closely related that marriage between them is legally or culturally prohibited.

incidence number of particular events occurring in a population in a given period of time, e.g. number of stillbirths per 1000 live births per annum.

incidental haemorrhage uncommon vaginal bleeding as a result of extra-placental causes, e.g. cervical polyps, erosion, acute vaginitis, cervical carcinoma; diagnosed on speculum examination and rarely leads to dangerous haemorrhage; treatment is that of the cause.

incompatibility state of being incompatible, applied to blood or chemicals, etc.

incompatible mutually repellent, unsuitable for combination.

incomplete abortion miscarriage in which some part of the products of conception – usually the placenta – is retained in the uterus; may cause serious haemorrhage. *See* ABORTION.

incontinence inability to control excretory functions. *I. of urine* enuresis. *Stress i.* involuntary escape of urine resulting from strain on the orifice of the bladder, as in coughing, sneezing or laughing. *Faecal i.* may occur after delivery if the mother sustains a third-degree tear involving the anal sphincter.

incoordinate lacking in harmony. *I. uterine action* failure of POLARITY, resulting in weak, ineffectual contractions with delay in the first stage of labour and poor, irregular cervical dilatation; oxytocic drugs are used to coordinate rather than accelerate uterine action.

incubate to place in an optimal situation for the development of living matter by providing a suitable temperature, humidity and oxygen concentration.

incubation, incubation period time elapsing between invasion of the body by pathogenic micro-organisms and clinical manifestation of disease, e.g. chickenpox, 14–15 days; diphtheria, 2–4 days; measles, 10–14 days; mumps, 14–28 days; rubella, 17–18 days; scarlet fever, 2–4 days; smallpox, 10–14 days; whooping cough, 7–14 days.

incubator 1. apparatus providing a suitable environment for low-birth-weight or sick babies. 2. heated apparatus used to culture micro-organisms in a laboratory.

independent midwife self-employed midwife, either working alone or in a partnership, who contracts directly with the mothers for whom she cares; practice must be contemporary, research based and of the highest standard; the midwife is personally accountable for her practice, required to notify intention to practise to the supervisor of midwives in each of the areas in which she works, and is advised to have adequate indemnity insurance cover.

indigenous occurring naturally in a certain locality. *I. midwife see* TRADITIONAL BIRTH ATTENDANT.

indirect antiglobulin test (IAT) used in the matching of blood products before blood transfusion. *See* COOMBS' TEST.

indomethacin anti-inflammatory, analgesic, antipyretic agent, used in arthritic disorders and degenerative bone disease; also a prostaglandin inhibitor, reducing uterine activity; may also be used in neonates to treat PATENT DUCTUS ARTERIOSUS.

induction causing to occur. *I. of labour* artificially starting labour with prostaglandin pessaries, amniotomy or intravenous oxytocin, performed when fetal or maternal health is endangered, e.g. poor fetal growth or well-being, maternal diabetes, hypertension, cardiac or renal disease, poor obstetric history, antepartum haemorrhage, breech presentation, postmaturity. If the cervix is assessed as favourable, i.e. a BISHOP'S SCORE of 6 or more, induction is likely to succeed; scores of below 6 indicate the need to deliver by Caesarean section.

inertia sluggishness. *Uterine i.* hypotonic uterine action; inability of the uterine muscle to contract efficiently; common cause of prolonged labour.

inevitable that which cannot be avoided. *I. abortion* irreversible vaginal bleeding in which miscarriage is unavoidable. *I. haemorrhage see* PLACENTA PRAEVIA.

infant baby from birth to 1 year of age. *I. feeding* breast and artificial feeding. *Preterm i.* baby born before 37 weeks' completed gestation.

infant mortality rate number of registered INFANT deaths for every 1000 registered live births in any given year.

infanticide murder of an infant.

infantile paralysis POLIOMYELITIS.

infarct area of necrosis in an organ caused by local ischaemia. *Placental i.* necrosis due to obstruction of the local circulation caused by fibrin deposits in the INTERVILLOUS spaces, so that any VILLI in the area die from ischaemia; initially deep red, subsequently changing through brown and yellow to white after about a week. Infarcts occur in ABRUPTIO PLACENTAE and hypertensive conditions, e.g. pre-eclampsia; large areas of infarct may cause the fetus to die or be SMALL FOR GESTATIONAL AGE.

infarction formation of an infarct. *Pulmonary i.* necrosis of lung tissue, caused by embolus.

infection invasion of tissues by pathogenic micro-organisms. For infection to occur there must be sufficient numbers of causative organisms and reservoirs in which they can thrive and reproduce; a portal through which the pathogen leaves the host, e.g. the intestinal or respiratory tract; a means of transfer, e.g. hands, air currents, FOMITES; a portal of entry for pathogens to enter the body or a susceptible host, e.g. open wounds, the respiratory, intestinal or reproductive tracts. The body responds to invading micro-organisms by forming ANTIBODIES and by INFLAMMATION. *Aerobic i.* infection caused by an AEROBE. *Airborne i.* infection by inhalation of organisms suspended in air on water droplets or dust particles. *Anaerobic i.* infection caused by an ANAEROBE. *Cross i.* infection transmitted between patients. *Droplet i.* caused by inhalation of respiratory pathogens suspended on liquid particles exhaled by someone already infected. *Endogenous i.* 1. infection caused by reactivation of organisms present in a dormant focus, e.g. as occurs in tuberculosis; 2. caused by organisms present in or on the body. *Exogenous i.* caused by organisms not normally present in the body but which have gained entrance from the body surface of others or the environment. *Hospital acquired i.* infections acquired during hospitalisation. *Nosocomial i.* hospital-acquired infection. *Opportunistic i.* caused by a micro-organism that does not normally cause disease but which may do so when a person's resistance is lowered, e.g. after severe postpartum haemorrhage. *Secondary i.* infection that occurs during or after treatment of another already existing infection. *Sexually transmitted i.* infection transmitted by intimate contact between genitals, mouth and rectum.

inferior longitudinal sinus venous sinus within tentorium cerebelli that, with the superior longitudinal sinus, drains blood away from the head; joins with the great vein of Galen and straight sinus at the *confluens sinuum*, which tears easily if excess or rapid moulding of the fetal skull occurs, leading to tentorial tears and intracranial haemorrhage; *See* FETAL SKULL.

infertility inability to conceive.

infestation animal parasites on or within the body.

infibulation process of fastening, e.g. joining wound edges with clasps during surgery; performed in FEMALE GENITAL MUTILATION when the labia are joined together to reduce the vestibular introitus.

infiltration entrance and diffusion of liquid. *I. analgesia* injection of lidocaine (lignocaine) into the tissues.

inflammation series of changes in tissues indicating their reaction to injury, whether mechanical, chemical or bacterial; characterised by heat, swelling, pain, redness and loss of function. *Acute i.* of sudden onset, with marked and progressive signs. *Chronic i.* inflammation with slow progress and formation of new connective tissue.

influenza acute, epidemic, viral respiratory tract infection, usually an acute general illness with fever, generalised aching, limb pain and minor respiratory symptoms; in severe cases pneumonia may follow as a result of secondary bacterial infection.

infra- prefix meaning 'below'.

infundibulum funnel-shaped structure; fimbriated end of the fallopian tube.

infusion 1. process of extracting the soluble principles of substances (especially drugs) by soaking in water. 2. treatment by introducing fluid into the body, e.g. dextrose or saline.

ingestion introduction of food and drugs by mouth.

inguinal relating to the groin. *I. canal* channel through the abdominal wall, above POUPART'S LIGAMENT, through which the spermatic cord and vessels pass to the testicle in the male; contains the round ligament of the uterus in the female. *I. hernia see* HERNIA.

inhalation breathing of air, vapour or volatile drugs into the lungs. *I. anaesthesia* anaesthesia induced by the inhalation of drugs. *I. analgesia* nitrous oxide and oxygen inhaled from specially designed machines, used as pain relief in labour. *See* ENTONOX.

inheritance transmission of characteristics or qualities from parent to offspring.

inhibin A biochemical MARKER used in second-trimester Down's syndrome screening: affected pregnancies have increased levels but levels may also be influenced by smoking. Inhibin A results are added to the results of the TRIPLE TEST to calculate the risk of Down's syndrome, i.e. the QUADRUPLE TEST.

inhibition arresting or restraining.

inhibitor agent that interferes with or inhibits a reaction.

iniencephaly congenital malformation with herniation of the brain in the occipital region.

injection introduction of liquid into the body via a syringe or other instrument. *Epidural i.* into the epidural space. *Intradermal i.* into the skin. *Intramuscular i.* into the muscles. *Intrathecal i.* into the theca of the spinal cord. *Intravenous i.* into a vein. *Subcutaneous i.* below the skin.

inlet (pelvic) brim, or entrance to the true pelvis. *See* PELVIS.

innate inborn; present in the individual at birth.

inner cell mass group of cells in the blastocyst cavity from which the amniotic membrane and the fetus develops.

innervation nerve distribution to an organ or part of the body.

innominate without a name. *I. artery* a branch of the arch of the aorta. *I. bone* the hip bone made up of fused ilium, ischium and os pubis. *See* PELVIS.

inoculation introduction into the body of a protective substance, e.g. antitoxin or vaccine.

inquest legal or judicial inquiry into some matter of fact. *Coroner's i.* held in all cases of sudden or unexplained death to determine the cause.

insemination introduction of semen into the vagina or cervix. *Artificial i.* insemination by other means than sexual intercourse.

insertion point of attachment, e.g. of a muscle to a bone or of the cord to the placenta.

insidious applied to a disease or condition developing almost imperceptibly.

insomnia inability to sleep.

inspection looking; initial part of the antenatal abdominal examination: the midwife observes the mother's abdomen for size, shape, scars, STRIAE GRAVIDARUM, presence of the LINEA NIGRA and fetal movements.

inspiration drawing in the breath.

instillation pouring a liquid into a cavity drop by drop, e.g. into the eye.

instruments *See* Appendix 3.

insufficiency inadequate function. *Placental i.* failure of the placenta to fulfil its function adequately, often associated with pre-eclampsia, essential hypertension, chronic nephritis, postmaturity and heavy smoking; causes the fetus to be SMALL FOR GESTATIONAL AGE or even to die *in utero*.

insufflation blowing of gas, fluid or powder into a cavity. *I. of the fallopian tubes* blowing of CARBON DIOXIDE via the uterus into the fallopian tubes to test their patency; methylene blue dye is now more often used for this purpose.

insulin HORMONE produced in the islets of Langerhans in the pancreas that regulates carbohydrate metabolism; deficiency causes DIABETES MELLITUS; overdosage of insulin preparations leads to HYPOGLYCAEMIA.

integrated medicine, integrative medicine combining complementary medicine with conventional health care; use of complementary therapies in pregnancy should be used in conjunction with conventional maternity care, rather than as an alternative, because only a midwife or doctor can legally take sole responsibility for a mother's care.

integrated test two-stage Down's syndrome screening test: maternal blood is assessed for PREGNANCY ASSOCIATED PLASMA PROTEIN-A (PAPP-A) and a NUCHAL TRANSLUCENCY ultrasound scan is performed; later, the TRIPLE or QUADRUPLE TEST is performed. Results of both stages are combined with the maternal age-related Down's syndrome risk for an overall result; the test is controversial, as parents are not informed of the results until the second stage is complete.

intention to practise statutory requirement of all UK-registered midwives intending to practise; a designated form is completed annually or at any time when a midwife intends to provide midwifery care in a health authority other than her usual one.

inter- prefix signifying 'between'.

interaction the quality, state or process of (two or more things) acting on each other. *Drug i.* action of one drug on the effectiveness or toxicity of another (or others).

intercellular between the cells, i.e. the tissue spaces.

intercostal between the ribs. *I. muscles* those of the chest wall.

intermittent having intervals or pauses, not continuous, e.g. intermittent uterine contractions to allow fetal oxygenation.

intermittent mandatory ventilation (IMV) method of weaning a baby from a ventilator by gradually reducing the ventilator pressure and then the respiratory rate settings.

intermittent positive pressure ventilation (IPPV) respiratory therapy using a VENTILATOR to treat patients with inadequate breathing, e.g. babies who are preterm or suffering from respiratory distress syndrome, severe apnoea, PO_2 of less than 5 kPa despite a high concentration of OXYGEN in inspired air, and PCO_2 greater than 12 kPa associated with acidosis that fails to respond to treatment. Very-low-birthweight babies may be routinely ventilated for 24 hours to prevent respiratory distress syndrome and complications, e.g. intraventricular haemorrhage. Complications of neonatal ventilation include pneumothorax, infection, bronchopulmonary dysplasia and retinopathy of the lens, caused by the high oxygen and CARBON DIOXIDE levels.

internal os cervical opening into the body of the uterus.

internal version method of turning a fetus by intrauterine manipulation, e.g. to change a transverse lie to a breech presentation, so enabling a vaginal delivery; rarely performed now when operative facilities are available.

International Code of Marketing of Breast Milk Substitutes *See* WHO INTERNATIONAL CODE OF MARKETING OF BREAST MILK SUBSTITUTES.

intersex abnormality of sex chromosomes, the gonads, the sex hormones or the genitalia. *See* KLINEFELTER'S SYNDROME *and* TURNER'S SYNDROME.

interspinous between the (ischial) spines. *See* PELVIS.

interstitial between body tissues.

intertrigo erythematous skin eruption on apposed surfaces, e.g. groin or armpit, caused by moisture, warmth, friction, sweat retention and infection; usually treated with good hygiene measures and application of zinc oxide talcum powder.

intervillous between (chorionic) villi; the intervillous spaces allow maternal arterial blood to cascade around the terminal placental villi where gaseous exchange and transport of amino acids, glucose, minerals and vitamins take place.

intestine part of the alimentary canal between the stomach and anus. *Small i.* first 7 m (20 ft) from the pylorus to caecum, consisting of the duodenum, jejunum and ileum. *Large i.* 2 m (6 ft) in length, consisting of the caecum, vermiform appendix, ascending, transverse, descending and pelvic colon and rectum; completes digestive processes and eliminates waste matter.

intra- prefix signifying 'within'.

intracellular within a cell. *I. organisms* those which invade cells, e.g. gonococci. *I. fluid* fluid within cells of the body.

intracranial within the cranium. *I. membranes* MENINGES covering the brain; a vertical fold in the midline between the cerebral hemispheres forms the falx cerebri, joining posteriorly the horizontal fold of the tentorium cerebelli, which separates the cerebellum and cerebrum. The membranes contain blood vessels (sinuses) and undue pressure or trauma during delivery may cause tearing of the membranes and sinuses leading to cerebral haemorrhage. *I. pressure* pressure exerted by cerebrospinal fluid within the subarachnoid space and ventricles of the brain, measured by monitoring pressure within the cerebral ventricles.

Intracranial membranes and sinuses

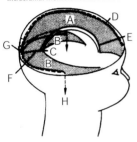

A, falx cerebri; **B,** tentorium cerebelli; **C,** great cerebral vein; **D,** superior longitudinal sinus; **E,** inferior longitudinal sinus; **F,** straight sinus; **G,** confluens sinuum; **H,** lateral sinuses leaving skull as internal jugular veins.

intragastric within the stomach. *I. tube feeding* artificial feeding, e.g. by nasogastric tube.

intrahepatic cholestasis of pregnancy idiopathic condition occurring in the second half of pregnancy, characterised by accumulation of bile in maternal blood; occurs in 1–2 per 1000 pregnancies, thought to be due to changes in bile metabolism, possibly as a result of inherited oestrogen hypersensitivity; geographical and environmental factors may also play a part. It is characterised by nocturnal pruritus without a rash, often starting in the extremities and becoming more general, fatigue and insomnia, followed about 2 weeks later by mild jaundice persisting until delivery, dark urine, pale stools, abdominal pain, nausea and vomiting. Increased serum bile acid levels affect placental blood flow and fetal steroid metabolism; there is risk of preterm labour, fetal compromise, meconium staining and stillbirth. Treatment involves administration of antihistamines, vitamin K to prevent hypoprothrombinaemia and elective delivery after 35 weeks' gestation. Usually resolves spontaneously within 3–14 days of delivery but likely to recur in subsequent pregnancies.

intramuscular within or into muscle.

intrapartum within or during parturition or labour.

intraperitoneal within the peritoneal cavity. *I. transfusion* introduction of Rhesus-negative red blood cells to replace haemolysed Rhesus-positive cells in cases of Rhesus isoimmunisation, to prolong the life of the affected fetus.

intrauterine within the uterus. *I. contraceptive device (IUCD)* device inserted into the uterine cavity for contraception; it increases tubal motility, rendering the endometrium less favourable for implantation, and possibly increases prostaglandin production, increasing the likelihood of expulsion of the conceptus. *I. death* death of fetus *in utero*, usually during pregnancy rather than labour. *I. growth restriction (IUGR) see* SMALL FOR GESTATIONAL AGE BABY. *I. transfer* transfer of a pregnant mother to a maternity unit with facilities for neonatal intensive care, e.g. a woman in very preterm labour. *I. transfusion* antenatal procedure used to treat severe fetal anaemia in cases of HAEMOLYSIS from maternal Rhesus

ALLOIMMUNISATION and anaemia due to PARVOVIRUS B19 infection; performed in specialist fetal medicine centres to avoid risk of miscarriage, preterm labour or fetal death. CORDOCENTESIS is performed to determine fetal haemoglobin levels and facilitate accurate calculation of transfusion requirements. May need to be repeated every 2–3 weeks until delivery becomes the safest option.

intravascular within a vessel, usually a blood vessel. *I. coagulation* clotting of blood within the circulation. *See* DISSEMINATED INTRAVASCULAR COAGULATION.

intravenous within a vein.

intraventricular haemorrhage (IVH) serious cerebral haemorrhage occurring in preterm infants below 34 weeks of gestation causing periods of APNOEA and death; the most common lethal condition in very-low-birth-weight infants (VLBW); diagnosed by COMPUTED TOMOGRAPHY (CT) or with a portable REAL-TIME ultrasound scanner.

intrinsic relating to a quality of a structure or substance, which is inherent within itself.

introitus entrance to any cavity of the body. *I. vaginae* entrance to the vagina.

intubation introduction of a tube. *Endotracheal i.* introduction of a catheter into the trachea; e.g. in an asphyxiated infant, with the aid of a direct-vision laryngoscope, followed by insufflation with oxygen or air at a controlled pressure.

intussusception prolapse of one part of the intestine into the lumen of an immediately adjacent part, causing intestinal obstruction; may occur during the first year of life.

inverse reverse of the normal.

inversion of the uterus rare partial or complete turning inside out of the uterus. *Acute i.* occurs spontaneously in third-stage labour or caused by attempting CRÉDÉ'S EXPRESSION or applying umbilical cord traction when the uterus is relaxed and placenta incompletely separated; results in extreme shock; the uterus must be replaced as soon as possible.

in vitro within a glass, observable in a test tube, in an artificial environment.

in vitro **fertilisation** artificial fertilisation of an ovum under laboratory conditions; the fertilised ovum is replaced in the woman's uterus.

in vivo within the living body.

involuntary independent of the will.

involution returning to normal size after enlargement, e.g. the uterus after labour by a process of ischaemia and AUTOLYSIS of muscle fibre: immediately post-delivery the uterus weighs 900 g and by the end of the puerperium (6–8 weeks) it weighs 60 g; length is reduced from 17.5 cm to about 7.5 cm. Soluble end products are removed by the bloodstream; thrombosed uterine blood vessels are self-digested and new vessels form; the placental site contracts and disappears below the pubic bone by the sixth or seventh week. *See also* SUBINVOLUTION.

iodide compound of iodine.

iodine non-metallic element with a distinctive odour, obtained from seaweed. *Tincture of i.* preparation most commonly used. Radioactive iodine is used to evaluate thyroid activity. *See also* ISOTOPE.

ion electrically charged atom(s) formed when an electrolyte dissolves in water. HYDROGEN ions carry a positive charge; hydroxyl ions a negative charge. The HYDROGEN ion concentration of a fluid determines its acidity, expressed as its pH.

iris coloured part of the eye made of two layers of muscle, the contraction of which alters pupil size.

iritis inflammation of the iris, causing pain, photophobia, contraction of the pupil and discoloration of the iris.

iron metallic element, an important constituent of haemoglobin. Iron compounds ingested in food are converted for use in the body by the action of hydrochloric acid in the stomach, which separates iron from food and combines with it in a form that is readily assimilated by the body; vitamin C enhances and administration of alkali hampers iron absorption. An adult requires 15 mg of iron daily. Iron deficiency anaemia is a common problem in pregnancy because of the increased demands on the mother's blood; iron-rich foods are advised and supplements may be prescribed.

ischaemia   local insufficiency of blood supply.

ischial   pertaining to the ischium.

ischiocavernosus   muscle   muscle extending from the ischium of the pelvis to the clitoris or penis, aiding in their erection.

ischiococcygeus   muscle   muscle extending from the pelvic ischium to the coccyx; the posterior portion of the levator ani muscle.

ischium   lower posterior part of the innominate bone of the pelvic girdle.

isoimmunisation   immunisation within the species, as occurs in a Rhesus-negative woman if Rhesus-positive cells from her fetus pass into her circulation via the placenta, causing sensitisation and the production of antibody (anti-D) against these red cells; when this antibody enters the fetal circulation, HAEMOLYSIS occurs.

isolation   separation of an infected person from those not infected.

isometric   maintaining, or pertaining to, the same length; of equal dimensions.

isoniazid   antibacterial compound used for treating tuberculosis.

isotonic   of the same strength or tension. *I. solution* of the same osmotic pressure as the fluid with which it is compared, e.g. normal saline is isotonic with blood plasma.

isotope   a form of an element having the same atomic number, i.e. number of protons in the nucleus, as another element, but a different number of NEUTRONS; leads to instability, often with emission of radioactivity, making even minute quantities identifiable with a Geiger counter.

isoxsuprine hydrochloride   beta-adrenergic stimulant used as a vasodilator in peripheral vascular disease and cerebrovascular insufficiency; used intravenously to arrest preterm labour by relaxing the myometrium.

ispaghula   oral laxative that works by increasing faecal mass.

isthmus   *See* UTERUS.

itching in pregnancy   pruritus; abdominal skin itching is common in pregnancy, but women with generalised itching or itching that starts on the palms should be referred to the obstetrician as it may be due to INTRA-HEPATIC CHOLESTASIS, hepatic or thyroid disease, lymphoma or scabies.

Jacquemier's sign blueness of the vaginal lining due to increased blood supply, observable in early pregnancy.

jaundice yellow discoloration of the skin, sclerotics and mucous membranes, due to excess bile pigments in the blood and tissues. It may be *haemolytic*, when the bile pigment is derived from the haemoglobin of haemolysed red blood cells, or *obstructive*, when the bile pigment is present as a constituent of bile. Maternal jaundice is rare but very serious in pregnancy and may be due to severe HYPEREMESIS GRAVIDARUM, pre-eclampsia or eclampsia, INTRA-HEPATIC CHOLESTASIS, acute liver atrophy, infective hepatitis, serum hepatitis or drugs. *Breast milk j.* elevated unconjugated bilirubin in some breastfed babies resulting from the presence of a steroid in the milk that inhibits glucuronyl transferase-conjugating activity. *Infectious j.* 1. infectious hepatitis. 2. leptospiral jaundice. *Physiological j.* mild icterus neonatorum. In the first days of life the baby no longer requires the high levels of circulating fetal haemoglobin that facilitate intrauterine oxygenation; excess red blood cells are broken down (haemolysed) into fat-soluble bilirubin and then conjugated into water-soluble bilirubin to be excreted; a liver enzyme, glucuronyl transferase, is required for this process, but as the baby's liver function is relatively immature the process is slow, allowing bilirubin to accumulate in the blood, leak into the tissues and cause yellow staining of the skin and sclerae. Treatment is unnecessary unless the serum bilirubin remains high, when phototherapy may be used to reduce the level of unconjugated bilirubin, to avoid the danger of KERNICTERUS.

jejunum small intestine from duodenum to ileum.

jelly a soft, coherent, resilient substance; generally a colloidal semi-solid mass. *Contraceptive j.* a non-greasy jelly used in the vagina for prevention of conception. *Petroleum j.* a purified mixture of semi-solid hydrocarbons obtained from petroleum. *Wharton's j.* soft, jelly-like intracellular substance of the umbilical cord, which insulates the vein and arteries, preventing occlusion and fetal hypoxia.

joint articulation; junction of two or more bones, providing motion and flexibility.

joule (J) international (SI) unit that measures the energy of food; 1 joule = 4.2 calories.

jugular concerning the neck. *J. veins anterior, external* and *internal* jugular veins, responsible for carrying blood away from the head.

justominor pelvis small gynaecoid pelvis with proportionately reduced diameters.

juxta- word element meaning 'situated near', 'adjoining'.

juxtaposition apposition; side by side or close together.

kalaemia presence of potassium in the blood.

kalium potassium; symbol K.

kanamycin broad-spectrum antibiotic effective against many gram-negative bacteria, and some gram-positive and acid-fast bacteria.

kaolin china clay used as a dusting powder and for poultices.

Kaposi's sarcoma multifocal, metastasising, malignant reticulosis with angiosarcoma features, involving mainly the skin; a major feature of AIDS, particularly in homosexuals.

karyo- word element meaning 'nucleus'.

karyotype number and structure of chromosomes within a cell nucleus, usually depicted on a photomicrograph of an individual's chromosomes, arranged in a standard format with the number, size and shape of each chromosome shown. The norm is 46 chromosomes: 22 AUTOSOMAL pairs and one pair of sex chromosomes (XX for females, XY for males). Karyotyping is used to diagnose chromosomal disorders such as DOWN'S SYNDROME.

Karyotype

keloid overgrowth of fibrous tissue in a scar.

keratin tough protein that forms the base of all horny tissues.

keratitis inflammation of the cornea.

kernicterus yellow staining of kernel cells in the basal ganglia of the brain; occurs in babies with severe jaundice, particularly that caused by Rhesus ISOIMMUNISATION, when unconjugated serum bile pigment rises above 350μmol/L (20mg/100mL) or at lower levels in preterm or seriously ill babies; manifested by irritability, fits and athetoid arm movements; may be fatal or cause mental or neurological disability; treatment is by one or more replacement transfusions or phototherapy.

Kernig's sign sign of meningitis in which the person is unable to straighten the leg at the knee joint when the thigh is supported at right angles to the trunk.

ketoacidosis state of electrolyte imbalance with ketosis and lowered blood pH.

ketones acetone, acetoacetic acid and β-hydroxybutyric acid. They are normal metabolic products of lipids and pyruvate within the liver, and are oxidised by muscles; acetone may also arise spontaneously from acetoacetic acid; excess ketones are excreted in urine, as in diabetes mellitus.

ketonuria presence of ketones in urine.

ketosis a condition in which excess ketones are formed in the body, as occurs in starvation or uncontrolled DIABETES MELLITUS as a result of an increase in fatty acid metabolism and impaired or absent carbohydrate metabolism. Often noticeable because of sweet or 'fruity' breath, which is produced by acetone. Ingestion of carbohydrate restores ketone body production to normal and ketoacidosis is reversed.

key worker social worker or other person who coordinates other agencies involved in an individual's or family's care; responsible for organising a CASE CONFERENCE.

kick chart fetal movement chart on which the mother subjectively records fetal movements over a given period of time; usually used in conjunction with other tests of fetal well-being.

kidneys two bean-shaped organs near the lower thoracic and upper lumbar vertebrae and behind the peritoneum, each consisting of a cortex and medulla with approximately one million nephrons. Functions include maintenance of water balance, solute content, osmotic pressure and constant plasma pH (between 7.35 and 7.45); excretion of waste products, especially nitrogen from protein metabolism; and regulation of blood pressure via the renin–angiotensin–aldosterone mechanism. Kidneys respond to ischaemia by secreting RENIN, which acts on a serum plasma protein to produce ANGIOTENSIN I, which is converted to angiotensin II by a lung enzyme, causing vasoconstriction, increased peripheral resistance and a rise in blood pressure. Angiotensin II also raises blood pressure through its influence on sodium and water retention, by increasing the secretion of aldosterone from the adrenal cortex.

Kielland's forceps obstetric forceps with a sliding lock and no pelvic curve, designed to enable rotation of the fetal head from any position in the pelvis to an occipitoanterior position. *See* Appendix 3.

kilo- prefix indicating 'one thousand', e.g. kilogram (kg), 1000 grams; kilometre (km), 1000 metres; kilopascal (kPa), 1000 pascals; kilocalorie (kcal), 1000 calories.

Klebsiella genus of Gram-negative bacteria.

Klebs–Löffler bacillus diphtheria bacillus.

Kleihauer test blood test used to confirm the presence of fetal cells in the maternal circulation following

ANTEPARTUM HAEMORRHAGE, placental ABRUPTION and other events; false-negative results may occur if there is haemolysis of fetal cells in the maternal circulation, e.g. following Rhesus sensitisation.

Klinefelter's syndrome (XXY syndrome) syndrome caused by additional X chromosome in males, occurring in approximately 1:500–1:1000 male births; detected antenatally from CHORIONIC VILLUS SAMPLING or AMNIO-CENTESIS or as a result of language or developmental delay in childhood. Adults are sterile and may develop gynecomastia (increased breast tissue), although some cases go undetected; clinical symptoms can be reduced by testosterone treatment and other therapies.

Klumpke's paralysis lower arm and hand paralysis, causing wrist drop; results from injury to the eighth cervical and first dorsal nerves, the lower BRACHIAL PLEXUS, which may occur when bringing down extended arms in a breech delivery or after applying undue traction to the anterior shoulder in a cephalic delivery.

knee presentation type of breech presentation with one or both knees below the buttocks.

Kocher's forceps artery forceps used to clamp the umbilical cord before separation and for artificial membrane rupture. *See* Appendix 3.

Konakion *See* PHYTOMENADIONE.

Koplik's spots small, irregular, bright red spots on the buccal and lingual mucosa with a minute bluish white speck in the centre of each; may be seen in the early stage of measles.

Korotkoff's sounds method of finding systolic and diastolic blood pressures by listening to sounds produced in an artery while pressure in a previously inflated cuff is gradually reduced, described by Korotkoff, a Russian surgeon in 1905. *Korotkoff 1* is the onset of clear rhythmical tapping as the cuff is deflated, representing systolic pressure. *Korotkoff 2* is a murmur or swishing sound. *Korotkoff 3* is a crisper, more intense tapping. *Korotkoff 4* is a muffled, low-pitched sound, easier to record in pregnancy than *Korotkoff 5*, the absence of sound, which represents diastolic pressure. During pregnancy, muffled tapping may be heard down to 0 when the cuff is fully deflated.

kraurosis vulvae dryness and atrophy of the vulva.

kwashiorkor severe protein deficiency; symptoms in babies and children include oedema, impaired growth and development, abdominal distension, pathological liver changes and pigmentation changes of skin and hair.

kyphosis posterior curvature of the spine; humpback.

labetalol hydrochloride oral or intravenous alpha- and beta-adrenergic receptor blocker used in hypertension.

labial pertaining to lips or labia.

labile unstable, liable to variation. *L. hypertension* blood pressure that varies between normal and an appreciably higher level.

labium lip. *L. majus pudendi* large fold of flesh surrounding the vulva. *L. minus pudendi* the lesser fold within. pl. *labia*.

labour parturition, childbirth. *Normal l.* occurs spontaneously between 37 and 43 weeks' gestation with a vertex presentation of a single fetus and is completed within 24 hours without maternal or fetal trauma; physiology depends on interaction between the uterus, maternal pelvis and fetus. During the *first stage* cervical effacement and dilatation occur; contractions are fundally dominant; uterine POLARITY facilitates contraction and RETRACTION in the upper uterine segment and contraction and dilatation in the lower uterine segment. The *second stage* is from full dilatation of the cervix until complete delivery of the baby. The *third stage* involves separation and expulsion of placenta and membranes and control of haemorrhage. *Obstructed l.* rare condition in which the fetus is unable to negotiate the pelvic canal, with no descent of the presenting part despite good uterine action. Maternal causes are a contracted bony pelvis or soft pelvic mass, e.g. fibroids or tumour; fetal causes are malpresentation, malposition or abnormality, e.g. hydrocephalus; dangers include uterine rupture, especially in multiparae, and fetal death.

Diagnosis: severe maternal pain, raised pulse rate, pyrexia, oliguria, ketonuria; on abdominal examination the uterus appears 'moulded' around the fetus, continuously hypertonic and fetal parts are not felt. Treatment consists of relieving pain, dehydration and shock, followed by Caesarean section or, if not possible, manipulative or destructive procedures to deliver the baby in order to save the mother's life. *Precipitate l.* labour that is completed in under 2 hours due to extremely strong uterine action of which the mother may be unaware; risks include haemorrhage, uterine inversion, and fetal trauma and birth injury because of rapid delivery and moulding of the head. *Preterm l.* labour occurring after 24 and before 37 weeks of pregnancy. *Spontaneous l.* labour occurring without induction or acceleration. *Spurious l.* contractions occurring without cervical dilatation, with no progress towards delivery; false labour.

laceration tear. *Perineal l. See* PERINEAL.

lacrimal pertaining to tears. *L. ducts* minute openings at the inner end of each eyelid, which convey lacrimal fluid into the nose via the nasolacrimal duct to mix with nose secretions. *L. glands* small bodies in the orbital cavity at the upper and outer surface of each eyeball which provide the fluid (tears) that keep the conjunctiva moist and free from infection through the action of LYSOZYME, except in the neonate.

lactalbumin main protein in human milk, easily digested by the baby.

lactase enzyme produced by cells in the small intestine, which splits

Physiological changes in the cervix during the first stage of labour

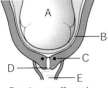

Cervix uneffaced

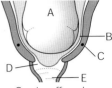

Cervix effaced
and partly dilated

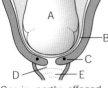

Cervix partly effaced

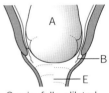

Cervix fully dilated

A, fetal head; **B,** membranes; **C,** internal os; **D,** external os; **E,** vagina.

LACTOSE into the MONOSACCHARIDES GLUCOSE and GALACTOSE.

lactation secretion of milk by the breasts. *L. period* period during which a baby is suckled.

lacteals the lymphatics of the intestine that absorb split fats.

lactic acid acid produced during hypoxia, e.g. in the blood of an asphyxiated baby, causing high ACIDAEMIA; also produced in the gut by fermentation of lactose through the action of bacilli.

lactiferous conveying milk.

Lactobacillus acidophilus Döderlein's bacillus; Gram-positive bacillus (*see* GRAM STAIN), normal inhabitant of the vagina during reproductive years; converts glycogen to lactic acid, inhibiting growth of other organisms; also predominates in the stools of breastfed babies.

lactoferrin iron-binding protein in human milk; bacteriostatic on *ESCHERICHIA COLI.*

lactogen substance that enhances lactation. *Human placental l. (hPL)* placental hormone with lactogenic, luteotrophic and growth-promoting activity; inhibits maternal insulin activity during pregnancy; disappears from the blood immediately after delivery.

lactoglobulin globulin occurring in milk.

lactose milk sugar, a DISACCHARIDE. *L. intolerance* inability of the baby to tolerate lactose because of insufficient LACTASE; causes diarrhoea; treated by giving milk that does not contain lactose, but another sugar; avoid confusion with GALACTOSAEMIA.

lactosuria lactose in the urine; must be distinguished from glycosuria; often occurs in the lactation period

Third stage of labour

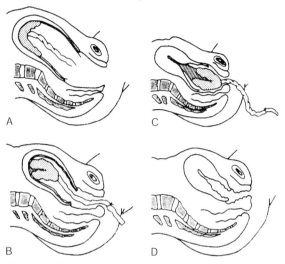

The placenta. **A,** before birth of child; **B,** partially separated immediately after birth; **C,** completely separated; **D,** contraction and retraction of uterus after expulsion.

and towards term; not clinically significant.

lactulose oral laxative; may take up to 48 hours to take effect.

laked blood in which haemoglobin has separated from the red blood cells.

La Leche League voluntary organisation that helps women to breastfeed.

Lamaze method method of preparation for natural childbirth by training mind and body to modify pain perception during labour and delivery; developed by French obstetrician Fernand Lamaze.

lambda posterior fontanelle of fetal skull, resembling the Greek letter lambda (λ).

lambdoidal suture suture between the occipital bone and the two parietal bones.

Lancefield's classification classification of haemolytic streptococci into groups on the basis of serological action.

Landsteiner's classification international designation of blood groups as O, A, B and AB, depending on the presence or absence of agglutinogens A and B in the erythrocytes.

Langerhans' islets collections of specialised pancreatic cells, producing insulin to control carbohydrate metabolism; disease of islet cells causes DIABETES MELLITUS.

Physiology of lactation

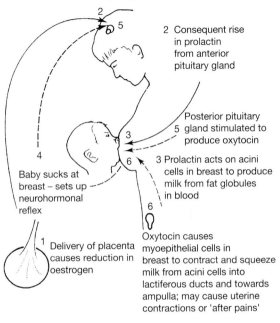

2 Consequent rise in prolactin from anterior pituitary gland

Posterior pituitary gland stimulated to produce oxytocin

3 Prolactin acts on acini cells in breast to produce milk from fat globules in blood

Baby sucks at breast – sets up neurohormonal reflex

Delivery of placenta causes reduction in oestrogen

Oxytocin causes myoepithelial cells in breast to contract and squeeze milk from acini cells into lactiferous ducts and towards ampulla; may cause uterine contractions or 'after pains'

Langhans' cell layer cytotrophoblast; inner layer of the TROPHOBLAST.

lanolin wool fat used as a basis for ointments.

lanugo fine hair covering the fetus *in utero*, mostly disappears by term.

laparoscope instrument for examining the peritoneal cavity.

laparoscopy examination of the interior of the abdomen with a LAPAROSCOPE.

laparotomy exploratory opening of the abdominal cavity.

Largactil *See* CHLORPROMAZINE.

large for gestational age baby baby whose weight is above the 90th centile.

laryngoscope endoscopic instrument used to inspect the larynx and vocal cords, and to aid insertion of an endotracheal tube.

larynx voice 'box' or organ at the upper end of the trachea; has a muscular and cartilaginous frame, lined with mucous membrane; vocal cords of elastic tissue are spread across it, with the glottis in the space between the cords.

laser device used in surgery, diagnosis and physiological studies to transfer electromagnetic radiation into an extremely intense, nearly non-divergent beam of monochromatic radiation; capable of mobilising immense heat and power at close range.

last menstrual period (LMP) determining the date of the first day of the last normal menstrual period assists in estimating the probable date of delivery; the mother may mistake implantation bleeding as a normal menstrual period so the midwife should check that the date refers to vaginal bleeding occurring when the mother expected a period and that the bleeding lasted the normal number of days.

latent hidden, not manifest. *L. period* apparently inactive period in early first-stage labour.

lateral relating to the side. *L. sinuses* sinuses in the FETAL SKULL passing from the confluence sinuum along the outer edge of the TENTORIUM CEREBELLI; carry blood to the internal jugular veins; the most vulnerable point is where the FALX CEREBRUM is attached to the tentorium, with a risk of tearing and bleeding from the great cerebral vein.

'laughing gas' NITROUS OXIDE.

lavage washing out a cavity. *Colonic l.* of the colon. *Gastric l.* of the stomach.

lavender oil *Lavandula angustifolia;* highly concentrated essential oil used by some midwives who are trained in its use to aid relaxation, ease labour pain and aid perineal healing; appears to facilitate uterine action and reduce blood pressure – not be used in large amounts with oxytocin or epidural anaesthesia; some types may be EMMENAGOGIC so use with caution in early pregnancy.

laxative medicine to loosen bowel contents, encouraging evacuation.

A mild laxative is an aperient and safe to use in pregnancy; a strong laxative is a cathartic or purgative, which may be dangerous in pregnancy as it may stimulate uterine activity and trigger bleeding.

lead professional professional who takes the principal responsibility for a mother's care, i.e. midwife, consultant obstetrician or general practitioner obstetrician, depending on the mother's needs and wishes; recommended by the CHANGING CHILDBIRTH REPORT.

learning difficulty learning disability, previously called mental handicap; affects babies with cerebral palsy resulting from birth injury or those with chromosomal disorders, e.g. Down's syndrome.

Leboyer method method of childbirth in which the baby is born gently and quietly in a darkened room, advocated by French doctor Leboyer; it is claimed that the baby born in a calm and tranquil environment, lifted onto the mother's abdomen and then put into a warm bath will cry less and be more contented because the shock of delivery is minimised.

lecithin complex molecule of protein and fatty acid in the alveoli of the lung; SURFACTANT is a lecithin that helps to keep the lungs open. Lecithin produced in the fetal lung flows into the amniotic fluid, where it can be measured to determine fetal maturity. *L-sphingomyelin (L/S) ratio* lecithin, but not sphingomyelin, increases in amount as pregnancy progresses, so the L/S ratio increases with fetal lung maturity; a ratio of 2 or more indicates little or no risk of respiratory distress in the neonate.

Lee–Frankenhauser plexus nerve network consisting of the third and fourth sacral, hypogastric and ovarian nerves, relating to the cervical area of the uterus.

leiomyoma smooth muscle tumour (fibroid), commonly occurring in the uterus.

length longest dimension of an object or measurement between two ends; internationally accepted (SI) unit of length is the metre (m). *Crown–heel l.* distance from crown of the head to the heel in the embryo, fetus and baby, equivalent to standing height. *Crown–rump l.* distance from crown of the head to the breech in the embryo, fetus and baby, equivalent to sitting height, measured by ultrasound in the first 14 weeks of pregnancy to assess fetal maturity; accurate to within 3–4 days.

lesion injury, wound or morbid structural change in an organ.

'let down' reflex neurogenic process that stimulates release of milk from the breasts, e.g., when the mother hears her baby crying.

leucine natural essential amino acid, vital for infant growth and adult nitrogen equilibrium.

leucocyte white blood corpuscle.

leucocytosis increased number of leucocytes in the blood, usually in response to infection.

leucopenia decreased number of leucocytes in the blood.

leucorrhoea white, mucoid, non-irritating vaginal discharge secreted by the cervical glands to moisten the vaginal membranes; often increased at ovulation, before a menstrual period and throughout pregnancy and stimulated by sexual excitement; normally white, inoffensive and non-irritating unless in the presence of infection.

leukaemia uncommon malignant blood disease characterised by increased numbers of abnormal leucocytes and reduced numbers of erythrocytes and blood platelets, resulting in anaemia and increased susceptibility to infection and haemorrhage.

levallorphan analogue of levorphanol, an antagonist to analgesic narcotics.

levator muscle that raises a part.

levator ani broad sheet of muscle forming the principal part of the pelvic floor.

levonorgestrel progestin used in combination with oestrogen as an oral contraceptive.

libido sexual desire.

Librium *See* CHLORDIAZEPOXIDE.

lidocaine (lignocaine) hydrochloride (Xylocaine) drug for infiltration analgesia and nerve block; 1% solution may be used by midwives for infiltration of the perineum before performing episiotomy and perineal repair.

lie, fetal relation of the long axis of the fetus to the long axis of the mother's uterus, normally parallel with a longitudinal lie; in an abnormal lie the fetus lies across the uterus, i.e. transverse or oblique lie, which, if not corrected, causes obstructed labour.

ligament tough fibrous band of tissue connecting bones or supporting internal organs. Supporting uterine ligaments are *transverse cervical* or *cardinal l.*, *pubocervical l.* and *uterosacral l.*; *round l's* extend from the uterine cornua to the labia majora; *broad l's* are not true ligaments but folds of peritoneum, adjacent to the uterus and covering the fallopian tubes.

ligamentum arteriosum vestiges of the ductus arteriosum.

ligamentum teres vestiges of the umbilical vein.

ligamentum venosum vestiges of the ductus venosus.

ligation process of applying a ligature.

ligature thread, usually of catgut, nylon or wire, used for tying blood vessels.

light for dates *See* SMALL FOR GESTATIONAL AGE BABY.

lightening relief experienced in late pregnancy as the presenting part sinks into the pelvis and the fundus no longer presses on the diaphragm, usually around 36 weeks' gestation in nulliparae but not until the onset of labour in multiparae.

linea line. *L. alba* tendinous central area of the abdominal wall into which the transversalis and oblique muscles are inserted. *L. nigra* temporarily pigmented linea alba of pregnancy between the umbilicus and pubis, and sometimes extending to the ensiform cartilage; caused by increased pituitary gland production of melanocytic hormone.

lint loosely woven cotton fabric with a fluffy and a smooth side, used for surgical dressings.

lipase ENZYME present in breast milk and pancreatic juice, which splits fat into fatty acids; pancreatic lipase is not present in large amounts, so a baby who is not breastfed is less able to digest fats.

lipid fatty substance insoluble in water but soluble in alcohol or chloroform; an important part of the diet, normally present in body tissues.

Lippe's loop intrauterine contraceptive device.

liquor amnii amniotic fluid filling the amniotic sac surrounding the fetus: about 99% water, with proteins, fats, carbohydrates, sodium and potassium in solution, and debris consisting of desquamated fetal epithelial cells, vernix caseosa, lanugo and various enzymes and pigments. It acts as a shock absorber; allows unhindered fetal growth; distributes pressure evenly around the whole fetus; permits free movement necessary for muscle function; and prevents diminution of the placental site. Volume is approximately 1 L at 37–38 weeks' gestation, reduced by half at term. *See also* AMNIOCENTESIS and AMNIOTIC FLUID.

liquor volume amount of amniotic fluid in the amniotic sac, which peaks at 28 weeks' gestation. *See* OLIGOHYDRAMNIOS, POLYHYDRAMNIOS and AMNIOTIC FLUID INDEX.

Listeria Gram-negative bacteria that causes upper respiratory tract disease, septicaemia and encephalitis; transmitted by eating infected unpasteurised dairy produce or by direct contact with infected animals or contaminated soil. Babies, pregnant women, elderly people and the immunosuppressed are more susceptible to infection.

lithopaedion very rare condition in which the fetus develops outside the uterus and dies and become petrified owing to lime salt deposition.

lithotomy position position in which the mother lies on her back with thighs and legs flexed and abducted, held in place with lithotomy poles; used for forceps or breech delivery and perineal suturing. The woman's legs must be lifted into or out of the stirrups together, preferably by two people, one on each side, to avoid possible hip dislocation due to joint laxity resulting from relaxin and progesterone effects.

litigation legal action or lawsuit, taken in the case of suspected negligence or malpractice; obstetrics is one of the clinical specialities most likely to result in court cases because of the emotive nature of childbirth.

litmus paper blotting paper impregnated with litmus, a pigment used to identify fluid reactions; blue litmus is turned red by acids; red litmus is turned blue by alkalis.

litre (L) measure of volume, 1000 mL or about 35 fl. oz.

live birth baby born alive.

liver large wedge-shaped gland in the right hypochondrium and epigastrium, essential for formation of bile; production of plasma proteins, except GAMMA GLOBULINS; storage of carbohydrates (as glycogen), iron and vitamins A, D, E and K; regulation of fat, protein and carbohydrate metabolism; detoxication of drugs and other substances; formation and destruction of

ERYTHROCYTES; production of PRO-THROMBIN and FIBRINOGEN; heat production; and phagocytosis of bacteria.

liver function tests (LFT) range of tests to assess liver function. Tests include albumin, with low levels possibly indicating liver disease, malnutrition or a low protein diet; liver enzymes, released into the general circulation when liver tissue is damaged or diseased; aminotransferases, e.g. aspartate aminotransferase (AST or SGOT) and alanine aminotransferase (ALT or SGPT), sensitive indicators of liver disease; alkaline phosphatase (ALP), elevated in hepatic or bone disease or in response to certain drugs; prothrombin clotting time, to identify prolonged clotting times and haemorrhagic disorders; bilirubin, which is excreted in bile.

livid cyanotic; bluene~~ ~~ with venous congest~~ ~~ quate OXYGEN.

lobe section of an o~~ ~~ from neighbouring pa~~ ~~

lobule small segment~~ ~~ cially one of the sm~~ ~~ making up a lobe. adj.

local authority local go~~ ~~

local supervising authorit~~ ~~ organisation, usually~~ ~~ monitors midwifery prac~~ ~~ by appointing supervi~~ ~~ wifery, facilitating their~~ ~~ training and enabling co~~ ~~ with the supervisors; developing systems to ensure eligibility to practise of each midwife working within the area; and, where necessary, suspending from practice any midwife who may have acted unsafely or negligently. The LSA nominates an officer, who is a practising midwife, to carry out its functions. *See also* SUPERVISOR OF MIDWIVES.

lochia uterine discharge occurring for about 2–6 weeks after labour or abortion, consisting of placental site blood, shreds of decidua, vaginal epithelial cells and, initially, uterine debris, e.g. amniotic fluid, vernix caseosa and meconium. *L. alba* (whitish) contains white blood cells and mucus. *L. rubra* (red) initially fresh, then staler blood. *L. serosa* (pinkish) contains fewer red and more white cells. Red, profuse lochia or sudden cessation of lochia may indicate subinvolution or, if combined with offensive odour, infection. sing. *lochium*.

locked twins rare cause of obstructed labour in which the bodies and heads of twins are caught together, precluding normal vaginal delivery for either baby.

locus place, site. In genetics, the specific site of a gene on a chromosome.

longitudinal study an investigation involving observations of the same group at sequential time intervals; valuable for studying human individual or organisational development or change.

lordosis exaggeration of the normal forward curve of the lumbar spine, common in pregnancy because of musculoskeletal laxity caused by relaxin and progesterone, but exacerbated by poor posture. The weight of the uterus pulls the body forwards; to compensate, the woman leans backwards, throwing extra strain on the relaxed sacroiliac joints and causing backache. Advice regarding posture, exercise and ergonomics may help to partially correct the problem, easing the discomfort.

Lövset's manoeuvre manoeuvre used in breech presentation to deliver the fetal shoulders when the arms are extended; the fetus is rotated through a half circle keeping the back uppermost, and the posterior arm is brought into an anterior position below the symphysis pubis to be delivered; the fetus is then rotated a half circle in the reverse direction and the other arm is similarly delivered.

low-birthweight baby   baby weighing 2.5 kg or less at birth; may be preterm or small for gestational age, or both.

lower uterine segment   part of the UTERUS between the vesicouterine peritoneal fold superiorly and the junction of the uterus and cervix inferiorly.

lubricant   cream, jelly or similar substance applied to the hands, gloves or instruments to make them slippery and to facilitate manipulations.

lumbar   pertaining to the loins. *l. puncture* introduction of a hollow needle into the subarachnoid space, usually between the fourth and fifth lumbar vertebrae, to withdraw cerebrospinal fluid for diagnostic purposes or to relieve pressure or introduce drugs.

lumbosacral   relating to both lumbar and sacral vertebrae or regions.

lumen   space inside a tube.

lumpectomy   surgical excision of only the local lesion (benign or malignant) of the breast.

lungs   two conical respiratory organs consisting of air tubes (bronchi and bronchioles) terminating in air spaces (alveoli) and occupying most of the thoracic cavity. During respiration the lungs supply the blood with oxygen inhaled from outside air and dispose of waste carbon dioxide in exhaled air.

lupus   chronic skin disease with many different manifestations.

luteal   pertaining to the CORPUS LUTEUM.

lutein   yellow pigment in the corpus luteum.

luteinising hormone   anterior pituitary gland hormone that, with follicle-stimulating hormone, causes ovulation of mature follicles and secretion of oestrogen by thecal and granulosa cells of the ovary; also concerned with corpus luteum formation. In the male, it stimulates development of the interstitial cells of the testes and secretion of testosterone.

luteotrophin   prolactin.

lymph   body fluid derived from interstitial fluid and carried in lymphatic vessels back to the bloodstream; lymph nodes occur at intervals throughout lymphatic vessels and act as filters.

lymphatics   vessels carrying lymph.

lymphocytes   white blood cells, formed mainly from lymphoid tissue in bone marrow and thymus.

lymphoedema   condition in which the intercellular spaces contain abnormal amounts of lymph due to obstruction of lymph drainage.

lyse   to cause disintegration of a cell or substance.

lysin   cell-dissolving substance present in blood serum.

lysis   1. gradual decline, e.g. of fever. 2. breaking down, as of red blood cells in haemolysis.

lysozyme   antibacterial (Gram-positive) agent present in all tissues and secretions, particularly tears and breast milk.

lytic cocktail   chlorpromazine, promethazine and pethidine, used to treat severe pre-eclampsia and eclampsia; promethazine and pethidine may also be used without chlorpromazine. Less commonly used now.

maceration softening of a solid by soaking, as with a dead fetus retained in the uterus for more than 24 hours; characterised by discoloration, softening of tissues, peeling fetal skin and eventual disintegration, indicating that a stillbirth has been dead *in utero* before labour; may lead to DISSEMINATED INTRAVASCULAR COAGULATION (DIC).

Mackenrodt's ligaments transverse or cardinal ligaments supporting the uterus in the pelvic cavity.

macro- prefix meaning 'large'.

macrocyte abnormally large red blood corpuscle found in megaloblastic anaemia of pregnancy resulting from folic acid deficiency.

macronutrient essential nutrient with daily requirement >100 mg, e.g. calcium, phosphorus, magnesium, potassium, sodium, chloride.

macrophage large, mononuclear, highly phagocytic cells derived from monocytes, occurring in blood vessel walls and loose connective tissue; components of the reticuloendothelial system. Become actively mobile when stimulated by inflammation; interact with lymphocytes to facilitate antibody production.

macroscopic discernible with the naked eye.

macrosomia large baby, birthweight >97th centile for gestation or more than 4–4.5 kg at term.

magnesium bluish-white metal, symbol Mg; found in intra- and extracellular fluids and excreted in urine and faeces; minute quantities are essential for enzyme activity, especially that concerned with oxidative phosphorylation. Normal serum level is approximately 1 mmol/L; deficiency causes nervous system irritability, tetany, vasodilatation, convulsions, tremors, depression and psychotic behaviour. *M. sulphate* saline purgative (Epsom salts) recommended by the World Health Organization for controlling eclamptic fits, and more effective than diazepam or phenytoin; administered intravenously: blood levels must be monitored regularly to ensure they remain between 2 mmol/L and 4 mmol/L; toxicity leads to loss of maternal reflexes, muscle paralysis, and respiratory and cardiac arrest. *M. trisilicate* antacid powder used to treat dyspepsia, peptic ulcer and heartburn, and reduce the acidity of gastric contents before general anaesthesia, particularly during labour to reduce the risk of MENDELSON'S SYNDROME.

magnetic resonance imaging (MRI) imaging technique that passes magnetic and radio waves through the body whilst the patient is in a cylindrical tunnel; this displaces cell nuclei and as they revert to normal a signal is generated that is converted into a computer image. Particularly useful for examination of brain and spinal cord – the fetal brain can clearly be seen *in utero*, although fetal movements may adversely affect image quality. May be used in conjunction with DOPPLER ULTRASOUND to investigate pelvic blood flow in gynaecological conditions, e.g. menstrual disorders, subfertility, cancer.

maintenance order court order requiring a person to give a regular payment to someone for whom they have responsibility, e.g. a father of a child.

mal- prefix meaning 'bad', 'wrong' or 'ill'. *Grand m.* generalised convulsive seizure with loss of consciousness. *Petit m.* momentary loss of consciousness without convulsive movements. *See also* EPILEPSY.

malabsorption impaired intestinal absorption of nutrients. *M. syndrome* group of disorders having subnormal intestinal absorption of dietary constituents, with excessive nutrient loss in stools.

malacia softening of tissues. *Osteomalacia* softening of bone tissue, one effect being deformity of the pelvic bones; uncommon in developed countries.

malaise feeling of general discomfort and illness.

malar pertaining to the malar bone of the face or the region adjacent to it.

malaria tropical infection contracted from mosquito bites, leading to the presence of protozoan parasites in red blood cells; periodic bouts of fever, sweating, chills and rigors may occur over several years. The incidence has increased greatly in non-affected countries because of increased travel, and prophylactic medication is essential before, during and after travelling to affected areas of the world.

male reproductive system consists of two sperm-producing testes within the scrotum; sperm are collected by the fine tubular epididymis and conveyed by the vas deferens to the seminal vesicles where they are stored. At ejaculation the prostate gland adds fluid to sperm, which are then passed into the urethra inside the erect penis; during intercourse sperm are deposited in the posterior vaginal fornix.

malformation anatomical abnormality or deformity, either congenital or acquired.

malignant tending to become progressively worse resulting in death, as in tumours; having the properties of anaplasia, invasiveness and metastasis.

malnutrition defective quantity or quality of nutrition, causing deficiency syndromes.

Malpighian body glomerulus and Bowman's capsule of the kidney.

malposition misplaced situation of any organ or part in relationship to neighbouring structures or parts; applied to a fetus with its occiput directed towards one or other posterior quadrant of the pelvis.

malpractice professional misconduct or negligence, unreasonable lack of skill or fidelity in professional duties, or illegal or immoral conduct, by either omitting to do something that a reasonable person would do or doing something a prudent person would not do. In midwifery malpractice results in injury, unnecessary suffering, or death of mother or baby.

malpresentation fetal presentation other than vertex, i.e. breech, face,

Male reproductive system

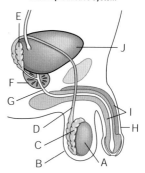

A, testes; B, scrotum; C, epididymis;
D, vas deferens; E, seminal vesicle;
F, prostate gland; G, urethra; H, penis;
I, erectile tissue; J, bladder.

brow or shoulder presentation; failure to diagnose the condition can lead to serious complications, e.g. obstructed labour, uterine rupture, fetal or maternal death.

maltase sugar-splitting enzyme that converts maltose to glucose, present in pancreatic and intestinal juice.

maltose sugar (disaccharide) formed when starch is hydrolysed by amylase.

mamma breast.

mammal member of a division of vertebrates, including all that possess hair and suckle their offspring.

mammary pertaining to the breasts.

mammilla nipple.

mammography breast radiography with or without injection of an opaque substance into the ducts; routine screening procedure to diagnose cancer and other breast disorders.

Manchester operation amputation of the cervix, with anterior and posterior colporrhaphy.

mandelic acid ketoacid used as a urinary antiseptic in nephritis, pyelitis and cystitis.

mandible horseshoe-shaped bone forming the lower jaw.

mania mental disorder characterised by acceleration of all mental processes, often with violence; may follow childbirth.

manipulation using the hands in a skilful manner, e.g. to change position of the fetus.

mannitol sugar alcohol occurring widely, especially in fungi; osmotic diuretic used for forced diuresis and in cerebral oedema; not recommended in pregnancy but may be used for acute tubular necrosis after postpartum haemorrhage. Not to be added to whole blood.

manoeuvre similar to MANIPULATION; procedure carried out with the hands, e.g. to facilitate delivery of baby or placenta. See LÖVSET'S MANOEUVRE *and* MAURICEAU–SMELLIE–VEIT MANOEUVRE.

manometer instrument used to measure pressure or tension of liquids or gases. See SPHYGMOMANOMETER.

Mantoux reaction reaction to the *M. test*, an intradermal injection of old tuberculin to determine susceptibility to tuberculosis; a weal developing within hours indicates a positive reaction, signifying that a previous infection has conferred some degree of immunity.

manual with the hand. *M. removal of the placenta* introducing a hand into the uterus to remove a retained placenta; may be necessary for a midwife to perform this procedure in isolated areas in an emergency when no medical aid is available. Antiseptic cream is applied to the gloved hand, which is introduced into the vagina; the umbilical cord is followed up to the uterus and placenta whilst the other hand supports the uterus through the abdominal wall. After finding a separated edge of the placenta the remainder is peeled off the uterine wall and withdrawn; bimanual compression may be required to control bleeding; risk of shock is greater when the procedure is performed without anaesthetic.

maple syrup urine disease genetic disorder caused by deficiency of an enzyme necessary for metabolism of branched-chain amino acids; marked clinically by physical and learning disabilities, feeding difficulties and a characteristic odour of urine.

marasmus severe malnutrition and weight loss in babies associated with protein-calorie deficiency, usually with normal appetite and mental alertness; related to KWASHIORKOR.

Marcain See BUPIVACAINE.

Marfan's syndrome hereditary disorder of connective tissue characterised by abnormal length of the extremities, especially fingers and toes, subluxation of the lens, congenital heart anomalies and other deformities.

marijuana, marihuana preparation of *Cannabis sativa* or hemp; also hashish. Contains several pharmacologically active principles, used therapeutically or recreationally for euphoric properties; more potent when smoked and inhaled than when ingested; hashish is more potent than marijuana. Possession is illegal in many countries, including the UK. May increase risk of miscarriage and birth defects.

marker indicator of increased risk of a disease or disorder; several markers are often combined to provide a more detailed clinical picture or to increase SENSITIVITY and SPECIFICITY of a screening test.

marrow soft, organic, sponge-like material in the bone cavities that assists in the manufacture of erythrocytes, leucocytes and platelets; occasionally subject to disease, e.g. aplastic anaemia, caused by destruction of the marrow by chemical agents or excessive X-ray exposure, leukaemia, pernicious anaemia, myeloma and metastatic tumours.

massage systematic therapeutic stroking or kneading of the body to aid relaxation, stimulate circulation and excretory processes and lower blood pressure; may be helpful to ease anxiety and fear in pregnancy and relieve pain in labour, as touch impulses reach the brain before pain impulses, although not all women like to be touched during labour; *see also* EFFLEURAGE. *Cardiac m.* intermittent heart compression by pressure applied over the sternum (closed cardiac massage) or directly to the heart through an opening in the chest wall (open cardiac massage). *Infant m.* has been shown to aid growth and physical and psychological development, especially in preterm babies.

mast cells large connective tissue cells in heart, liver and lungs containing granules that release heparin, serotonin and histamine in response to inflammation or allergy.

mastitis inflammation of the breast. *Puerperal m.* infection caused by staphylococci or streptococci, which enter through cracked nipples; a wedge-shaped area of breast becomes tender, red and warm and the mother feels generally unwell; responds quickly to antibiotic treatment but delay may lead to breast abscess.

MAT B1 maternity certificate certificate signed by midwife or doctor confirming expected date of delivery; must be presented when claiming financial and employment benefits related to pregnancy.

materia medica science of the source and preparation of drugs used in medicine. *Homeopathic m.m.* resources detailing actions and effectiveness of homeopathic remedies after they have been thoroughly tested on healthy volunteers, used by homeopaths to determine precisely the most appropriate remedy for the client.

maternal pertaining to the mother. *M. mortality* death due to pregnancy or childbearing, the commonest causes of which are hypertensive and haemorrhagic disorders. *M. mortality rate* number of maternal deaths due to pregnancy and childbearing per 1000 registered live births and stillbirths; the CONFIDENTIAL ENQUIRY into maternal deaths is a triennial report detailing all deaths that have occurred in the UK.

maternity pertaining to childbearing. *M.Alliance* charity comprising various maternity-related organisations, which campaigns for improved conditions for mothers and babies, provides education, undertakes and supports research and publishes numerous books and leaflets. *M. benefits see* Appendix 12 for summary. *M. care assistant* auxiliary practitioner who is not a midwife but is specifically trained to assist mothers and midwives.

maternity services liaison committee local committees set up to serve the interests of maternity service consumers through two-way communication between obstetric, paediatric, anaesthetic and midwifery representatives and prospective and retrospective users of the services, including Community Health Council members.

matrix intercellular substance of a tissue, e.g. bone matrix, or the tissue from which a structure develops, e.g. hair or nail matrix.

Matthews Duncan expulsion of placenta placental expulsion in which the maternal side appears first at the end of the third stage of labour, often due to a low-lying placenta; more severe haemorrhage is likely than with SCHULTZE EXPULSION.

maturation process of ripening or developing, as in cell division when the number of chromosomes in the germ cell is reduced to half the number characteristic of the species.

Mauriceau famous French male midwife. *M.-Smellie-Veit manoeuvre* method of delivering the aftercoming head in breech delivery; flexion is increased and jaw and shoulder traction applied; allows for better control over the delivery of the head than BURNS–MARSHALL TECHNIQUE in cases in which forceps delivery is not possible.

Maxolon *See* METOCLOPRAMIDE.

mean average; numerical value intermediate between two extremes. *M. corpuscular haemoglobin (MCH)* indicator of the mean (average) amount of haemoglobin in red blood cells. Low levels indicate reduced oxygen-carrying capacity of the blood; MCH concentration of <25 pg may indicate ALPHA THALASSAEMIA trait. *M. corpuscular volume (MCV)* measurement of red blood cell size, usually decreased (microcytic) in iron deficiency anaemia and increased (macrocytic) in vitamin B12 deficiency anaemia.

measles highly infectious viral disease; also called rubeola or morbilli. *See* Appendix 14.

meatus opening or passage. *Auditory m.* opening leading into the auditory canal. *Urinary m.* where the urethra opens to the exterior.

mechanism of labour sequence of movements made by the fetus during labour to facilitate passage through the maternal pelvis.

meconium greenish-black material in the fetal intestinal tract, passed *per rectum* in the first few days of life; contains bile pigments and salts, mucus, intestinal epithelial cells and amniotic fluid. *M. aspiration* inhalation of fluid containing meconium, as occurs in babies who have been hypoxic *in utero*, especially those who are growth-retarded. *M. ileus* gross distension of the bowel with inspissated meconium found in CYSTIC FIBROSIS.

median situated in the median plane or midline of a body or structure. *M. nerve* nerve originating in the brachial plexus that innervates muscles of the wrist and hand. *M. plane* imaginary plane passing longitudinally through the body from front to back, dividing it into right and left halves.

mediastinum 1. median septum or partition. 2. mass of tissues and organs separating the sternum in front and vertebral column behind, containing the heart and large vessels, trachea, oesophagus, thymus, lymph nodes and other structures and tissues; divided into anterior, middle, posterior and superior regions.

medical herbalism *See* HERBAL MEDICINE.

medicine 1. any drug or remedy. 2. art and science of diagnosis and treatment of disease and maintenance of health. 3. non-surgical treatment of disease, as opposed to surgery.

Medicines Act 1968 Act that established administrative and licensing systems to control the sale and supply of medicines to the public and retail pharmacies, and the packing and labelling of medicinal products.

Medicines (Prescription Only) Order 1983 schedule 3 order detailing the medicines, normally only available on prescription issued by a doctor, that may be supplied to midwives who have notified their intention to practise for use in their practice, including analgesics, oxytocics, sedatives and drugs for neonatal resuscitation.

medium 1. agent by which something is accomplished or an impulse is transmitted. 2. substance providing correct nutritional environment for growth of micro-organisms; also called culture medium.

medium-chain acyl-coenzyme A dehydrogenase deficiency (MCADD) inherited autosomal recessive metabolic disorder, occurring in 1:6000 UK births and having a 25% cot death rate; carried by 1:40 to 1:68 people in the UK. Caused by lack of medium-chain acyl-coenzyme A dehydrogenase, an enzyme required to break down stored fat into energy; fats cannot be completely broken down, causing hypoglycaemia and accumulation of toxins. Acute symptoms, often with concomitant infection, include hypoglycaemia, poor feeding, drowsiness and lethargy, seizures and unconsciousness. Screening is available in some areas of the UK via the NEWBORN BLOOD-SPOT SCREENING test.

medroxyprogesterone acetate (Depo-Provera) single-dose intramuscular contraceptive, effective for 12 weeks, given to women after rubella vaccination, to those whose partners have had a vasectomy and to women unable to manage other methods of contraception; risk of heavy bleeding if used before the fifth postnatal week.

medulla central or inner portion of an organ. *M. oblongata* lowest part of

the brainstem between the pons varolii and spinal cord, seat of the vital centres, i.e. the cardiac, respiratory and vasomotor centres.

mega (M) word element meaning 'large'; used in units of measurement to designate an amount that is 10^6 (one million) times the size of the unit to which it is joined, e.g. megacuries, 10^6 curies.

megalo- prefix meaning 'great'.

megaloblastic anaemia anaemia in which immature red cells circulate in the blood, caused by folic acid deficiency; epileptic women and those on long-term administration of PHENYTOIN are more prone.

megaloblasts large, nucleated, immature red blood cells, normally present in bone marrow.

meiosis process by which the germinal epithelium in either ovary or testis gives rise to a gamete containing only one CHROMOSOME from each pair, i.e. haploid number (23 in humans); the normal number is the diploid (46 in humans).

melaena dark, altered blood in the stools, occurring in haemorrhagic disease of the newborn; may be accompanied by HAEMATEMESIS.

melanin dark pigment found in hair, choroid coat, etc., sometimes deposited in malignant tumours. Increased pigmentation occurs during pregnancy because of raised melanocytic hormone levels; results in the LINEA NIGRA, darkening of the areolae of the nipples and, in some women, facial CHLOASMA.

melanocyte-stimulating hormone (MSH) anterior pituitary gland peptide that influences formation or deposition of melanin in the body.

membrane thin tissue covering the surface of certain organs and lining body cavities. *Mucous m.* contains secreting cells and lines all cavities connected directly or indirectly with the skin. *Fetal m.'s* the CHORION and AMNION.

menarche onset of menstruation at puberty.

Mendel's laws the pattern, first demonstrated by the Moravian monk, Gregor Mendel, whereby inherited characteristics are transmitted, some being dominant and others recessive.

Mendelson's syndrome marked irritation of bronchi and alveoli, characterised by extreme dyspnoea, cyanosis and tachycardia, causing severe bronchospasm and pulmonary oedema and sometimes leading to hypotension and death; occurs when acidic gastric juice is inhaled during general anaesthesia; the midwife may be asked by the anaesthetist to apply CRICOID pressure to prevent it.

meninges the membranes covering the brain and spinal cord: dura mater, arachnoid and pia mater.

meningitis inflammation of the meninges, either viral, developing after common childhood illnesses, e.g. chickenpox or measles, or bacterial, a much more serious form with a mortality rate of 5% and a 25% risk of long-term problems in survivors, including deafness, epilepsy or permanent brain damage. Children are offered vaccination at 3, 4 and 12 months of age. Symptoms are initially flu-like, making diagnosis difficult, and include constant generalised headache, confusion and drowsiness, pyrexia with cold extremities, abdominal pain, vomiting and diarrhoea, rapid respirations, and joint or muscle pain; three cardinal signs and symptoms are neck stiffness, sensitivity to light and a red/purplish rash of spots, which, when pressed, does not fade. In babies symptoms include fever, vomiting, muscle dystonia, high-pitched moan or whimpering cry, irritability when handled, refusal to feed, neck retractions, arching of back, lethargy, convulsions and a tense, bulging fontanelle. Urgent treatment including hospital admission, good nursing care and antibiotics (for bacterial meningitis) is required, with prognosis being better the earlier medical treatment is sought.

meningocele congenital deformity; protrusion of the meninges through the skull or spinal column, appearing as a cyst filled with cerebrospinal fluid. *See also* SPINA BIFIDA.

meningoencephalocele hernial protrusion of the meninges and brain substance through a defect in the skull.

meningomyelocele hernial protrusion of the meninges and spinal cord through a defect in the vertebral column.

meniscocyte sickle cell.

menopause normal cessation of menstruation. *Artificial m., induced m.* cessation induced by operation or irradiation.

menorrhagia excessive menstrual discharge.

menses menstruation.

menstrual pertaining to menstruation. *M. cycle* cyclical event, normally occurring every 28 days. Menstrual bleeding begins on day 1 as a result of falling progesterone levels and normally lasts 4–5 days, during which the endometrium is shed down to the basal layer. In the secretory phase that follows, increasing oestrogen levels from the pituitary gland trigger the ovary to stimulate one of the graafian follicles to mature while at the same time the endometrium thickens in anticipation of receiving a fertilised ovum. Once the follicle has ripened (usually 14 days *before* the next cycle) it bursts to release the ovum (ovulation), which begins its journey along the fallopian tube towards the uterus. At the same time progesterone levels now rise; if fertilisation occurs levels are maintained to assist embedding and development of the embryo; if conception does not occur the ovum passes to the uterus and a fall in hormone activity causes the thickened endometrium to be shed with the ovum and some blood. Changing hormone levels also cause the ruptured uterine follicle to degenerate, when it becomes known as the corpus luteum.

Endometrial and follicular changes during the menstrual cycle (from Weller B. 2000 *Baillière's Nurses' Dictionary*, Baillière Tindall, p. 140, with permission)

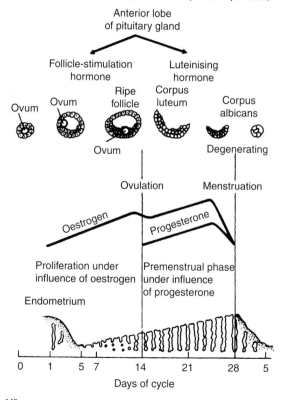

menstruation discharge of blood from the uterus at approximately 4-week intervals, commencing at puberty and lasting until the menopause.

mental 1. pertaining to the mind. 2. pertaining to the chin.

mentoanterior fetal position with the chin directed anteriorly in the pelvis; similarly, mentolateral and mentoposterior.

mentum chin; denominator in face presentation.

meptazinol narcotic analgesia claimed to cause less respiratory depression than pethidine with a relatively quick onset but short duration of action of 2–4 hours; nausea and vomiting are common side effects.

Meptid See MEPTAZINOL.

mercury element; symbol Hg. Liquid heavy metal used in thermometers as it expands with heat, and in SPHYGMOMANOMETERS as it is heavier than water, meaning that only a short tube is needed to record a wide variation in pressure.

meridian imaginary line; in traditional Chinese medicine, the energy lines throughout the body along which are situated the points for acupuncture or acupressure.

mesentery a membranous fold attaching various organs to the body wall, especially the peritoneal fold attaching the small intestine to the dorsal body wall. adj. *mesenteric.*

mesoderm cells lying between ectoderm and endoderm cell layers in the embryo, from which bone, muscle, heart, blood, blood vessels, gonads, kidneys and connective tissues develop.

mesosalpinx peritoneum covering the fallopian tubes.

mesovarium fold of peritoneum connecting the ovary to the broad ligament.

meta-analysis analysis and evaluation of results of all accessible research trials on a given subject.

metabolism process of life, by which tissue cells are broken down by combustion (catabolism) and new protein is built up from the end products of digestion (anabolism). *Basal m.* See BASAL METABOLIC RATE. *Inborn error of m.* genetically determined biochemical disorder in which a specific enzyme defect produces a metabolic block that may have pathological consequences at birth, as in phenylketonuria, or in later life.

metastasis transfer of disease from one organ to another not directly connected with it. pl. *metastases*; growth of malignant cells or pathogenic micro-organisms distant from the primary site.

metatarsum part of the foot between ankle and toes; five bones (metatarsals) extending from the tarsus to the phalanges.

methadone hydrochloride synthetic compound with pharmacological properties similar to those of morphine and heroin; may be prescribed for drug addicts in pregnancy as a maintenance drug.

methicillin-resistant *Staphylococcus aureus* (MRSA) strain of *S. aureus* resistant to 'methicillin-like' antibiotics; carried in the nose or on skin without symptoms; spread by direct contact and cause of severe, contagious, hospital-acquired infection.

methohexitone sodium intravenous anaesthetic.

methotrexate folic acid antagonist used as an anti-neoplastic agent and to treat psoriasis.

methyldopa hypotensive drug, sometimes used in essential hypertension in pregnancy; crosses the placenta but there is no evidence that it affects the fetus.

metoclopramide drug that increases gastric action, used to treat nausea and vomiting and heartburn.

metopic suture frontal suture.

metra uterus.

metra-, metro- word element meaning 'uterus'.

metre (m) international (SI) unit for measuring length and distance; 1 metre = 39.4 inches.

metritis inflammation of the uterus.

metronidazole (Flagyl) antimicrobial drug effective against anaerobic infections, e.g. *Trichomonas vaginalis*.

metropathia haemorrhagica painless excessive menstrual and intermenstrual bleeding and failure of ovulation, hence failure of corpus luteum development.

metrorrhagia haemorrhage from the uterus independent of menstruation.

metrostaxis persistent slight haemorrhage from the uterus.

Michel's clips small metal clips for closing skin wounds.

miconazole antifungal agent used topically for dermatophytic infections, e.g. athlete's foot, vulvovaginal candidiasis; orally for candidiasis of the mouth and gastrointestinal tract; and systemically by intravenous infusion for systemic fungal infections.

micro- 1. prefix meaning 'small', of microscopic size. 2. prefix indicating 'one-millionth', e.g. microgram (µg), one-millionth of a gram.

microbe micro-organism, especially a pathogenic bacterium. adj. *microbial, microbic*.

microcephaly abnormally small head; a microcephalic baby has ossified skull bones and always has learning difficulties.

microcytic having unusually small cells. See ANAEMIA.

micrognathia unusually small mandible or lower jaw, with a receding chin. See PIERRE–ROBIN SYNDROME.

Microgynon 30 combined oral contraceptive pill containing oestrogen and progesterone. See ETHINYLOESTRADIOL.

Micronor contraceptive minipill of progesterone only, used during breastfeeding and for women with thrombosis risk or who suffer severe side effects from oestrogen.

micro-organism minute living organism, animal or vegetable, e.g. virus or bacterium, visible under a microscope.

microphage small phagocyte; actively mobile neutrophilic leucocyte capable of phagocytosis.

micturition act of passing urine.

middle cerebral artery (MCA) flow blood flow through the middle cerebral artery, measurable with ultrasound; increased velocity indicates severe fetal anaemia. Valuable test in the investigation and management of haemolytic disease from maternal red cell ALLOIMMUNISATION as it may indicate when INTRAUTERINE TRANSFUSION is required.

midwife the International Confederation of Midwives 1972 and International Federation of Gynaecologists and Obstetricians 1973 defined a midwife as 'a person who, having been regularly admitted to a midwifery education programme, duly recognised in the country in which it is located, has successfully completed the prescribed course of studies and acquired the requisite qualifications to be registered and/or legally licensed to practise midwifery, able to give the necessary supervision, care and advice to women during pregnancy, labour and the postpartum period, conduct deliveries on her [or his] own responsibility and care for the newborn and the infant; care includes preventative measures, detection of abnormal conditions in mother and child, procurement of medical assistance and execution of emergency measures in the absence of medical help. She [or he] has an important task in health counselling and health education, ... antenatal education and preparation for parenthood and ... certain areas of gynaecology, family planning and child care. She [or he] may practise in hospitals, clinics, health units, domiciliary conditions or in any other service.'

midwifery art and science of caring for women undergoing *normal* pregnancies, labours and puerperia; OBSTETRICS deals with *abnormal* pregnancies, labours or postnatal periods.

miliaria cutaneous condition involving retention of sweat, which is extravasated at different levels in the skin; also called prickly heat or heat rash.

military attitude attitude of the fetus that is neither flexed nor extended.

milk secretion of the mammary gland. *Human breast m.* contains lipids, 98% as triglycerides, which provide more than 50% of the calorific requirements; carbohydrates, mainly lactose, giving 40% of the calorific needs; whey-dominant protein; vitamins; minerals; trace elements; and anti-infective factors, such as leucocytes, immunoglobulins, lysozyme, lactoferrin, bifidus factor, hormones and growth factor. *Pasteurised m.* milk held at 73°C for 15 seconds or at 63–66°C for 30 minutes, then rapidly cooled and bottled. *Sterilised m.* milk heated to 100°C for 15 minutes to render it free from bacteria. *Tuberculin-tested m.* milk from cows certified free from tuberculosis and subject to strict bacteriological tests.

milk flow mechanism, milk ejection reflex oxytocin released from the posterior pituitary gland in response to nervous stimulation causes contraction of MYOEPITHELIAL CELLS; milk is forced out of the ALVEOLI into the ducts and lacteal sinuses and is available to the baby; occurs about 30–40 seconds after the baby takes the AREOLA of the breast in his mouth.

milli- prefix indicating 'one-thousandth', e.g. milligram (mg), one-thousandth of a gram; millilitre (mL), one-thousandth of a litre; millimetre (mm), one-thousandth of a metre.

Milton proprietary antiseptic, 1% solution of electrolytic sodium hypochlorite, used for sterilisation of babies' feeding bottles.

mineral naturally occurring non-organic homogeneous solid substance; 19 occur in the body, with at least 13 essential to health; obtained from a mixed and varied diet of animal and vegetable products.

Minilyn combined oestrogen and progesterone contraceptive pill.

Minovlar, Minovlar ED combined oestrogen and progesterone contraceptive pills.

miscarriage ABORTION; expulsion of the fetus before 24 weeks of pregnancy, i.e. before the fetus is legally viable.

misoprostol oral uterotonic, a prostaglandin E$_1$ analogue, approved for use in gastric ulcer but has also been shown to be suitable for use in active management of the third stage of labour, especially in developing countries.

missed abortion former term for MISSED MISCARRIAGE.

missed miscarriage non-viable pregnancy in which products of conception remain *in utero*; miscarriage may occur several weeks after fetal death; ultrasound appearance is consistent with ANEMBRYONIC PREGNANCY or there may be fetal evidence but no fetal heart beat.

Misuse of Drugs Act 1971 controls possession and supply of narcotic drugs, e.g. papaveretum (Omnopon), cocaine, morphine, diamorphine and those that affect the central nervous system (e.g. LSD and amphetamines).

mitosis normal process of cell multiplication in which nuclear division occurs with each chromosome dividing into two, so that two identical cells are formed. cf. MEIOSIS.

mitral shaped like a mitre. *M. incompetence* defective mitral valve, usually the result of scar tissue following endocarditis. **M. regurgitation** result of mild endocarditis, when the valve is puckered and closes imperfectly. **M. stenosis** more serious condition in which fibrous tissue causes a narrowed orifice, the commonest cardiac lesion occurring in childbearing women. **M. valve** bicuspid valve between the left atrium and left ventricle of the heart. **M. valvotomy** cutting into and widening of the narrowed mitral valve, performed to relieve mitral stenosis.

mittelschmerz abdominal or pelvic pain occurring between menstrual periods, possibly related to ovulation.

mobile epidural low concentration of bupivacaine, sometimes with an opiate, administered into the epidural space by a patient-controlled epidural analgesic system (PCEAS) pump so that the mother can be mobile during labour; pain relief may not be as complete as with conventional epidural anaesthesia; normal labour observations should be continued and monitoring of the mother's respiratory rate undertaken.

mole dead and degenerate ovum.

molecule smallest particle of a substance having a varying number of atoms, e.g. water, H_2O, is a molecule consisting of two HYDROGEN atoms and one OXYGEN atom.

mongolian blue spot smooth, brown to grey-blue sacral naevus with excess melanocytes sometimes found at birth in babies of African and Asian parents and occasionally in those of Mediterranean origin; usually disappears during childhood.

mongolism *See* DOWN'S SYNDROME.

Monilia *See* CANDIDA ALBICANS, THRUSH.

moniliasis candidiasis.

Monitor adaptation of the USA Rush Medicus system of assessing quality of nursing care. It consists of 'checklists' for quality leading to a scoring system: the closer the score to 100%

the better the care being given. The master list has over 200 criteria, which are divided into four categories based on patient dependency levels.

monoamine amine with only one amino group. **M. oxidase inhibitors (MAOIs)** substances inhibiting the activity of monoamine oxidase, increasing catecholamine and serotonin levels in the brain; used as antidepressants and antihypertensives; not to be given concurrently with pethidine as they potentiate its action by about 10 times.

monoclonal derived from a single cell. **M. antibodies** are derived from a single clone of cells, all with identical molecules and reacting with the same antigenic site.

monosaccharide simplest form of sugar, e.g. dextrose, glucose.

monozygotic pertaining to or derived from a single zygote (fertilised ovum). **M. twins**, uniovular twins, developing from one ovum and one spermatozoon that divide; they are the same sex, with one placenta and one chorion but two amniotic sacs; developmental abnormalities are more common in monozygotic twins than DIZYGOTIC. *See also* MULTIPLE PREGNANCY.

mons veneris area covered with hair over the pubes in a woman.

Montgomery's glands or tubercles sebaceous glands around the nipple, which enlarge during pregnancy.

morbid diseased, relating to diseased parts.

morbidity relating to morbid.

moribund dying.

morning sickness *See* NAUSEA *and* VOMITING.

Moro reflex response of the newborn baby to any sudden movement or noise nearby, with quick extension of arms then bringing them together again; 'embrace' or 'startle' reflex. In sick and preterm babies the reflex may be absent.

Moulding

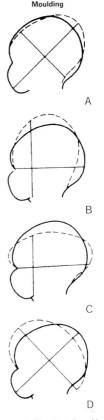

morphine sulphate principal alkaloid obtained from opium, used hypodermically as an analgesic for severe pain, e.g. placental abruption, only on medical orders; may cause respiratory depression.

mortality death. *M. rate* death rate of a given population, e.g. maternal, neonatal or infant mortality rates.

morula fertilised ovum about 4 days after fertilisation, resembling a small mulberry.

mosaicism person with several different types of cell within the body, e.g. in some types of DOWN'S SYNDROME not all cells have 47 chromosomes.

motor nerves nerves conveying impulses of motion from a nerve centre to a muscle.

mould fungus, e.g. *Penicillium*.

moulding process of overriding of the fetal cranial bones at the sutures and fontanelles during passage through the maternal pelvis; the head is squeezed, changing its shape and the length of various diameters. *Normal m.* in a vertex presentation the fetal head is well flexed; suboccipitobregmatic and biparietal diameters present and decrease as the bones overlap, and the mentovertical diameter lengthens. *Abnormal m.* excessive or extremely rapid alterations in the diameters due to abnormal position in a cephalic presentation may cause tearing of the falx cerebri and tentorium cerebelli, leading to intracranial haemorrhage and possible death. *See diagram.*

movements (fetal) *See* 'QUICKENING'.

moxibustion traditional Chinese medicine technique involving moxa sticks made from the herb mugwort, which act as a heat source when held over appropriate ACUPUNCTURE points; may turn breech presentations to cephalic.

mucoid resembling mucus.

mucopolysaccharidosis gargoylism; inborn error of metabolism in which

The unmoulded head is indicated by the heavy line **A,** moulding in the occipitoanterior position; **B,** moulding in the persistent occipitoposterior position; **C,** face moulding; **D,** brow moulding.

mucopolysaccharide builds up within the body; the child has distorted features with a large spleen, difficulty in joint movements and learning difficulties.

mucopurulent containing mucus and pus.

mucosa mucous membrane.

mucous pertaining to or secreting mucus. *M. membrane see* MEMBRANE.

mucoviscidosis *See* CYSTIC FIBROSIS.

mucus viscid secretion of mucous membranes.

müllerian ducts two embryonic ducts developing into the vagina, uterus and uterine tubes in the female, and becoming largely obliterated in the male; paramesonephric ducts.

multicultural society community or country in which a number of different cultural and/or ethnic groups reside together.

multidisciplinary involving two or more professional disciplines.

multifactorial 1. of, pertaining to, or arising through the action of many factors. 2. in genetics, arising as a result of the interaction of several genes.

multigravida pregnant woman who has previously had more than one pregnancy. *Grande m.* pregnant woman who has had four or more previous pregnancies. *See also* MULTIPARA. adj. *multigravid.*

multipara woman who has borne more than one VIABLE infant. adj. *multiparous.* pl. *multiparae.*

multiple of the median (MOM) measurement commonly used in biochemistry reports, 1 indicating the median or middle range of scores; considered to be more accurate than the mean as it is less likely to be skewed by extreme results; 0.5 indicates half the median and 2 indicates twice the median amount.

multiple pregnancy pregnancy with more than one fetus. Twins occur in approximately 1 in 80 pregnancies,

although increasingly successful assisted conception rates mean that this number is increasing; triplets occur in 1 in 80^2 pregnancies (i.e. 1 in 6400); quadruplet pregnancies occur in 1 in 80^3 pregnancies (i.e. 1 in 512 000). Early ultrasound diagnosis of amnionicity and chorionicity is important; monoamniotic (shared amniotic cavity) and monochorionic (common placenta with vascular connections) twins have a higher risk of morbidity and mortality, e.g. PRETERM LABOUR, PREGNANCY-INDUCED HYPERTENSION, GESTATIONAL DIABETES.

multivariate analysis analysis of data collected on several different variables but all having relevance to the study; data analysis indicates the effects of each of these variables and their interactions.

mumps communicable paramyxovirus disease that attacks one or both of the parotid glands and occasionally the submaxillary glands; immunisation in the first 2 years of life (with measles and rubella – MMR) is recommended.

Munro Kerr's manoeuvre *See* HEAD FITTING.

murmur auscultatory sound, particularly a periodic sound of short duration of cardiac or vascular origin, often associated with disease or abnormality.

muscle bundle of long, slender cells, or fibres, having the power to relax and contract, producing movement; uterine muscle, myometrium, is also capable of retraction, whereby the muscle fibres retain some of the shortening that occurs with contractions; this assists in the progressive passage of the fetus down the birth canal.

muscular dystrophy genetically determined, painless, degenerative myopathy resulting in gradual muscle weakening and eventual atrophy. *Duchenne m. d.* gradually-developing sex-linked recessive disease carried by women; sons have a 50% chance of inheriting the disease.

mutation change in form or other characteristic; in genetics, a change in a gene from parent to offspring.

myasthenia muscular debility or weakness. *M.gravis* autoimmune disease manifested by mild to life-threatening muscle weakness, fatigue and exhaustion, aggravated by activity and relieved by rest; characteristically affects ocular and other cranial muscles, tends to fluctuate in severity and responds to cholinergic drugs.

mycobacterium Gram-positive bacterium (*see* GRAM STAIN) distinguished by acid-fast staining, e.g. *Mycobacterium tuberculosis*.

myocardium middle, thickest layer of the heart wall, composed of cardiac muscle. adj. *myocardial*.

myoepithelial cells branched contractile epithelial cells surrounding each ALVEOLUS in the breast tissue. *See also* MILK FLOW MECHANISM, BREAST *and* LACTATION.

myoma benign tumour of muscle tissue.

myomectomy removal of a myoma, e.g. uterine fibroids.

myometrium uterine muscle.

myxoedema hypothyroidism; deficient thyroid hormone secretion from the thyroid gland, characterised by oedematous swelling of face, limbs and hands; dry rough skin; loss of hair; slow pulse; subnormal temperature; slowed metabolism; and mental dullness; treated with preparations of thyroid gland. Congenital hypothyroidism causes CRETINISM.

Naboth's (Nabothian) cysts (follicles) cyst-like formations resulting from occlusion of the lumina of glands in the cervical mucosa causing them to be distended with retained secretion.

Naegele's pelvis very rare asymmetrical pelvis due to congenital failure of one sacral ala to develop fully.

Naegele's rule rule for calculating the estimated date of labour: subtract 3 months from the first day of the last normal menstrual period and add 7 days.

naevus birthmark; circumscribed area of dilated superficial blood vessels.

naloxone (Narcan) antidote to narcotic drug, e.g. pethidine; 0.01 mg/kg of estimated body weight is administered to the baby if the APGAR SCORE is low and the mother had a narcotic drug in labour; the baby should be observed for respiratory difficulties for the first 24 hours.

nano- prefix indicating 'one-thousand-millionth', e.g. nanogram (ng), one-thousand-millionth of a gram.

napkin/nappy rash skin rash developing on the buttocks, commonly ammoniacal dermatitis, which produces erythema and vesicles; other causes are thrush, psoriasis and peri-anal erythema.

Narcan *See* NALOXONE.

narco- prefix denoting 'stupor'.

narcosis state of unconsciousness produced by a narcotic drug.

narcotic drug that produces narcosis, insensibility or stupor, obtainable only on prescription. Legally it refers to habit-forming drugs, e.g. morphine, heroin, pethidine. Misuse of Drugs Act 1971 prohibits sale or possession of narcotics other than for medical purposes.

nares nostrils. *Posterior n.* opening of the nares into the nasopharynx. sing. *naris.*

nasal pertaining to the nose.

nasogastric tube soft rubber or plastic tube inserted via the nostril into the stomach to enable instilling of liquid food or other substances, or for with-drawing gastric contents.

nasojejunal feeding method of feeding a baby on a ventilator or one receiving CONTINUOUS INFLATING PRESSURE (CIP) by mask or nasal tube, in which a silicone-coated catheter is passed via the nose to the jejunum; used to avoid aspiration dangers of nasogastric tube feeding.

nasopharynx part of the pharynx above the soft palate.

National Childbirth Trust (NCT) charitable organisation offering education for pregnancy, birth and parenthood, with over 300 UK branches and groups providing antenatal classes, breastfeeding counselling and post-natal support.

National Health Service (NHS) established in 1948 to provide free accessible health care to all in the UK.

National Institute for Clinical Excellence (NICE) special health authority responsible for assessing the clinical and cost-effectiveness of new and existing health technologies, and providing guidance to the NHS on their adoption.

National Screening Committee (NSC) government advisory body that assesses, implements and monitors UK screening programmes; specific sub-groups oversee antenatal, newborn and child health screening programmes. Decisions regarding risks, benefits and effectiveness of screening programmes are largely based on evidence from the Health Technology Assessment (HTA) programme.

National Service Frameworks (NSFs) templates or blueprints for care in major service areas, developed nationally by NICE; used locally by the NHS Executive and other health-care organisations to review and reshape local service provision.

natural childbirth, active birth approach to labour and delivery advocating avoidance of medical interference and technology and analgesia in labour, and encouraging both parents to participate in and share the experience of childbirth.

nausea sensation of sickness with inclination to vomit; common physiological disorder of pregnancy possibly associated with hormonal or metabolic changes, *Helicobacter pylori* infection, vestibular apparatus sensitivity or structural adaptations. *See also* VOMITING.

navel umbilicus.

Necator genus of HOOKWORM.

necro- prefix meaning 'dead'.

necrobiosis degeneration and death of tissue, as occurs with uterine fibroids in the second trimester; bed rest and analgesia are required.

necropsy post-mortem examination.

necrosis death of tissue.

necrotising enterocolitis inflammatory bowel disease associated with septicaemia in the newborn baby, especially those with a history of asphyxia, respiratory distress, hypoglycaemia, hypothermia or cardiovascular disease, thought to be due to bacteria proliferating in the bowel and penetrating the bowel wall at points where it has suffered ischaemic damage. Oedema, ulceration and haemorrhage of the bowel wall occur and may progress to perforation and

peritonitis; treated with parenteral nutrition, antibodies and, in cases of perforation, surgery.

negligence in law, the failure to do something that a reasonable person of ordinary prudence would do in a certain situation; may provide the basis for a lawsuit when there is a legal duty, as in midwifery, to provide reasonable care to clients, and when negligence results in damage to the client.

Neisseria gonorrhoeae micro-organism that causes GONORRHOEA; difficult to culture outside the human body.

nem unit of nutrition equivalent to the nutritive value of 1 g of breast milk.

neo- prefix meaning 'new'.

neomycin broad-spectrum antibiotic; used as an intestinal antiseptic.

neonatal pertaining to the first 4 weeks after birth. *N. mortality rate* number of deaths of infants up to 4 weeks old per 1000 live births in a year.

neonate newborn baby up to 4 weeks old.

neonatology branch of paediatric medicine dealing with disorders of the newborn baby.

neoplasm new growth, e.g. tumour.

nephrectomy excision of a kidney.

nephritis inflammation of the kidneys. *Acute n.* kidney lesion, often following streptococcal infection, e.g. scarlet fever or tonsillitis, characterised by lumbar pain, pyrexia and oedema. Renal function is impaired, the urine contains albumin, blood and renal tubule casts but little urea, while serum urea rises; some patients develop chronic nephritis. *Chronic n.* permanently impaired renal function with oedema, proteinuria, hypertension and raised blood urea. *N. in pregnancy* severe nephritis increases the risk of spontaneous abortion and PRE-ECLAMPSIA; women with chronic nephritis are often infertile or subfertile.

nephron the functioning unit of the kidney, consisting of glomerulus, Bowman's capsule and the tubule system; there are about one million nephrons in each kidney.

nephropathy any disease of the kidneys.

nephrosis any renal disease.

nephrotic syndrome kidney disease marked by degenerative lesions of the renal tubules; may follow acute nephritis; characterised by excessive accumulation of fluid resulting from loss of protein in the body and decreased serum albumin. Treatment is with diuretics, high protein diet and, possibly, steroids and immuno-suppressive drugs.

nerve bundle of fibres enclosed in a sheath called the epineurium, which transmits impulses between any part of the body and a nerve centre. *Motor (efferent) n.* conveys impulses causing movement from a nerve centre to a muscle. *N. fibre* prolongation of the nerve cell, which conveys the impulse to or from the part that it controls. *Sensory (afferent) n.* conveys sensations from sense organs to a nerve centre. *Vasomotor n.* either a dilator or constrictor of blood vessels.

nerve block local analgesic blocking impulses passing along nerves, e.g. EPIDURAL ANALGESIA.

nervous 1. pertaining to, or composed of, nerves. 2. unduly excitable. *N. breakdown* generic lay term for mental illness that interferes with a person's normal activities. *N. system* organ system that, with the endocrine system, correlates adjustments and reactions of an organism to internal and environmental conditions; the central nervous system is composed of the brain and spinal cord; and the peripheral nervous system is subdivided into the voluntary and autonomic systems.

neural tube defect structural anomaly of the brain or spinal cord causing anencephaly – absence of the cranium with exposure of brain tissue, incompatible with life – or spina bifida; spina bifida occulta, in which a defect of the posterior laminae and spinous processes of one or more vertebrae presents as a hairy patch or dimple on the midline of the baby's back, requires no treatment; if the defect allows herniation of the meninges (meningocele), corrective surgery is required; herniation of both meninges and spinal cord (meningomyelocele) is a serious condition that may be incompatible with life.

neuritis inflammation of a nerve.

neuroblast embryonic nerve cell.

neuroblastoma malignant tumour of immature nerve cells, most often occurring in children.

neurohormonal pertaining to nerves and hormones and their coordination. *N. reflex* physiology of LACTATION involves a process in which nerves and hormones work in harmony to control the 'LET DOWN' REFLEX.

neurological assessment of newborn performed shortly after birth with the baby awake and alert but not crying; assessed for neck retraction, limb posture, limb hyperextension or hyperflexion, jittery or abnormal involuntary movements, and high-pitched or weak cry, any of which may indicate a possible antenatally acquired or perinatal neurological disorder.

neuromuscular pertaining to nerves and muscles and their coordination. *N. harmony* relationship between upper and lower segments of the uterus in labour, i.e. efficient uterine action occurs when the upper uterine segment contracts and RETRACTS and the lower segment and cervix contracts and dilates.

neuron, neurone nerve cell; conducting cell of the nervous system, with a cell body, nucleus and surrounding cytoplasm, axon and dendrites. *N. thermal environment* environmental temperature in which energy losses and OXYGEN consumption required to maintain body temperature within normal limits will be minimal.

neurosis functional nervous system disturbance characterised by emotional instability but without any obvious structural change in the nerve substance.

neutral neither acid nor alkaline, e.g. hydrogen ion concentration (pH) of 7.

neutron neutral particle found with protons in the nucleus of an atom.

Neville Barnes forceps obstetric forceps for operative vaginal delivery with rarely used axis traction handle attachments to allow downward traction of a high head into the pelvis. *See* Appendix 3.

newborn blood-spot screening programme national programme to screen neonates for disorders benefiting from early diagnosis; a blood-spot sample is taken on about the sixth day of life and tested for a range of disorders including PHENYLKETONURIA, congenital HYPOTHYROIDISM, SICKLE CELL disease and CYSTIC FIBROSIS. Other tests may be added in the near future.

niacin water-soluble B complex vitamin found in liver, yeast, bran, peanuts, lean meats, fish and poultry; required for synthesis of some enzymes.

nicotine poisonous alkaloid in tobacco that can cause indigestion, appetite suppression, hypertension and vasoconstriction.

nidation embedding of the fertilised ovum in the endometrium of the uterus.

nipple small conical projection in the centre of the AREOLA of the breast that gives outlet to the milk from the breast; the tip contains 15–20 small openings of the lactiferous ducts. *Accessory n.* rudimentary nipple anywhere in a line from the breast to the groin. *Retracted n.* nipple drawn inwards; may be a sign of breast cancer.

nitrazepam hypnotic and sedative drug used to treat insomnia with early morning wakening.

nitrofurantoin antibacterial agent used to treat urinary tract infection; may cause neonatal haemolysis if given to the mother at term.

nitrogen element, symbol N; gas that forms nearly 80% by volume of atmospheric air; constituent of all protein foods and substances.

nitrous oxide (N_2O) 'laughing gas'; gas that is combined with oxygen (50% of each; Entonox) and used to relieve pain in labour without loss of consciousness; premixed in a single blue and white cylinder with a simple valve, tubing and face mask for self-administration by the mother and approved by the Nursing and Midwifery Council for use by midwives. Excreted via the lungs; may cause giggling, loss of control and nausea.

node small swelling, knot or protuberance of tissue, either normal or pathological. adj. *nodal*.

nodule small solid boss or node that can be detected by touch.

non-accidental injury (NAI) injury caused by a 'battered baby' including bone fractures, especially of the skull, intracranial haemorrhage, the giving of poisons and dangerous drugs, sexual abuse, starvation and any other physical assault; most commonly inflicted by the parents or other adult responsible for the child's care; careful investigation and handling is needed.

non-maleficence health-care concept of the legal duty to avoid harming the interests of others.

non-shivering thermogenesis neonatal use of brown adipose tissue, stored in the mediastinum, around the nape of the neck, between the scapulae and around the kidneys and suprarenal glands, to produce heat in times of cold stress.

non-specific urethritis (NSU) common sexually transmitted disease caused by various organisms, notably *Chlamydia trachomatis*.

noradrenaline (norepinephrine) catecholamine neurotransmitter of most sympathetic postganglionic neurons and certain tracts in the nervous system, released from the adrenal medulla in response to sympathetic stimulation, primarily hypotension, and producing vasoconstriction, an increase in heart rate and elevation of blood pressure.

norethisterone progesterone-only contraceptive pill, useful for mothers who are breastfeeding.

Noriday progesterone-only contraceptive pill suitable for use while breast-feeding.

Norinyl combined oestrogen and progesterone contraceptive pill.

normoblasts immature nucleated red blood cells normally remaining in the bone marrow until maturity, but released into the circulation in certain anaemias.

normotensive having a normal blood pressure.

notifiable applied to certain transmit-table diseases, including ophthalmia neonatorum, infective jaundice, lepto-spirosis, scarlet fever, whooping cough, measles, smallpox, diphtheria and tuberculosis, the occurrence of which must be statutorily notified by the doctor to the director of public health in the health authority; mid-wives suspecting any notifiable dis-ease must inform a doctor.

notification See INTENTION TO PRACTISE.

notification of birth See BIRTH, NOTIFI-CATION OF.

nucha nape of the neck.

nuchal pertaining to the back of the neck. *N.fold* fat pad at the back of the fetal neck, measured on ultrasound scan after 14 weeks' gestation and at the 18- to 20-week fetal anomaly scan. Measurements of ≥6 mm increase the chances of DOWN'S SYNDROME and may also be associated with other disorders, e.g. TURNER'S SYNDROME. *N. translucency (NT)* subdermal col-lection of lymphatic fluid at the back of the fetal neck, best visualised

between 11 and 14 weeks' gestation. Increased levels are associated with chromosomal abnormalities, structural abnormalities (e.g. cardiac), neuro-muscular problems and various syn-dromes. See PREGNANCY-ASSOCIATED PLASMA PROTEIN-A, COMBINED TEST *and* INTEGRATED TEST.

nuchal displacement complication of breech labour, when an arm is dis-placed behind the baby's neck.

nuclear family parents and their chil-dren living together in a household, without members of the extended family, such as grandparents, living with them or in the same locality.

nuclear magnetic resonance (NMR) phenomenon exhibited by atomic nuclei, which behave as if they are tiny bar magnets; when disturbed from equilibrium by a radiofrequency pulse their alignment changes but, at the ter-mination of the pulse, the nuclei return to their position of equilibrium. Signals elicited can be used for chemical analy-sis (NMR spectroscopy) or imaging (MAGNETIC RESONANCE IMAGING; MRI).

nucleic acids extremely complex, long-chain compounds of high molecular weight occurring naturally in cells of all living organisms, forming the genetic material of the cell and direct-ing the synthesis of protein within the cell. See DEOXYRIBONUCLEIC ACID (DNA) *and* RIBONUCLEIC ACID (RNA).

nucleus essential part of a cell con-taining the chromosomes, its division being vital for the formation of new cells. *Basal n.* group of nerve cells in the brain that, in severe jaundice in the newborn, may become stained with bilirubin, causing KERNICTERUS.

nullipara woman who has never given birth to a viable child, although she may have been pregnant previously but suffered miscarriage or termin-ation of pregnancy. adj. *nulliparous.*

nurse 1. professional qualified in nursing, meeting certain prescribed standards of education and clinical competence. 2. to provide services that are essential to or helpful in the promotion, maintenance or restoration of health and well-being. 3. to nourish at the breast. *Day nursery* nursery for children under school age of working mothers – especially those who are unsupported or sick – provided by the local authority social services department and by private or voluntary bodies registered and supervised by the local authority. *N. school* school for children between 2.5 and 5 years provided by the local education authority; there are limited places available so priority is given to children with special needs.

Nursing and Midwifery Council (NMC) organisation designated by statute to regulate the nursing, midwifery and health visiting professions in the UK in order to protect the public. Responsible for quality assurance of education programmes leading to registration and recordable qualifications; maintains registers of practitioners; and publishes professional conduct rules and other documents to guide professional practice.

nutrition process by which food is assimilated into the body for nourishment, particularly food that builds sound bodies and promotes health; good nutrition means a balanced diet containing adequate amounts of the essential nutritional elements, i.e. proteins, vitamins, minerals, fats and carbohydrates. Depending on need, the body can manufacture sugars from fats, and fats from sugars and proteins, but it cannot manufacture proteins from sugars and fats. *N. therapy* complementary therapy focusing on the quantity, quality, absorption, assimilation and utilisation of nutrients, the effects of deficiencies and the use of dietary changes and supplements to correct them.

nylon synthetic material of exceptional strength, used for sutures.

nystagmus involuntary, rapid, rhythmic movement – horizontal, vertical, rotatory or mixed – of the eyeball.

Nystan *See* NYSTATIN.

nystatin antibiotic used to treat superficial fungal infections, e.g. candidiasis, administered orally or as a vaginal pessary.

obesity excessive fat storage throughout the body; increase in weight beyond the norm in relation to gender, age, height and bone structure. May cause menstrual and fertility problems; pregnancy complications such as hypertension are more common.

oblique slanting. *See* PELVIS. *O. lie* abnormal lie in which the long axis of the fetus lies between the oblique diameters of the pelvis; may progress to shoulder presentation and obstructed labour with the risk of cord or arm prolapse, ruptured uterus, haemorrhage and fetal or even maternal death.

oblongata *See* MEDULLA OBLONGATA.

observational study epidemiological study of events without intervention of the investigator.

obstetric pertaining to obstetrics. *O. cholestasis* intrahepatic cholestasis of pregnancy; third-trimester condition characterised by pruritus, dark urine, anorexia, fat malabsorption and increased bile, probably caused by genetic oestrogen hypersensitivity, associated with high fetal morbidity and mortality, and maternal coagulopathies. Women complaining of severe itching, especially on the palms, should have liver function assessed; treatment involves administration of vitamin K to prevent coagulation defects, fetal monitoring and early delivery; antihistamines may be given to relieve itching. There is a 50% risk of recurrence in subsequent pregnancies. *O. conjugate* pelvic diameter from the sacral promontory to the upper inner border or the symphysis pubis, measuring approximately 11 cm; the first narrow strait through which the fetal head has to pass. *Emergency o. unit* emergency team from a consultant maternity unit comprising obstetrician, midwife, anaesthetist and/or paediatrician, who go by ambulance to emergencies in the home or in small maternity hospitals taking O-negative blood and emergency equipment for blood transfusion, operative delivery, manual removal of the placenta, anaesthesia (if required) and maternal and neonatal resuscitation. *O. history* detailed information about all previous pregnancies, including abortions, labours, puerperia and babies, recorded when a woman books with her midwife or doctor for a subsequent pregnancy. *O. pulsar* appliance used for transcutaneous electrical nerve stimulation (TENS). *O. shock* collapse associated with childbirth and caused by circulatory failure, occurring most commonly as a result of haemorrhage or trauma, e.g. acute uterine inversion, or septicaemia caused by Gram-negative organisms.

obstetrician doctor who specialises in the care of women with abnormal pregnancies, labours and puerperia. cf. MIDWIFE.

obstetrics branch of medicine dealing with pregnancy, labour and the puerperium.

obstipation intractable constipation.

obstructed labour situation in which there is no advance of the presenting part despite strong uterine contractions; most commonly occurs at the pelvic brim but may occur at the outlet, e.g. deep transverse arrest in an android pelvis; situation is avoidable with diligent midwifery care. When advanced the mother is distressed and anxious and has tachycardia, pyrexia, ketonuria and oliguria, vomiting and persistent abdominal pain; the uterus appears 'moulded' around the fetus; on palpation it is continuously hard, fetal parts cannot be felt and fetal heart sounds are absent; fetal death from anoxia occurs. BANDL'S RING can be seen as a ridge running obliquely around the abdomen marking the junction between the thickened upper segment and the dangerously thinned and overdistended lower uterine segment. On examination the vagina is hot and dry with oedematous vaginal walls, a high presenting part with excessive caput succedaneum and a thick 'curtain' of cervix hanging around and below it. A multipara is in imminent danger of death from uterine rupture and exhaustion; a primigravida may develop secondary uterine inertia. Medical aid should be summoned urgently; intramuscular pethidine is administered to relieve pain; intravenous fluids are commenced to combat shock and dehydration; and blood is taken for cross-matching. Caesarean section should be performed immediately whenever possible, whether the fetus is alive or dead; in isolated areas it may be necessary to undertake a fetal destructive operation as the only means of emptying the uterus and saving the mother's life, although this also carries the risk of rupturing the thinned overstretched lower uterine segment.

obturator anything that closes an opening. *O. foramen* opening in the anterolateral aspect of the innominate bone closed by fascia and muscle.

occipital relating to the occiput.

occipitoanterior when the occiput or back of the fetal head is directed to the front of the mother's pelvis.

occipitolateral, occipitotransverse the fetal occiput is to the side of the mother's pelvis as it enters the brim, either on the right or the left side; if the uterine contractions are efficient it will usually turn to an occipitoanterior position as it reaches the resistance of the pelvic floor.

occipitoposterior the fetal occiput is directed towards the right or left sacroiliac joint of the mother's pelvis, the commonest of all mechanical difficulties in labour; caused by an abnormal maternal pelvic shape, e.g. android or anthropoid; the fetal attitude is often a military (erect) one or deflexed; occurs in about 10% of all pregnancies. On examination the abdomen appears flattened below the umbilicus and a high deflexed fetal head is palpated with limbs felt over a large area on both sides of the midline; fetal heart sounds are heard in the middle and over the flank. Vaginal examination reveals a high head with the bregma lying anteriorly or centrally. In many cases the fetal head will flex as it meets the pelvic floor, so that it makes a long rotation to an occipitoanterior position with delivery following normally. Risks include prolonged labour, difficult delivery, cord prolapse, infection, fetal hypoxia and intracranial haemorrhage from the upwards moulding of the fetal skull. In the second stage, DEEP TRANSVERSE ARREST may occur, requiring Kielland's forceps delivery, or the head is born FACE-TO-PUBES.

occiput back of the head, extending from the lambdoidal suture to the nape of the neck.

occlusive cap rubber contraceptive cap to cover the cervix and mechanically obstruct the entrance of spermatozoa, used with spermicidal gel or cream to increase effectiveness.

occult obscure or hidden from view. *O. blood test* microscopic or chemical examination of faeces, urine, gastric juice, etc. to determine the presence of blood not otherwise detectable.

ocular pertaining to the eye.

odds of being affected given a positive result (OAPR) term to describe the chances of a positive screening test result being correct, i.e. proportion of people with a positive screening result who have the condition; a positive predictive value.

oedema excess fluid, either due to excess formation or failure of absorption, often first recognised by excess weight gain (occult oedema), then by pitting on pressure. Approximately 50% of pregnant women develop mild physiological ankle oedema towards term, which is normal unless accompanied by other signs and symptoms, e.g. hypertension. In the puerperium ankle oedema often worsens temporarily, as the kidneys are unable to cope immediately with excretion of the excess fluid resulting from the autolytic process of INVOLUTION. Pathological oedema occurs with chronic renal disease, PRE-ECLAMPSIA, ECLAMPSIA, severe heart disease, severe anaemia and malnutrition. *Pitting o.* severe oedema in which pressure leaves a persistent depression in the tissues.

oesophageal pertaining to the oesophagus. *O. atresia* absence of the oesophageal opening; often suspected by the presence of maternal POLYHYDRAMNIOS because the fetus is unable to swallow saliva; in the neonate saliva comes out of the mouth continuously as clear mucus; a stiff tube should be passed immediately after birth via the mouth to ensure patency of the oesophagus; often accompanied by TRACHEO-OESOPHAGEAL FISTULA.

oesophagus canal extending from the pharynx to the stomach, about 22.5 cm (9 in) long in the adult.

oestradiol (also estradiol) ovarian hormone; the most potent naturally occurring OESTROGEN in humans.

oestriol (also estriol) ovarian hormone; a relatively weak human oestrogen.

oestrogen (also estrogen) hormone with OESTROGENIC activity, including oestradiol, oestriol and oestrone, produced by the ovary, adrenal gland, testis and fetoplacental unit; responsible for development of female secondary sexual characteristics and act on the female genitalia during the menstrual cycle to produce an environment suitable for fertilisation, implantation and nutrition of the early embryo. During pregnancy oestrogens stimulate growth of the uterus and duct system of the breasts. Oestrogens also influence water and electrolyte retention, for the suppression of ovulation and inhibition of lactation in pregnancy.

Oesophageal atresia with tracheo-oesophageal fistula

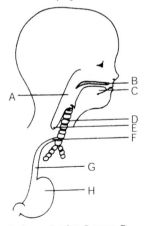

A, pharynx; **B,** palate; **C,** tongue; **D,** trachea; **E,** oesophageal atresia; **F,** tracheo-oesophageal fistula; **G,** distal oesophagus; **H,** stomach.

oestrogenic (also estrogenic) hormonal effects producing secondary sexual characteristics in a female at puberty, and menstrual and pregnancy changes, particularly development of uterine muscle and breast ducts.

oestrone (also estrone) OESTROGEN isolated from urine in pregnancy and from the human placenta; also prepared synthetically.

olfaction sense of smell.

oligaemia deficiency in volume of the blood.

oligohydramnios reduced amount of amniotic fluid, associated with fetal malformations, e.g. renal agenesis, limb deformities and intrauterine growth retardation of the fetus.

oligomenorrhoea scanty menstruation.

oligospermia deficiency of spermatozoa in the semen.

oliguria diminished secretion of urine, possibly associated with impaired renal function following severe abruptio placentae, postpartum haemorrhage, pre-eclampsia or eclampsia.

ombudsman person appointed to receive and investigate complaints about unfair administration and failures in the health services; the person appointed as ombudsman or Health Service Commissioner does not pass judgement on clinical matters.

omentum fold of peritoneum extending from the stomach to adjacent abdominal organs.

omnivorous eating both plant and animal foods.

Omnopon *See* PAPAVERETUM.

omphalocele umbilical hernia.

omphalus umbilicus.

onco- word element meaning 'tumour', 'swelling', 'mass'.

oncology study of tumours.

onych(o)- word element meaning 'the nails'.

onychia inflammation of the nail bed.

ooblast primitive cell from which an ovum ultimately develops.

oocyte immature ovum.

oophor(o)- word element meaning 'ovary'.

oophorectomy removal of an ovary.

oophoritis inflammation of an ovary.

oophorosalpingectomy surgical removal of an ovary and its associated fallopian tube.

operant conditioning form of behaviour therapy in which a reward is given when the subject performs the action required of them, serving to encourage repetition of the action.

operative delivery instrumental delivery; forceps delivery of the baby, ventouse or vacuum extraction, or Caesarean section.

operculum plug of mucus filling the cervical canal during pregnancy; shed at the beginning of labour. *See* 'SHOW'.

ophthalmia neonatorum any purulent discharge from the eyes of an infant within 21 days of birth; most commonly caused by CHLAMYDIA TRACHOMATIS but also by GONOCOCCI (leading to blindness), *Escherichia coli* or staphylococci. NOTIFIABLE to the Director of Public Health.

ophthalmic pertaining to the eye.

ophthalmoscope instrument for inspecting the interior of the eye.

opiate class of powerful analgesic and narcotic drugs that produce drug tolerance and dependence, including naturally occurring opiates derived from the opium poppy, e.g. opium, morphine, codeine; semi-synthetic opiates, e.g. heroin; synthetic opiates, e.g. methadone, pethidine, phenazocine; and narcotic antagonists, which when used in conjunction with an opiate block its effects but when used alone have opiate-like properties. Naloxone is an important exception being an opiate antagonist but having no narcotic properties.

opium substance derived from poppy juice used to relieve pain. *Alkaloids of o.* morphine and codeine. *Tincture of o.* laudanum.

opportunistic micro-organism not normally causing disease but capable of so doing under certain circumstances; disease or infection caused by such an organism.

opsonin substance that coats bacteria making them more easily phagocytosed, e.g. antibody.

optic pertaining to vision.

oral pertaining to the mouth. *O. contraceptive pill* combined oral contraceptive pill containing both oestrogen and synthetic progesterone and with a low failure rate of 0.1–1 per hundred women years (HWY), i.e. the number who would become pregnant if 100 women used the method for 1 year; progestogen-only pill, often prescribed for breastfeeding women, women over 35 years and in other cases when the combined pill is contraindicated, having a failure rate of 0.3–5 per HWY.

orbit bony cavity containing the eyeball.

orbital ridge bony rim of the orbit.

orchi(d)(o)- word element meaning 'testis'.

orchidopexy operation to release an undescended testis and place it in the scrotum.

orchitis inflammation of a testis.

organ part of the body with a particular function.

organic pertaining to the structure of an organ.

organism individual animal or plant.

organogenesis origin or development of organs.

orgasm apex and culmination of sexual excitement.

orifice any opening in the body, e.g. mouth, vagina.

oropharynx part of the pharynx between the soft palate and upper edge of the epiglottis.

-orrhaphy suffix meaning 'repair' or 'suturing', e.g. perineorrhaphy.

orthostatic standing erect. *O. albuminuria* albuminuria occurring when the individual is upright but not after rest in bed.

Ortolani's test method of diagnosing CONGENITAL DISLOCATION OF THE HIP; a 'click' or popping sensation is felt on reversing the movements of abduction and rotation of the hip while the baby is lying with knees flexed.

os 1. bone. *O. calcis* heel bone or calcaneum. *O. innominatum* nameless bone; the right and left innominate bones articulate with the sacrum to form the pelvic girdle. 2. mouth or opening. *External o.* opening of the cervix into the vagina. *Internal o.* junction of the cervical canal with the cavity of the uterus. *O. uteri* opening of the uterus into the vagina, which dilates progressively as labour advances.

Osiander's sign pulsation of the uterine arteries through the lateral fornices, which can be felt on examination *per vaginam* in early pregnancy; may assist in the diagnosis of pregnancy.

osmolality concentration of a solution in terms of osmoles of solutes per kilogram of solvent. *Serum o.* measure of the number of dissolved particles per unit of water in serum, used to assess status of hydration. *Urine o.* measure of the number of dissolved particles per unit of water in the urine.

osmosis passage of a solvent through a semipermeable membrane into a more concentrated solution; clinically important in maintaining adequate body fluids and for proper balance between volumes of extracellular and intracellular fluids.

osmotic pressure power of a fluid, dependent on its molecular content, to draw another fluid towards it.

ossification formation and hardening of bone. *O. centres* seen on radiography at the distal end of the fetal femoral epiphysis between 35 and 40 weeks' gestation and the proximal tibial epiphysis at 37–42 weeks; may help to determine fetal maturity.

See also ULTRASOUND. *Centres of o.* on the fetal head include the frontal bosses, occipital protuberance and parietal eminences.

osteoblasts cells that mature and form bone.

osteogenesis formation of bone. *O. imperfecta* inherited dominant condition of extreme fragility of the bones, in which spontaneous fractures are liable to occur.

osteomalacia adult rickets, characterised by painful softening of bones, caused by severe vitamin D deficiency.

osteomyelitis localised or generalised bone inflammation caused by pyogenic infection; may cause bone destruction, stiffening of joints if the infection spreads, and shortening of limbs if it occurs in children.

osteopathy statutorily regulated profession supplementary to medicine in which manipulation of the musculoskeletal system is used to restore structural and functional balance within the body; may be effective in treating disorders of pregnancy, e.g. backache and carpal tunnel syndrome, assisting the mother in labour and for postnatal problems. *See also* CRANIOSACRAL THERAPY.

otitis inflammation of the ear. *O. externa* inflammation of the external ear. *O. media* infection of the middle ear, occasionally occurring in newborn babies. *O. interna* labyrinthitis.

otoacoustic emissions (OAE) test one of two tests within the Newborn Hearing Screening Programme, based on the fact that a healthy cochlea produces a faint echo when stimulated with sound. Failure to detect the cochleic echo when an earpiece is inserted in the baby's ear and a clicking sound is played requires the baby to undergo further testing. The test is difficult to interpret if the baby is unsettled or there is fluid in the ear from the birth.

-otomy suffix meaning 'cutting into', e.g. hysterotomy, incision into the pregnant uterus.

ounce (oz) measure of weight. *Fluid o.* unit of liquid measure of the apothecaries' system, being 8 fluid drams or 29.57 mL.

outlet means or route of exit. *Pelvic o.* inferior opening of the pelvis bounded by the ischial spines, lower border of the symphysis pubis and sacrococcygeal joint.

output yield or total production. *Cardiac o.* effective volume of blood expelled by either ventricle of the heart per unit of time (usually volume per minute), equal to the stroke output multiplied by the number of beats per time unit used in the computation. *Fluid o.* amount of urine passed, usually compared with oral fluid intake.

outreach clinic clinic, e.g. antenatal clinic, situated some distance from the main maternity department, perhaps in a smaller hospital, general practitioner's surgery or public building such as a village hall, enabling women to access consultant care without having to make a long or inconvenient journey to hospital.

ova plural of ovum.

ovarian pertaining to an ovary. *O. cyst* tumour of the ovary containing fluid. *O. pregnancy* fertilised ovum that develops in the ovary. *O. vein syndrome* obstruction of a ureter, most commonly the right, due to compression by an enlarged or varicosed ovarian vein; typically the vein becomes enlarged during pregnancy, symptoms being those of obstruction or infection of the upper urinary tract.

ovariotomy incision of an ovary.

ovaries two glandular organs in the cavity of the female pelvis, attached to the posterior fold of the broad ligament near the fimbriated end of the fallopian tube; produce ova and oestrogens and progesterone, which cause various changes in the body at the time of puberty and in pregnancy.

oviduct passage through which ova leave the maternal body or pass to an organ communicating with the exterior of the body.

oviferous producing ova.

ovulation release of an ovum from the ovary by rupture of a graafian follicle, normally occurring about every 28 days and alternating between the two ovaries; occasionally ovulation produces two or more ova, which, if fertilised, may result in multiple births.

ovum egg; reproductive cell of the female. pl. *ova*.

oxidase enzymes that catalyse the reduction of molecular oxygen independently of hydrogen peroxide.

oxidation process of combining with oxygen.

oxprenolol beta-blocking drug used to treat angina, hypertension and cardiac arrhythmias.

oxygen element, symbol O; colourless, odourless gas, essential to life. Constitutes 21% of the atmosphere; obtained from the air and drawn into the lungs by the process of respiration. For therapeutic purposes it is stored in black and white cylinders. Lack of oxygen (hypoxia) causes CYANOSIS and ANOXIA leading to neonatal death; oxygen is administered during resuscitation via an endotracheal tube. Careful monitoring of oxygen concentration is necessary in newborn preterm babies to ensure that they receive sufficient oxygen to prevent brain damage but not so much as to cause retinopathy of prematurity leading to blindness.

oxyhaemoglobin haemoglobin combined with molecular oxygen, the form in which oxygen is transported in the blood.

oxytetracycline broad-spectrum antibiotic of the tetracycline group.

oxytocic any drug that stimulates contractions of the uterus, used for induction or acceleration of labour.

oxytocin hormone secreted by the posterior pituitary gland causing stimulation, i.e. contraction, of the uterine myometrium and, during breastfeeding, expulsion of milk from the alveoli into the lactiferous ducts. Synthetic oxytocin (Syntocinon) may be administered intravenously to induce or accelerate labour, or intramuscularly or intravenously to contract uterine muscle after delivery of the placenta and control haemorrhage. Synthetic oxytocin is combined with ergometrine to produce Syntometrine.

pack large swab or tampon used to control bleeding in a wound or abdominal contents during surgery.

packed cells fresh blood for transfusion from which some of the plasma has been removed to facilitate cell haemolysis; given when it is necessary to replace blood cells without overloading the circulation with fluid.

packed cell volume (PCV) percentage of blood cells to PLASMA; normal PCV is about 45%.

paediatrician doctor specialising in the study of infant and child health and disease.

paediatrics branch of medicine dealing with the care of babies and children.

paedophilia abnormal fondness for children; sexual activity of adults with children. adj. *paedophiliac*.

pain suffering and distress, resulting from stimulation of free nerve endings in small myelinated or unmyelinated nerve fibres in the superficial skin layers and some deeper tissues, which transmit impulses along sensory nerve fibres to the spinal cord and then along the sensory pathways to the thalamus, the main sensory relay station of the brain. Conscious perception of pain probably occurs in the thalamus and lower centres; interpretation of pain intensity occurs in the cerebral cortex. *Labour p.* increasingly frequent and intense intermittent lower abdominal pain caused by contractions of the upper uterine segment dilating the cervix and expelling the fetus through the birth canal; sacral back pain originates in the cervix and, if severe, may indicate poor cervical dilatation and prolonged labour. *See also* GATE CONTROL THEORY OF PAIN.

palate roof of mouth. *Hard p.* bony palate at the front. *Soft p.* muscular area behind the hard palate *See also* CLEFT PALATE.

palliative agent that relieves but does not cure disease.

pallor pale skin, may be mottled; in the newborn, a sign of poor peripheral perfusion; associated with low circulating blood volume or circulatory adaptation and compensation for hypoxaemia; also occurs in anaemia.

palpation physical examination by touch; using light finger pressure on the skin surface to determine the condition of the parts beneath the surface, thereby aiding diagnosis. *See* ABDOMINAL EXAMINATION *and* VAGINAL EXAMINATION.

palpitation abnormally rapid beating of the heart of which the person is conscious.

palsy paralysis. *Bell's p.* facial paralysis due to a lesion of the facial nerve, resulting in characteristic facial distortion. *Cerebral p.* persistent qualitative motor disorder appearing before the age of 3. *Erb's p.* limp inwardly-rotated arm with half-closed hand turned outwards; caused by damage to the upper roots of the brachial plexus. *Klumpke's p.* paralysis of the hand and wrist drop caused by damage to the eighth cervical and first thoracic nerve roots.

Panadol *See* PARACETAMOL.

pancreas racemose gland about 15 cm (6 in) long, located behind the stomach with its head in the curve of the duodenum and its tail in contact with the spleen; secretes INSULIN from the islets of Langerhans and digestive juice, which enters the duodenum through the pancreatic duct and the common bile duct.

pancreatic duct main excretory duct of the pancreas, uniting with the common bile duct before entering the duodenum at the major duodenal papilla.

pancuronium neuromuscular blocking agent used to relax muscle during surgery, or during mechanical intermittent positive pressure ventilation, when it prevents pneumothorax in babies actively expiring against ventilator inflation.

pandemic epidemic spreading over a wide area.

panhysterectomy total hysterectomy, i.e. removal of the body and cervix of the uterus.

Papanicolaou test (smear) simple test used to detect uterine and cervical cancer. A wooden spatula (Ayre's spatula) is passed through the cervix and rotated 360° near the internal os to scrape off surface cells; these cells are transferred on to a glass slide and examined microscopically.

papaveretum (Omnopon) analgesic drug; a mixture of opium alkaloids.

papilla small nipple-like eminence. pl. *papillae.*

papilloma benign tumour derived from epithelium. *P. virus* sexually transmitted infection causing anogenital warts (condylomata acuminata), associated with increased incidence of cervical carcinoma. *Laryngeal p.* rare neonatal condition caused by infection acquired during vaginal delivery.

papule small solid raised elevation of the skin.

papyraceous like parchment. *Fetus p.* very rare abnormality of multiple pregnancy in which one fetus dies very early in pregnancy and becomes flattened; usually delivered with the placenta.

para woman who has produced one or more VIABLE offspring, i.e. all babies delivered over 24 weeks' gestation including stillbirths. Number of viable offspring are designated by numbers: *para 0* NULLIPARA, woman who has not delivered a viable baby; *para 1* PRIMIPARA, woman who has delivered one viable baby; *para 2* or more, MULTIPARA woman who has delivered two or more viable babies. Miscarriages and terminations are not counted but usually identified by adding +1 after the number designating viable deliveries, e.g. para 3^{+1}. adj. *parous.*

para- prefix meaning 'near', e.g. parametrium, connective tissue near the uterus.

paracentesis puncture of a cavity wall to draw off fluid. *P. uteri* amniocentesis; puncture of the abdominal and uterine walls to draw off amniotic fluid in pregnancy. *See* POLYHYDRAMNIOS.

paracervical block infiltration of the LEE–FRANKENHAUSER PLEXUS with local anaesthetic through the lateral fornices to relieve cervical dilatation pain in labour, effective for up to 3 hours. Inadvertent injection into the uterine artery, which is in close proximity to the plexus, may cause fetal bradycardia and intrauterine fetal death.

paracetamol oral analgesic and antipyretic drug used instead of aspirin to relieve moderate pain and reduce pyrexia; acute paracetamol overdosage can cause severe, potentially fatal, hepatic necrosis.

paraesthesia disorder of sensation, e.g. a feeling as of 'pins and needles'; may occur with CARPAL TUNNEL SYNDROME and is occasionally felt in the feet following epidural analgesia. pl. *paraesthesiae.*

paraldehyde powerful, fast-acting, relatively safe hypnotic, sedative and anticonvulsant drug with a strong, unpleasant smell.

paralysis palsy; failure of nerve function, especially of a motor nerve, leading to impairment of voluntary or involuntary muscles supplied by the affected nerve. *Facial p. see* BIRTH INJURY. *Infantile p.* POLIOMYELITIS.

See also ERB'S PARALYSIS *and* KLUMPKE'S PARALYSIS.

paralytic pertaining to or affected by paralysis.

paramedical, paramedic related to the science or practice of medicine; adjunctive to medical practice. Paramedical services include physiotherapy, occupational and speech therapy, and those of social workers and ambulance service personnel with specialist training to perform in emergency settings certain procedures normally undertaken by doctors.

parametric 1. near the uterus; parametrial. 2. pertaining to or defined in terms of a parameter.

parametritis inflammation of the PARAMETRIUM; pelvic cellulitis.

parametrium pelvic connective tissue surrounding the lower part of the uterus, filling the spaces between the uterus and related organs.

paranoia chronic uncurable mental disorder developing over months or years, characterised by well-systematised delusions of persecution, illusions of grandeur, or a combination of both. adj. *paranoiac*.

paranoid 1. resembling paranoia. 2. person suffering paranoia.

paraplegia central nervous system paralysis of the legs and, occasionally, the lower body, affecting all muscles within the local area. adj. *paraplegic*.

parasite plant or animal living in or on another living organism (host), from which it satisfies all its needs.

parasympathetic nervous system part of the autonomic NERVOUS SYSTEM; post-ganglionic nerve fibres with almost 75% being in the VAGUS nerves, which serve the thoracic and abdominal regions; the remainder are distributed to the heart, smooth muscles, head and neck glands and pelvic viscera; acetylcholine is screted from the nerve endings, acting either to excite or inhibit certain activities.

parathyroid glands four small endocrine (hormonal) glands associated with the thyroid gland; help to maintain plasma calcium levels.

paratyphoid notifiable infection caused by *Salmonella*.

parent–infant relationship 'bonding'; relationship that develops between parents and their baby.

parenteral outside the alimentary tract. *P. feeding* introduction of nutritional substances by any route other than the alimentary tract.

parenthood education health education to help parents prepare for labour and parenthood and provide a social environment for couples approaching parenthood, usually offered as a series of classes.

paresis partial paralysis affecting muscular action but not sensation.

parietal related to or attached to the wall of a cavity. *P. bone* one of two thin flat bones forming the major part of the vault of the skull. *See also* FETAL SKULL.

parity 1. para; condition of a woman with respect to her having borne viable babies. 2. equality; close correspondence or similarity.

Parlodel bromocriptine mesylate, a dopamine receptor agonist.

paronychia commmon neonatal inflammation of the folds of skin surrounding the fingernail, almost always staphylococcal in origin.

parotid near the ear. *P. glands* largest of the three main pairs of salivary glands, located on either side of the face, just below and in front of the ears.

parous having borne one or more viable offspring. *See also* NULLIPARA *and* PRIMIPAROUS.

paroxysm 1. sudden recurrence or intensification of symptoms. 2. spasm or seizure. adj. *paroxysmal*.

partial pressure *See* PO₂.

partogram graphical record of labour progress obtained by performing

CARDIOTOCOGRAPHY, enabling assessment of visual patterns of cervical dilatation and descent of the presenting part in conjunction with records of maternal and fetal well-being. *See* Appendix 5.

parturient being in labour; relating to childbirth.

parturition giving birth to a child.

parvovirus B19 (human parvovirus B19) causes fifth disease, also called slapped cheek or erythema infectosum; droplet-spread viral infection attacking mainly schoolchildren in 3-yearly outbreak cycles, characterised by facial rash, giving rise to the appearance of 'slapped cheeks', general malaise and fever. Approximately 50% of adults show evidence of previous infection. Maternal antenatal infection can cause miscarriage and fetal death as a result of the virus attacking erythroid progenitor cells, which causes fetal anaemia. HYDROPS FETALIS may also occur, detectable on ultrasound scan. Diagnosis is confirmed from maternal serum; INTRAUTERINE TRANSFUSION may be necessary to correct the fetal anaemia, leading to recovery in 85% of cases.

pascal (Pa) international (SI) unit of pressure, corresponding to a force of 1 newton per square metre.

passive not active. *P. immunity see* IMMUNITY. *P. movements* manipulation by a physiotherapist without active movement by the patient.

pasteurisation heating of milk or other liquids to 60°C for 30 minutes, which kills pathogenic bacteria and delays other bacterial development.

Patau's syndrome (trisomy 13) congenital disorder due to an additional chromosome 13, occurring in approximately 1 in 10 000 live births, with the risk increasing with advancing maternal age. Affected babies may have weak muscle tone, CLEFT LIP/PALATE, heart defects and skeletal abnormalities, and rarely survive

infancy. Mosaic Patau's syndrome, in which only some cells have the additional chromosome, is usually less severe.

patella small, circular, sesamoid bone forming the kneecap.

patent open. *P. ductus arteriosus* abnormal persistence after birth of an open lumen in the ductus arteriosus between the aorta and pulmonary artery, which burdens the left ventricle of the heart and causes diminished blood flow in the aorta. In preterm infants administration of a prostaglandin inhibitor, indomethacin, may help to close the ductus; however, in those with severe congenital heart defects in which an open ductus arteriosus could be beneficial, prostaglandins are given to keep the channel open.

paternity biological fatherhood; analysis of DNA in blood will confirm paternity in cases in which an unsupported mother applies for maintenance payments from the baby's biological father.

patho- prefix denoting 'disease'.

pathogen micro-organism or material that causes disease.

pathogenic causing disease.

pathological pertaining to the study of disease.

pathology branch of medicine diagnosing and treating the essential nature of disease, especially the structural and functional changes in tissues and organs in the body.

Patients' Charter charter detailing standards of care that health-care consumers can expect and have a right to receive; an attempt to improve service quality, e.g. hospital waiting times, hospital environment, ambulance, dental, optical and pharmaceutical services. There is a special charter for maternity services.

patulous distended, open, as in the external os of a multiparous woman or cervical incompetence.

Paul–Bunnell test   test for presence of serum heterophil antibodies, used to diagnose infectious mononucleosis.

Pawlik's grip   use of one hand to palpate the lower pole of the uterus during abdominal examination to estimate mobility and engagement/non-engagement of the fetal presenting part, especially in obese women; uncomfortable if not performed gently and slowly.

Pawlick's grip

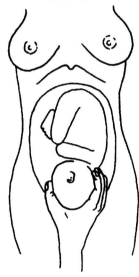

pectineal   pertaining to the os pubis.

pectoral   1. of, or pertaining to, the chest or breast. 2. relieving disorders of the respiratory tract, as an expectorant.

pedicle   stem of a tumour.

pediculosis   lice infestation of the skin or hair.

pediculus   louse.

pedigree   chart or diagram of an individual's ancestors, used in genetics to analyse mendelian inheritance.

peduncle   large stalk or pedicle.

peer review   system of ensuring quality, in which midwifery care or professional publications, for example, are evaluated according to defined criteria established by professional peers.

pellagra   syndrome caused by niacin deficiency usually resulting from inadequate vitamin B intake or the inability of the body to convert tryptophan to niacin, as in alcohol and drug abuse; other vitamin deficiencies often co-exist, e.g. vitamin B2 (riboflavin).

pelvic   pertaining to the pelvis. *P. bone* hip bone, comprising the ilium, ischium and pubis. *P. cellulitis see* PARAMETRITIS. *P. diameter* any diameter of the bony pelvis. *P. floor* or *diaphragm* strong sheets of muscle fibres, principally the LEVATOR ANI muscles, forming support for the pelvic organs. *See also* PERINEUM. *P.girdle* innominate bone and sacrum. *P. inflammatory disease* (**PID**) infection involving the uterine tubes, ovaries, parametrium and, occasionally, the gut.

pelvimeter   calipers for measuring the diameters of the pelvis, rarely used now.

pelvimetry   internal and/or external measurement of the pelvic capacity and diameters, manually or by radiography.

pelvis   bony girdle formed anteriorly and laterally by the innominate bones, and posteriorly by the sacrum and coccyx, with a muscular floor and containing the uterus, fallopian tubes, ovaries, urinary bladder and rectum. *False p.* part lying above the brim bounded by the iliac fossae laterally,

Caldwell and moloy's classification of the brim of the pelvis

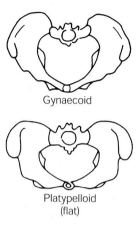

Gynaecoid

Anthropoid

Platypelloid
(flat)

Android

lumbar spine posteriorly and abdominal wall anteriorly, of little importance in obstetrics. *True p.* bony pelvis from the level of the brim and below, forming the bony canal through which the fetus must pass to be born normally. Consists of the *brim* or *inlet*, bounded by the sacral promontory and alae, upper sacroiliac joints, iliopectineal lines, upper inner borders of the upper pelvic rami and symphysis pubis; *cavity*, bounded by the sacral hollow, sacrospinous ligaments, ischial and pubic bones and symphysis pubis; and anatomical *outlet*, bounded by the coccyx, sacrotuberous ligaments, ischial tuberosities and pubic arch. The *obstetrical outlet* is bounded posteriorly by the lower aspect of the sacrum and laterally by the ischial spines and is the lowest level of bone surrounding the fetus in the birth canal. *Inclination of p.* the brim slopes at approximately

Pelvic brim

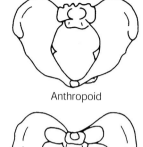

A–A, anteroposterior diameter;
B–B, oblique diameters; **C–C,** transverse diameter.

55° to the horizontal, and the bony outlet slopes at about 15°. *See also* CURVE OF CARUS. Normal pelvic shapes include the *android p.* pelvis with masculine characteristics, including a roughly triangular or heart-shaped brim and a narrow funnel shape, with

an outlet that is narrower than in the gynaecoid pelvis; *anthropoid p.* pelvis with a brim that is long anteroposteriorly and narrow transversely; *gynaecoid p.* normal female pelvis, almost round at the brim, cavity and outlet, roomy, shallow and ideally shaped for childbearing; *platypelloid* or *flat p.* pelvis with an oval brim, small anteroposteriorly and wide transversely. Pelvic deformities resulting from disease, accident or rare inherited characteristics include the asymmetrical *Naegele p.*, in which one sacral alae has failed to develop; the extremely rare *Robert p.*, in which both sacral alae are undeveloped and the symphysis pubis is sometimes split; the *spondylolisthetic p.*, in which the fifth lumbar vertebra has slipped forwards on the sacrum, creating a false promontory; and the *rachitic p.*, the brim of which is markedly flattened and kidney-shaped. *Assessment of p.* undertaken through observation of the mother's gait, by consideration of previous obstetric history, measurement of the pelvic capacity manually or by ultrasound scan or, most accurately, by VAGINAL EXAMINATION.

Pelvic outlet

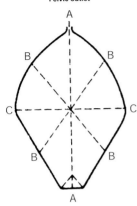

A–A, anteposterior diameter;
B–B, oblique diameters; **C–C,** transverse diameter.

Table of average measurements of pelvis: internal measurements

	ANTEROPOSTERIOR (cm)	RIGHT AND LEFT OBLIQUE DIAMETERS (cm)	TRANSVERSE (cm)
Brim	11	12	13
Cavity	12	12	12
Outlet	13	12	10–11

Diagonal conjugate: 12–12.5 cm measured from the apex of the pubic arch to the sacral promontory; 11 cm.
Obstetric conjugate: extends from the inner upper border of the symphysis pubis; 11 cm.
True or anatomical conjugate: measures slightly more than the obstetric conjugate as it extends from the sacral promontory to the centre of the upper surface of the symphysis pubis, but the extra space is not available for the passage of the fetus.

pemphigus acute or chronic skin disease characterised by watery blisters. *P. neonatorum* bullous impetigo; extremely infectious, usually caused by infection with *Staphylococcus aureus*; requires immediate medical attention and isolation of the baby. *Syphilitic p.* may, rarely, occur in the neonate.

pendulous hanging down. *P. abdomen* condition of multigravid women with extremely lax abdominal muscles in which the uterus falls forwards and the abdomen hangs below the symphysis pubis, causing discomfort and, often, fetal malpresentation.

penicillin antibiotic substance obtained from cultures of the mould *Penicillium*.

penicillinase enzyme that inactivates penicillin, produced by many bacteria, particularly staphylococci.

penis male organ of copulation.

pentazocine hydrochloride (Fortral) synthetic narcotic analgesic taken orally and intravenously for moderate to severe pain, although relief is variable.

pepsin proteolytic enzyme, the principal digestive component of gastric juice; acts as a catalyst in the chemical breakdown of protein to form polypeptides; has a milk-clotting action similar to that of RENNIN and thus facilitates the digestion of milk protein.

peptides constituent parts of proteins: di-, tri-, tetrapeptides, etc., according to the number of amino acids in the molecule.

per through (Latin), e.g. *per vaginam*, through the vagina.

percentile statistical term used to show the incidence of a characteristic; diagrammatic line representing the percentage of the population with the specific characteristic, e.g. in terms of babies weights or lengths, the 90th percentile/centile means that 90% of the population will have measurements below that figure; the 50th percentile is the median or average.

percussion tapping a surface with the fingers to elicit a sound, which helps to determine the condition of the underlying organs.

percutaneous umbilical cord blood sampling (PUBS) *See* CORDOCENTESIS.

perforation hole or break in the wall or membranes of an organ or structure, occurring when erosion, infection or other factors create a weak spot in the organ and internal pressure causes a rupture.

performance indicators 'package' of routine statistics derived nationally and presented visually to highlight the relative efficiency of health services in each health authority compared with other authorities.

peri- prefix meaning 'around'.

pericardium smooth membranous sac around the heart, with an outer fibrous and inner serous coat.

pericranium external periosteum of the cranial bones.

perimenopause the time approaching and immediately after cessation of menstrual periods, during which some women experience symptoms, e.g. MENORRHAGIA and hot flushes.

perimetrium peritoneum of the uterus.

perinatal around birth. *P. period* first week of life. *P. mortality rate* number of stillbirths plus deaths of babies under 1 week old per 1000 total births in any 1 year.

perineal pertaining to the perineum. *P. laceration* tear occurring in the perineum at delivery. *First-degree p. laceration* involves skin only, the muscle remaining intact. *Second-degree p. laceration* involves skin and muscle, but not the anal sphincter. *Third-degree* or *complete p. laceration* tear extends through the whole of the perineal body and through the anal sphincter into the rectum. *P. repair* suturing of perineal lacerations or episiotomy by a doctor or by a midwife trained and assessed as competent; involves inserting a

Perineal repair (commonly used method)

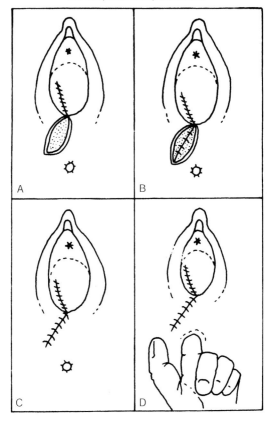

A, vagina sutured with continuous catgut; **B,** muscle layer sutured with interrupted catgut; **C,** perineal skin sutured with interrupted catgut or silk; **D,** rectal examination to exclude rectal involvement.

tampon to ensure a clear visual field followed by suturing of the vagina with interrupted sutures, commencing just above the apex of the incision or tear; suturing of deep and superficial muscle layers, starting in the centre of the incision to give good approximation; and suturing of perineal skin. The tampon is then removed and a gloved finger is passed into the rectum to ensure no sutures encroach into it. *See also* Appendix 3.

perineorrhaphy repair of the perineal body following injury sustained during childbearing.

perineum anatomically, the area extending from the pubic arch to the coccyx, with the underlying tissues; obstetrically, the fibromuscular pyramid between the lower third of the vagina anteriorly, anal canal posteriorly and ischial tuberosities laterally. *See also* PELVIC FLOOR.

periosteum specialised connective tissue covering all bones of the body, possessing bone-forming potentialities; serves as a point of attachment for certain muscles.

peripheral relating to the periphery.

periphery outer surface or circumference.

peristalsis wave-like contraction that travels along the walls of a tubular organ, pressing its contents onwards; occurs in the muscle layer of the alimentary canal and fallopian tubes; visible peristalsis may occur in PYLORIC STENOSIS.

peritoneum serous membrane lining the abdominal cavity and covering the abdominal organs. *Parietal p.* lines the abdominal cavity. *Pelvic p.* covers the pelvic organs, in the female forming the pouch of Douglas between the rectum and uterus and the shallow uterovesical pouch between the uterus and bladder; peritoneum hanging over the fallopian tubes is the broad ligament. *Visceral p.* inner layer closely covering the organs, including the mesenteries. adj. *peritoneal.*

peritonitis inflammation of the peritoneum caused by infection. *General p.* affecting the whole abdominal cavity. *Pelvic p.* restricted to peritoneum of the pelvic cavity; an occasional complication of puerperal sepsis.

periventricular haemorrhage serious complication of preterm babies, notably those under 34 weeks' gestation; haemorrhage is graded from 0 to 3, with 3 being the most extensive.

periventricular leukomalacia cystic, ischaemic lesions in the periventricular region, diagnosed on ultrasound scan; associated with periventricular haemorrhage and a high incidence of spastic cerebral palsy.

permeable able to be penetrated, as in membranes that allow fluids to pass through, e.g. the walls of the capillaries (also semipermeable).

pernicious highly destructive; fatal. *P. anaemia* megaloblastic anaemia occurring in middle age, caused by failure of the gastric secretion of intrinsic factor; treated with vitamin B12; not to be confused with megaloblastic anaemia caused by lack of folic acid.

peroxide compound of any element with more than the normal quantity of oxygen required to form an oxide. *P. of hydrogen* compound of hydrogen and oxygen.

perphenazine (Fentazin) oral antiemetic; avoid in the first trimester.

persistent mentoposterior face presentation in which the sinciput rotates forwards and the chin rotates backwards to the sacral hollow; rare cause of obstructed labour, when the thorax must present at the pelvic brim with the head.

persistent occipitoposterior deflexed vertex presentation with the sinciput rotated forwards and the occiput rotated backwards to the hollow of the sacrum; common cause of delay in the second stage of labour;

spontaneous FACE-TO-PUBES delivery is possible.

personality factors that constitute, distinguish and characterise an individual as a separate identity, determined by inheritance and shaped and modified by the individual's environment.

perspiration 1. sweating; excretion of moisture through the pores of the skin. 2. sweat; salty fluid, largely water, excreted by sweat glands in the skin; in cystic fibrosis the sweat has raised sodium chloride levels.

pertussis whooping cough; potentially serious respiratory tract infection caused by *Bordetella pertussis*, particularly serious in babies under 3 months and children with asthma; incidence has risen in recent years because of the fall in uptake of immunisation programmes.

pessary object inserted into the vagina, e.g. antifungal or contraceptive drug in a solvent base, device to maintain anteversion of the uterus in early pregnancy. *Prostaglandin p.* pessary of prostaglandins, inserted into the posterior vaginal fornix to facilitate cervical ripening and onset of labour.

petechiae small spots caused by minute subcutaneous haemorrhages, seen in purpura and sometimes on the face of the normal neonate as a result of venous congestion during delivery; feature of congenital RUBELLA, TOXOPLASMOSIS and CYTOMEGALOVIRUS when it covers the entire body.

pethidine hydrochloride analgesic, antispasmodic drug used to relieve labour pain; midwives may carry and administer it under the Misuse of Drugs Regulations 1973; may cause respiratory depression if the baby is delivered shortly after maternal administration, so less popular now.

petit mal relatively mild epileptic attack with momentary loss of consciousness, as opposed to GRAND MAL.

Pfannenstiel's incision transverse abdominal incision just above the symphysis pubis.

pH symbol expressing hydrogen ion concentration or reaction of a fluid on a scale from 0 to 14; neutral pH is 7, acid pH is below 7 and alkaline pH is above 7; the pH of blood is 7.4, slightly alkaline. pH can be measured with an Astrup machine to ascertain whether the body is maintaining a normal ACID–BASE BALANCE; favourable pH is essential for enzyme function and other biological systems.

phaeochromocytoma rare, usually benign, adrenal tumour, or occasionally found elsewhere, e.g. bladder, associated with increased adrenaline (epinephrine) production leading to hypertension with wide diurnal variations; diagnosis is by direct assay of plasma and urine adrenaline and noradrenaline (norepinephrine), or by measuring urinary vanillylmandelic acid (VMA), metanephrine and normetanephrine, which increase to almost twice the normal upper limits in the presence of the tumour; the tumour should be surgically removed.

phage virus that kills certain microorganisms.

phagocytes polymorphonuclear leucocytes and monocytes that engulf and digest bacteria and foreign particles.

phagocytosis action of PHAGOCYTES.

phalanx any bone of a finger or toe. adj. *phalangeal*.

phallic pertaining to the penis.

phantom 1. image or impression not evoked by actual stimuli. 2. model of the body or of a specific part thereof. 3. device for simulating the *in vivo* interaction of radiation with tissues. *P. pregnancy* pseudocyesis or false pregnancy.

pharmaceutical relating to drugs.

pharmacokinetics study of drug metabolism and actions, especially absorption, duration of action, distribution within the body and method of excretion.

pharmacology science of the nature and preparation of drugs.

pharmacopoeia authoritative publication giving the standard drug formulae and preparation as used in a given country. *British Pharmacopoeia (BP)* that authorised for use in Great Britain.

pharmacy 1. art of preparing, compounding and dispensing medicines. 2. shop in which medicines are dispensed and sold.

pharynx back of the mouth leading to the oesophagus and larynx, communicating with the nose through the posterior nares and the ears through the Eustachian tubes.

Phenergan *See* PROMETHAZINE HYDROCHLORIDE.

phenindione oral anticoagulant similar to warfarin; should be avoided in pregnancy and breastfeeding.

phenobarbital barbiturate drug that depresses the cerebral cortex, used to treat epilepsy and eclampsia, but should be avoided in early pregnancy.

phenol powerful, very poisonous antiseptic, which may also cause severe skin irritation in mild dilutions.

phenomenology inductive descriptive approach to research developed from phenomenological philosophy, involving an understanding of the response of the whole human being; focuses on describing experiences as they are lived by a person, such as describing a person's pain as they perceive it.

phenothiazines group of major tranquillisers, the phenothiazine derivatives.

phenotype 1. outward, visible expression of the hereditary constitution of an organism. 2. individual exhibiting a certain phenotype; a trait expressed in a phenotype.

phenoxymethylpenicillin oral antibiotic commonly used for mild streptococcal infections (penicillin V).

phenylalanine essential amino acid, normally converted to tyrosine by an enzyme from the liver.

phenylketonuria presence in the urine of phenylketones resulting from incomplete breakdown of PHENYLALANINE to tyrosine; a high blood level of phenylalanine causes learning disabilities, fits and poor muscular coordination; autosomal RECESSIVE inherited condition with an incidence of 1:10 000. The GUTHRIE TEST performed on day 7 of life enables early diagnosis; treatment is by giving a low phenylalanine diet. Those affected are usually blue-eyed, blond, with defective pigmentation and excessively sensitive skin, tending to eczema.

phenylpyruvic acid abnormal constituent excreted in the urine of those with PHENYLKETONURIA.

phenytoin sodium (Epanutin) anticonvulsant drug used to control epilepsy; should be avoided in early pregnancy unless the potential benefits outweigh the risk of congenital abnormality.

phimosis constriction of the orifice of the prepuce so that it cannot be drawn back over the glans of the penis.

phlebitis inflammation of a deep or superficial vein, usually in the leg; may lead to THROMBOSIS or EMBOLISM.

phlebothrombosis formation of a blood clot loosely attached to a vein wall, not associated with infection; risk of separation of all or part of the clot, leading to EMBOLISM. cf. THROMBOPHLEBITIS.

phlebotomist one who performs phlebotomy, i.e. obtaining samples of blood for testing.

phlebotomy venesection.

phlegmasia inflammation. *P. alba dolens* white leg; uncommon puerperal femoral THROMBOPHLEBITIS or PHLEBOTHROMBOSIS, associated with venous obstruction and/or reflex arterial spasm in which the leg is swollen and very painful; treatment involves elevating the leg without immobilisation and giving antibiotics if the condition is caused by thrombophlebitis; in other cases anticoagulants may also be given.

phlegmatic of dull and sluggish temperament.

phobia persistent abnormal dread or fear appearing to result from repressed inner conflicts of which the affected person is unaware; trigger uncontrollable and unreasonable reactions to the feared situation, e.g. acrophobia, fear of heights; claustrophobia, morbid fear of enclosed places.

phocomelia congenital absence of the proximal portion of a limb or limbs, the hands or feet being attached to the trunk by a small, irregularly shaped bone.

phospholipid lipid containing phosphorus, including phosphoglycerides, plasmalogens, sphingomyelins; major lipids in cell membranes.

phosphorus essential chemical element required for almost all metabolic processes; major component, as phosphates, of the mineral phase of bone; obtained from milk products, cereals, meat and fish, and its use by the body requires vitamin D and calcium. Symbol P.

photophobia intolerance of light; a symptom of meningitis.

photosensitivity abnormal degree of skin sensitivity to sunlight, caused during pregnancy by increased levels of melanocytic hormone; also caused by certain drugs, e.g. chlorpromazine.

phototherapy fluorescent light treatment, used to reduce unconjugated bilirubin levels of over 340 μmol/L at term, 210 μmol/L at 34 weeks and 150 μmol/L at 28 weeks in the jaundiced skin of a neonate; complex changes occur and the non-toxic photodegradation products result without the help of the enzyme system in the liver. Side effects include loose green stools, which require an extra fluid intake of about 30 mg/kg per 24 hours to compensate, and skin rashes; the baby's eyes and gonads are covered to prevent problems from light exposure. Used prophylactically in preterm babies with bruising and in Rhesus incompatibility.

phrenic pertaining to the diaphragm or to the mind. *P. nerve* major branch of the cervical plexus, carrying nerve impulses from the inspiratory centre in the brain, causing contraction of the diaphragm to aid inspiration.

phthisis pulmonary tuberculosis.

physiological third stage non-interventionist management of the third stage of labour in which the placenta is allowed to separate from the uterine wall without the use of oxytocic drugs to expedite the process; the signs that the placenta has separated are the uterus rising in the abdomen, feeling small, hard and mobile, lengthening of the cord and a small gush of blood from the vagina; the placenta and membranes may then be delivered with maternal effort or CONTROLLED CORD TRACTION, in which case it is imperative to await signs of separation and descent. *See also* ACTIVE MANAGEMENT OF LABOUR.

physiology science of the function of living organisms.

physiotherapist practitioner of physiotherapy who uses massage, manipulation, remedial exercises and heat, light and electrical impulses to treat and rehabilitate. *Obstetric p.* specialises in treating pregnant women.

physique organisation, development and structure of the body.

phytomenadione (Konakion) vitamin K preparation used to treat haemorrhage occurring during anticoagulant therapy and caused by vitamin K deficiency; given prophylactically to newborn babies, orally or intramuscularly, to prevent haemorrhagic disease.

phytotherapy treatment using plant substances, such as herbal medicine and aromatherapy.

pia mater innermost membrane enveloping the brain and spinal cord.

pica craving to eat unnatural substances, sometimes occurring during pregnancy, thought to be related to nutritional deficiencies.

pie chart circular diagram divided into segments showing the proportional distribution of observations of particular events.

Pierre–Robin syndrome congenital abnormality involving MICROGNATHIA and cleft palate; if not recognised at birth severe respiratory obstruction may occur as the tongue occludes the pharynx, the baby is nursed prone, with the tongue pulled forwards if necessary to clear the airway.

pigment dye or colouring agent. *Bile p.* BILIRUBIN and biliverdin. *Blood p.* haematin.

piles HAEMORRHOIDS.

pilonidal having a nest of hairs. *P.cyst* dermoid cyst implanted in the natal cleft; results from penetration of hairs through the skin of the natal cleft fold causing a sinus and epithelium cell implantation; prone to recurrent infection. *P.depression* non-significant depression in the midline near the coccyx, seen in the newborn baby. *P. sinus* small pericoccygeal sinus, seen on routine examination of the baby, a remnant of the neural canal; may become infected, necessitating excision.

pilot study small-scale version of a planned investigation or observation, used to test the design of the larger study.

Pinard's stethoscope trumpet-shaped fetal (monaural) stethoscope; placed on the mother's abdomen over the fetal chest to hear the fetal heart sounds.

pineal pertaining to the pineal body. *P.body, p. gland* small conical structure attached by a stalk to the posterior wall of the third ventricle of the cerebrum, believed to be an endocrine gland.

pinna projecting part of the ear lying outside the head.

Piriton *See* CHLORPHENAMINE (CHLORPHENIRAMINE) MALEATE.

pituitary gland endocrine gland in the pituitary fossa of the sphenoid bone; the anterior lobe produces GONADOTROPHIC hormones, GROWTH HORMONE, lactogenic hormone (prolactin), ADRENOCORTICOTROPHIC HORMONE and thyrotrophic hormone; the posterior lobe secretes OXYTOCIN and antidiuretic hormone.

place of safety order court order by which a child is arbitrarily removed from parental care for his or her safety.

placebo substance given to, or procedure performed on, a patient or a research subject, as in controlled clinical trials of new drugs, that is effective because the person expects it to be, yet it has no intrinsic therapeutic value.

placenta afterbirth; a flat organ of 17.5–20 cm in diameter and 2.5 cm thick, tapering to 1.2 cm at the periphery; weighs approximately one-sixth of the baby's birthweight at full term; formed by 12 weeks' gestation, developed from trophoblastic layers with a lining of mesoderm in which the blood vessels develop; composed of numerous chorionic villi grouped together in cotyledons, embedded in the uterine decidua basalis. The villi contain fetal blood vessels, ultimately joining together as the umbilical vessels, separated by intervillous spaces through which the maternal blood circulates. The fetal surface reveals the fetal blood vessels radiating from the cord insertion, usually central, covered by amnion; the chorion is continuous with the edge of the placenta. *Abruptio placentae* premature separation of a normally situated placenta. *Battledore p.* cord is attached to placental margin and not the centre. *Bipartite p.* has two main lobes.

P. accreta abnormally adherent placenta attached to the myometrium, with partial or complete absence of the decidua basalis. *P. circumvallata* encircled with a dense, raised, white nodular ring of attached membranes doubled back over the placental edge. *P. fenestrata* one having a gap or 'window' in its structure. *P. membranacea* abnormally thin placenta spread over an unusually large area of the uterus, sometimes occurring in PLACENTA PRAEVIA. *P. percreta* abnormal insertion in which the chorionic

Functions of the placenta

Glycogen storage
Respiration
Excretion
Endocrine
Nutrition
Partial barrier

villi invade the perimetrium causing total adherence – hysterectomy is usually required to control haemorrhage. *Succenturiate p.* one with a separate or accessory lobe joined to the main placenta by blood vessels, which may cause serious postpartum haemorrhage if it separates from the main placenta and is retained.

placenta praevia placenta situated abnormally in the lower uterine segment, leading to unavoidable, painless, recurring haemorrhage towards the end of pregnancy as the lower uterine segment stretches in preparation for labour. *Grade 1 p. p.* only the edge of the placenta encroaches into the lower uterine segment; *grade 2 p. p.* the whole placenta is in the lower segment; *grade 3 p. p.* the placenta reaches to the internal cervical os; *grade 4 p. p.* the entire placenta covers the central cervical os. Hospital admission is necessary to control bleeding, confirm the exact location of the placenta on ultrasound scan and determine the safest mode of delivery of the baby. Fetal malpresentations, e.g. oblique lie, are common and vaginal delivery is unsafe unless the degree of placenta praevia is minimal; occasionally, in grades 3 or 4, examination under anaesthetic is performed to attempt controlled membrane rupture and induction of labour, with preparations made for

Manual removal of the placenta

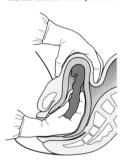

Placenta with succenturiate lobe

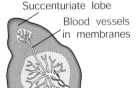

Succenturiate lobe

Blood vessels in membranes

immediate Caesarean section in the event of tumultuous haemorrhage.

placental lactogen hormone affecting breast growth and development in pregnancy; also affects glucose metabolism in pregnancy; similar to pituitary GROWTH HORMONE but does not actually promote growth.

placentography radiological visualisation of the placenta after injection of a contrast medium.

placentophagy eating of the placenta, in the belief that its hormones prevent postnatal depression.

plagiocephaly asymmetry of the head resulting from irregular closure of the sutures.

planned parenthood birth control.

plantar pertaining to the sole of the foot.

plasma straw-coloured fluid accounting for 55% of the blood; made up of 92% water containing plasma proteins, inorganic salts, foods, gases, waste materials, hormones, secretions and enzymes, which are transported to and from body tissues by the plasma; may be transfused to increase plasma proteins or in cases of shock.

plasmapheresis method of removing a portion of the plasma from the circulation in cases of disease caused by circulating antibodies in the plasma; venepuncture is performed, plasma is removed from the blood sample and red cells are returned to the circulation.

plasmin FIBRINOLYSIN; enzyme that dissolves the fibrin in a thrombus, present in blood as plasminogen before activation.

Plastibell pre-sterilised plastic device used for circumcision. The bell is slipped inside the foreskin and a string tied around it; the foreskin becomes gangrenous and drops off with the bell.

platelets thrombocytes; disc-shaped, non-nucleated blood elements with a very fragile membrane, which adhere to uneven or damaged surfaces; formed in red bone marrow and average about 250×10^9 per litre of blood; assist in coagulation and may occlude small breaks in blood vessels and prevent escape of blood.

platypelloid flat. See PELVIS.

plethora excess; in medicine, excess of blood.

plethoric florid colouring; may be seen in a baby with a large placental transfusion or in one of the twins with TWIN-TO-TWIN TRANSFUSION syndrome.

pleura serous membrane lining the thorax and surrounding each lung, the two layers enclosing a potential space, the pleural cavity.

pleurisy inflammation of the pleura.

plexus network of veins or nerves. *Brachial p.* network of nerves of the neck and axilla. *Solar* or *coeliac p.* network of nerves and ganglia at the back of the stomach, supplying the abdominal viscera.

pneumococcal disease infective disease caused by the bacteria *Streptococcus pneumoniae*, commonly carried in the nose and throat, especially in children, who are particularly at risk when mixing with others; infection is spread by coughing and sneezing, causing non-bacteraemic pneumonia, otitis media, sinusitis or, more seriously, leading to meningitis, septicaemia or bacteraemic pneumonia; children under 5 years, particularly those under 2, are most at risk, as are the elderly and individuals with some chronic diseases or a non-functioning spleen; there is a 10–15% mortality rate and, of those who survive, 50% develop chronic problems including hearing loss, learning impairment, cerebral palsy or epilepsy. The bacteria has become resistant to penicillin and erythromycin and prophylaxis is now advocated through vaccination with pneumococcal conjugate vaccine (PCV) at 2 and

4 months of age, with a booster at 13 months; to avoid giving infants too many injections at one time, this has led to changes in the existing immunisation schedule. *See* Appendix 14.

pneumonia inflammation of the lung. *Lobar p.* pneumococcal infection of one or more lobes of the lung. *Bronchopneumonia* caused by *Staphylococcus aureus*, streptococcus or *Haemophilis influenzae* and affecting the bronchioles. *Viral p.* RESPIRATORY DISTRESS SYNDROME predisposes the neonate to viral pneumonia.

pneumonitis inflammation of the lungs.

pneumothorax accumulation of air or gas in the pleural cavity, causing collapse of the lung on the affected side; may occur spontaneously, as in pulmonary disease, follow trauma and perforation of the chest wall, be a complication of vigorous resuscitation, ventilation or CONTINUOUS INFLATING PRESSURE, or follow MECONIUM ASPIRATION. pl. *pneumothoraces*.

PO₂ partial pressure of oxygen; about 100 mmHg in an adult and 60–90 mmHg in a baby; if it exceeds 100 mmHg in a preterm baby there is a danger of RETROLENTAL FIBROPLASIA.

podalic version internal correction of a transverse lie by grasping a foot, converting it to a longitudinal lie and breech presentation.

polarity gradient of strength of uterine contractions from the upper fundal pole, where the activity is strongest, to the lower segment and cervix, where contractions are weak or absent, which causes cervical dilatation.

pole one extremity or end of an organ of the body, e.g. the uterus, or of the fetus.

policy plan of action; written plan of action for specific situations, e.g. clinical or managerial.

poliomyelitis viral infection causing inflammation of anterior cells of the spinal cord, leading to infantile paralysis; a notifiable disease, preventable by vaccination.

poly- prefix meaning 'much' or 'many'.

polycystic containing numerous cysts. *P. kidneys* congenital malformation having enlarged kidneys containing numerous cysts, often remaining undiagnosed and allowing normal pregnancy although urinary tract infections and hypertension may occur in the woman; the baby's kidneys are enlarged at birth and survival is unlikely. *P. ovarian syndrome (PCOS)* Stein–Leventhal syndrome; affects 6–10% of women, often asymptomatically; characterised by irregular or absent menstrual periods, numerous ovarian cysts, hypertension, acne, infertility, hirsutism and obesity, and may lead to diabetes; treatment involves lifestyle changes to control weight and diabetes, and ovulation stimulation when pregnancy is desired.

polycythaemia excess of red blood cells, as occurs in the neonate because of high levels of fetal haemoglobin.

polydactyly supernumerary fingers.

polygraph apparatus for simultaneously recording several mechanical or electrical impulses, e.g. blood pressure, pulse, respiration and variations in electrical resistance of the skin.

polyhydramnios HYDRAMNIOS; excess amniotic fluid, usually over 1500 mL, associated with maternal diabetes, congenital abnormalities, especially of the central nervous system, uniovular twins and a rare tumour of the placenta (CHORIOANGIOMA).

polymerase chain reaction (PCR) molecular technique for amplifying deoxyribonucleic acid (DNA), widely used in medical and biological research; also used to identify genetic fingerprints, diagnose infectious diseases, clone genes and for paternity testing. *See also* QUANTITATIVE FLUORESCENCE POLYMERASE CHAIN REACTION (QF-PCR).

polymorphonuclear possessing multi-lobed nuclei as in most of the white blood cells.

polyneuritis multiple neuritis.

polyp, polypus small pedunculated tumour arising from any mucous surface. *Cervical p.* occurs in the cervical canal. *Fibroid p.* occurs in the uterus, contains fibrous myomatous tissue. *Placental p.* consists of remains of the placenta. pl. *polypi.*

polysaccharide complex carbohydrate, e.g. starch.

polyuria excess secretion of urine, caused by diuretics or diabetes; normal in the first few days of the puerperium because of autolysis occurring as part of the process of INVOLUTION.

pons 1. part of the metencephalon between the medulla oblongata and midbrain, ventral to the cerebellum. 2. any slip of tissue connecting two parts of an organ.

popliteal relating to the posterior part of the knee, described as the *p. fossa* or *p. space.*

pore minute circular opening on a surface, e.g. of sweat glands.

port-wine stain naevus flammeus.

portal vein large vein carrying nutritive material from digestive tract to liver, formed from gastric, splenic and superior mesenteric veins.

portfolio collection of competency evidence assembled by the practitioner to demonstrate professional development, e.g. marked assessments, evidence of reflective practice, certificates of attendance at conferences or study days.

position attitude or posture. *Dorsal p.* lying flat on the back. *Genupectoral* or *knee-chest p.* resting on the knees and chest with arms crossed above the head or resting on knees and elbows; traditional position to relieve pressure on a prolapsed cord. *Left lateral p.* lying on the left side, right knee drawn up towards the chin. *Lithotomy p.* lying on the back with thighs raised and knees supported and held widely apart; used for instrumental delivery and operative procedures performed via the vagina. *Prone p.* lying face down. *Recumbent p.* lying down. *Sim's p.* similar to *left lateral* but almost on the face, semi-prone with the right knee and thigh drawn up and resting on the bed in front of the left one. *Trendelenburg p.* lying on the back on a tilted plane (usually an operating table at an angle of 30° to the floor), with the head lowermost and the shoulders supported.

position of the fetus eight positions relating the fetal DENOMINATOR to the mother's pelvis. In a vertex presentation the denominator is the occiput, thus in *occipitoanterior p.*, the commonest and most favourable position, the fetal occiput is directed to the symphysis pubis, either to the right or left iliopectineal eminence; in *occipitolateral* or *occipitotransverse p.* the occiput is directed to the midpoint of the left or right iliopectineal line; in *occipitoposterior p.* the occiput is directed to the left or right sacroiliac joint; in *direct* or *persistent occipitoposterior p.* the occiput is directed towards the sacrum. The breech positions are similar but with the sacrum as the denominator. *See* Appendix 4.

positive end-expiratory pressure (PEEP) in mechanical ventilation, positive airway pressure maintained until the end of expiration.

positive predictive value *See* ODDS OF BEING AFFECTED GIVEN A POSITIVE RESULT.

posseting regurgitation of a small amount of milk immediately after a feed.

post- prefix meaning 'after', e.g. postnatal clinic.

postcoital contraceptive contraceptive method used as an emergency

measure after unprotected sexual intercourse; may be a hormonal oral contraceptive pill, taken within 72 hours of
unprotected sex, or an intrauterine
contraceptive device, inserted within
5 days of unprotected intercourse to
prevent the embedding of a fertilised
ovum.

posterior at the back.

posthumous occurring after death.
P. birth birth of baby after the father's
death or by Caesarean section after
the death of the mother.

postmaturity pregnancy prolonged
after the expected date of delivery
(EDD), usually considered as being
41–42 weeks after the last menstrual
period, although first-trimester ultrasound scans are now considered
more accurate; EDD is used as a
marker to define when induction of
labour may be necessary, because
placental deterioration after term
may lead to fetal hypoxia.

post mortem after death. *P-m. exam-
ation* autopsy.

postnatal after childbirth, referring to
the mother. *P. examination* 1. maternal
examination undertaken frequently
during the first 10 days of the
puerperium to ensure that INVOLU-
TION is taking place, lactation is
becoming established and the mother
is adapting physically, emotionally
and psychologically to motherhood.
2. medical/midwifery examination at
the end of the 6-week puerperium to
ensure the mother's body has
returned to the non-pregnant state
without complications. *P. exercises*
exercises taught by the midwife or
physiotherapist for the mother to perform several times daily during the
puerperium and, ideally, for the rest
of her life; aimed specifically at
strengthening the pelvic floor and
abdominal muscles, but also include
deep breathing and leg exercises as
preventative measures against respiratory tract infection and deep vein

thrombosis. *P. period* phase of the
puerperium of between 10 and 28
days after labour ends, during which
the midwife is required by Nursing
and Midwifery Council rules to attend
the mother and baby regularly.

postpartum after labour. *P. haemorrhage (PPH)* excessive genital tract
bleeding at any time from the birth
of the baby up to 6 weeks after
delivery. *Primary PPH* occurs within
the first 24 hours, usually referring to
blood loss of more than 500 mL
or any amount detrimental to the
mother's health; *secondary PPH*
occurs after the first 24 hours. *See*
Appendix 6. *P. shock* collapse due
to circulatory failure, occurring after
delivery, which may be haemorrhagic (ante- or postpartum haemorrhage) or non-haemorrhagic (uterine
inversion or rupture, acid aspiration
syndrome, pulmonary or amniotic
fluid embolism, hypotension or
endotoxic shock as a result of septicaemia); characterised by hypotension, tachycardia, cold, clammy,
white skin and air hunger; the
mother must be resuscitated urgently
by maintaining the airway and
administering oxygen, as well as
intravenous fluids to increase blood
volume and antibiotics if shock is
endotoxic.

post-traumatic stress disorder immediate or delayed reaction to extremely
stressful events, e.g. rape, drowning
or major natural or man-made disas-
ters; can occur after a very traumatic
birth experience such as extremely
urgent Caesarean section or forceful
forceps delivery, or when the mother
feels she has been abused as a result
of her delivery experience. Signs and
symptoms are acute anxiety, insomnia, nightmares, flashbacks, depression, loss of concentration, apathy,
guilt and difficulties with sexual relationships; support and counselling
are needed. Adequate debriefing of

181

mothers by the midwife or doctor who conducted each delivery may help to prevent the condition.

posture general attitude of body and limbs.

potassium metallic element, symbol K; forms one of the electrolytes of blood and tissue fluids; essential for maintenance of acid–base and water balance and for proper cardiac function, in conjunction with plasma sodium, calcium and potassium.

potential possible. *P. diabetic* someone with normal glucose tolerance but an increased risk of developing clinical DIABETES, e.g. woman who has one or both parents as diabetics or who delivers a baby weighing 4.5 kg (10 lb).

Potter's syndrome congenital condition of renal agenesis, pulmonary hypoplasia, low-set ears, furrows under the eyes (Potter's facies); commonly associated with only two umbilical cord vessels; fatal if both kidneys are absent.

pouch pocket-like space or cavity. *P. of Douglas* lowest fold of peritoneum between uterus and rectum. *Uterovesical p.* fold of peritoneum between uterus and bladder.

Poupart's ligament inguinal ligament; tendinous lower border of the external oblique muscle of the abdominal wall, passing from the anterior superior spine of the ilium to the pubis bone.

practitioner person who practises a profession.

prandial pertaining to a meal, e.g. *postprandial* after a meal.

pre- prefix meaning 'before', e.g. prenatal, premature.

precipitate 1. settling in solid particles of a substance in solution. 2. occurring with undue rapidity, as in *p.labour,* in which the mother may suffer severe perineal lacerations and the baby may have intracranial trauma due to rapid passage through the birth canal.

preconception before conception. *P. care* health education, medical examination and investigation for the purpose of detecting and treating problems before conception, promoting optimum maternal and paternal health at conception and during first-trimester organogenesis and reducing risks of congenital malformations. Includes taking a detailed personal, medical, family, reproductive and lifestyle history, e.g. diet, smoking, alcohol and drug intake and occupational hazards; gynaecological examination and cervical smear; full urinalysis and blood tests for rubella antibodies, haemoglobin, haemoglobinopathies, syphilis and HIV antibodies; hair and domestic water analysis to test for toxic metals; semen analysis; and stool tests for infestation. Referral to appropriate physician or genetic counsellor may follow.

precursor something that precedes; in medicine, a sign or symptom that heralds another.

pre-diabetes state preceding diabetes mellitus, before the condition is clinically manifested; the diabetes may become evident during pregnancy or it may present no signs and symptoms but the baby's birthweight may be above the norm, usually more than 4.5 kg in a term baby.

predisposition latent susceptibility to disease, which may be activated under certain conditions.

prednisone, prednisolone synthetic glucocorticoid, anti-inflammatory and anti-allergic preparations, which act in the same way as adrenocortical hormones.

pre-eclampsia pregnancy hypertension (diastolic blood pressure of 80 mmHg or a rise of more than 15–20 mmHg above the booking baseline) combined with oedema, proteinuria and other system changes, usually occurring in the second half of the pregnancy and resolving within 48–72 hours of delivery. Manual recording of blood pressure is important because electronic blood pressure devices tend to undermeasure true blood pressure. Untreated or severe cases may develop into ECLAMPSIA.

Pregaday iron preparation specifically used to prevent and treat iron deficiency and megaloblastic anaemia in pregnancy.

pregnancy from conception to delivery of the fetus; normal duration is 280 days (40 weeks or 9 months and 7 days), counted from the first day of the last normal menstrual period to delivery, or 265 days, from conception to delivery. *Ectopic p.* extrauterine pregnancy, occurs relatively frequently in the fallopian tube and very rarely in the ovary or the abdominal cavity. adj. *pregnant*.

pregnancy-associated plasma protein-A (PAPP-A) plasma protein originating from placental syncytiotrophoblasts, levels rising as pregnancy advances. Average first-trimester levels are significantly reduced in DOWN'S SYNDROME pregnancies. *See also* COMBINED TEST and INTEGRATED TEST.

pregnancy-induced hypertension (PIH) asymptomatic rise in blood pressure without proteinuria after the 20th week of pregnancy, most commonly in primigravidae and multiple pregnancy. Should be monitored closely to detect PRE-ECLAMPSIA; must also be distinguished from ESSENTIAL HYPERTENSION. Complications include placental abruption, renal and cardiac failure, cerebral haemorrhage, placental insufficiency and intrauterine growth retardation.

pregnancy tests urinary or blood tests that measure HUMAN CHORIONIC GONADOTROPHIN (hCG), used to detect pregnancy or monitor abnormal hCG levels. *See also* IMMUNOLOGICAL PREGNANCY TEST.

pregnanediol derivative of pregnane, formed by reduction of progesterone, present in urine of pregnant women.

pregnant with child; gravid; having a developing embryo or fetus within the uterus.

pre-implantation genetic diagnosis (PGD) form of genetic diagnosis performed after *in vitro* fertilisation and before embryo implantation in couples with a high risk of having a child with an inherited condition; preferred by some as it avoids selective termination of pregnancy. *See also* ANEUPLOIDY diagnosis.

premature early.

premedication drugs given before general anaesthesia, e.g. atropine, hyoscine or papaveretum; opiates are not used before Caesarean section to avoid neonatal respiratory depression.

premenstrual preceding menstruation. *P.syndrome* condition affecting many women in the 7–10 days before menstruation as a result of fluctuating hormone levels; characterised by numerous symptoms, e.g. irritability, aggression, anxiety, mood changes, headache, breast tenderness, oedema, cravings, particularly for sweet or salty foods, lack of coordination or concentration; subsides once menstruation commences.

premonition forewarning. *See* AURA.

prenatal occurring before birth.

preoperative preceding an operation.

prepuce foreskin; a loose fold of skin covering the glans penis.

preregistration midwifery education theoretical and practical education to prepare those wishing to practise as midwives; in the UK it involves a 3-year diploma or degree course, shortened to 18 months for those who are already nurses.

prescription doctor's written or verbal instruction for administration of drugs; UK NHS prescriptions are free during pregnancy and for 1 year after delivery.

presentation fetal part entering the pelvis first, occupying the lower pole of the uterus; normally cephalic (vertex), breech or, occasionally, face, brow or shoulder.

presenting part fetal part lying lowest in the birth canal, the first part felt on examination *per vaginam*; the occiput in a vertex presentation.

pressor increases blood pressure.

pressure stress or strain, by compression, expansion, pull, thrust or shear. *Arterial p.* blood pressure in the arteries. *See also* BLOOD PRESSURE.

preterm before term, i.e. before 37 completed weeks of pregnancy. *P. infant* baby born before 37 weeks' gestation, with low birthweight and, possibly, being SMALL FOR GESTATIONAL AGE, which is assessed using the DUBOWITZ SCORE. Complications include RESPIRATORY DISTRESS SYNDROME, feeding difficulties caused by immature sucking, swallowing and coughing reflexes, hypothermia, jaundice and infection, and poor a maternal–infant relationship because of the prolonged stay in the neonatal intensive care unit. *P. labour* labour occurring before 37 weeks' gestation; spontaneous labour is caused by changing hormone levels, overstretched uterus, weak cervix or infection and is treated with tocolytic drugs, e.g. ritodrine hydrochloride to delay delivery; labour is induced before term when the extrauterine environment is considered to be less hazardous for the fetus because of poor maternal or fetal well-being, and is followed by controlled delivery with obstetric forceps to protect the delicate fetal head.

prevalence total number of cases of a specific disease in existence in a given population at a certain time.

preventive prophylactic; means of preventing something.

previable before viability; baby born before 24 weeks' gestation.

primary first, in order of time or importance. *P. postpartum haemorrhage see* POSTPARTUM HAEMORRHAGE.

primary care group (PCG) group of general practitioners and services in a defined geographical area with a community of approximately 100 000 people; commissions services, promotes good health and combats health inequalities; a direct means for general practitioners, community nurses, etc. to secure appropriate high-quality care for local people.

primary care trust (PCT) organisation that plans, secures local services, improves local community health and integrates health and social care.

primary health care community-based medical, midwifery and nursing care.

primary health-care team team providing community primary health care: general practitioner, community midwife, community nurse, health visitor and social worker based in a health centre or general practice area.

primigravida woman pregnant for the first time.

primipara woman who has given birth to a viable baby, alive or stillborn.

primiparous having borne one viable baby.

probability (*P*) statistical term indicating the likelihood of an association between variables being due to chance.

probe blunt, malleable instrument for exploring sinus tracks, wounds, cavities or passages.

procaine local anaesthetic; hydrochloride salt is used in solution for infiltration.

procaine benzylpenicillin intramuscular antibiotic, commonly used to treat syphilis and gonorrhoea.

process 1. prominence or projection, as from a bone. 2. series of operations or events leading to achievement of a specific result. *Midwifery/nursing p.* systematic, problem-solving approach to the task of meeting the needs of clients/patients.

prochlorperazine tranquilliser and antiemetic, sometimes administered in labour with pethidine.

procidentia complete uterine prolapse with the cervix protruding through the vulva.

procreation act of begetting young.

proctalgia pain in the rectum.

proctitis inflammation of the anus or rectum.

proctoscope instrument for examination of the rectum.

prodromal preceding. *P. symptom* warning symptom, e.g. visual disturbances occurring before ECLAMPSIA.

profession specialised knowledge, skills and attitudes pertinent to the practice of a specific role, usually requiring academic preparation in the underlying scientific and historical principles; members are required to undertake continuing study to expand the body of knowledge, to practise autonomously and to behave in accordance with expected standards.

professional development portfolio individual resumé of personal professional education and other relevant experiences, including learning acquired through reflection on and in practice; mandatory requirement of the Nursing and Midwifery Council (NMC) for all midwives, nurses and health visitors; supervisors of midwives or an officer from the NMC can request to examine the profile to ensure it is being maintained.

profibrinolysin plasminogen, precursor of fibrinolysin.

profile 1. simple outline, e.g. side view of head or face. 2. graph representing quantitatively a set of characteristics determined by tests. 3. record of achievements developed during or after a course of study. *See* PROFESSIONAL DEVELOPMENT PORTFOLIO.

progeny issue; descendants.

progesterone female sex hormone essential for maintaining pregnancy, produced from the corpus luteum and placenta; promotes formation and maintenance of the decidua, development of the glandular breast tissue, relaxation of plain muscle throughout the body and retention of water and electrolytes in the tissues. During the menstrual cycle it regulates endometrial secretory changes in preparation for the reception of a fertilised ovum.

progesterone-only contraceptive continuous daily oral contraceptive pills prescribed when combined oestrogen and progesterone contraceptive pills are contraindicated, e.g. during breast-feeding; should be taken at the same time every day to reduce the higher risk of failure that occurs than with the combined pill.

progestogen any substance having progestational activity.

prognosis forecast of the course and duration of a disease.

projectile vomiting *See* VOMITING.

prolactin anterior pituitary gland hormone that stimulates and sustains milk production.

prolapse descent of an organ or structure. *Umbilical cord p.* cord that lies below the fetal presenting part, occurring after rupture of the membranes; danger of fetal HYPOXIA or ANOXIA due to cord compression and immediate

Uterovaginal prolapse

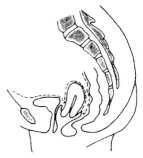

185

delivery of the baby is required. *Rectal p.* protrusion of rectal mucosa and muscle through the anal canal to the exterior. *Arm p.* serious complication of uncorrected shoulder presentation in which the fetal arm falls into or through the vagina. *Uterine p.* protrusion of the uterus into the lower part of the vagina due to weakening of ligaments and the pelvic floor; the uterus, vaginal walls, bladder or rectum may be involved.

proliferation rapid multiplication of cells, as in a malignant growth.

prolonged labour labour lasting more than 24 hours, resulting from inadequate or incoordinate uterine action, cephalopelvic disproportion or a poorly fitting presenting part, as in malpresentation or malposition. The midwife must ensure that the mother receives adequate pain relief, that progress is being made and that maternal and fetal conditions are satisfactory. Fetal risks include hypoxia and trauma, especially excessive skull moulding causing intracranial haemorrhage; maternal risks include exhaustion, dehydration, uterine rupture and physical trauma, leading to long-term uterine, cervical or urinary tract problems.

prolonged pregnancy pregnancy lasting 42 weeks (294 days) or more from the first day of the last normal menstrual period; induction of labour is only necessary when either the maternal or fetal condition is compromised.

promazine hydrochloride tranquilliser, phenothiazine derivative; often given with pethidine in labour to combat nausea and vomiting, in doses of 25–50 mg intramuscularly.

promethazine hydrochloride (Phenergan) antihistamine, phenothiazine derivative; often allied with pethidine in labour; also used to treat vomiting in pregnancy.

promontory projection. *Sacral p.* important pelvic landmark formed by the projection of the upper border of the first sacral vertebra.

pronation turning downwards. *P. of the hand* downwards flexion of the hand.

prone lying face downwards.

pronucleus haploid nucleus of a sex cell.

prophylactic pertaining to prophylaxis, preventative.

prophylaxis measures taken to prevent a disease; preventive treatment.

propranolol beta-adrenergic blocking agent used to treat hypertension and some cardiac conditions.

propylthiouracil thyroid inhibitor used to treat thyrotoxicosis.

prostacyclin potent vasodilator and inhibitor of platelet aggregation; an intermediate in the metabolic pathway of arachidonic acid, formed from prostaglandin endoperoxides in the artery and vein walls.

prostaglandins oxytocic substances present in menstrual blood, amniotic fluid, semen and many other cells; used to induce abortion before 10 weeks and to ripen the cervix and induce labour.

prostate gland male gland surrounding the bladder neck and prostatic urethra, which contributes secretions to seminal fluid.

prosthesis artificial replacement of, or substitute for, a missing part. adj. *prosthetic.*

Prostin E *See* PROSTAGLANDINS.

protamine sulphate antidote to heparin overdosage.

protease proteolytic enzyme in the digestive juices, which causes protein breakdown.

protein material composed of carbon, hydrogen, nitrogen and oxygen; the essential constituent of body tissue, obtained from dietary sources, e.g. meat, fish, milk, eggs, peas, beans and lentils, and broken down into 20 amino acids, e.g. PHENYLALANINE and TYROSINE, which facilitate growth of new cells and repair of others; excess amino acids are broken down by the liver and excreted in the urine as urea. Proteins in blood plasma are classified as specific protein carriers, involved in transport of hormones and other substances; acute-phase reactants, e.g. alpha-1-antitrypsin or fibrinogen, involved in inflammation or clotting; complement components; and immunoglobulins. Albumin helps to maintain normal water distribution by exerting osmotic pressure at the capillary membrane, preventing plasma fluid from leaking out of the capillaries into the intercellular spaces.

proteinuria protein, usually albumin, in urine.

proteus Gram-negative bacteria in faecal and other putrefying matter.

prothrombin plasma protein synthesised in the liver, vital for blood clotting: when activated by thromboplastin, which is released when tissues are damaged and platelets broken down, and in the presence of calcium it forms thrombin; the thrombin, with fibrinogen, then forms insoluble fibrin. *P.time* time, in seconds, required for a specimen of blood brought into contact with thromboplastin to clot.

prothrombinase thromboplastin.

protocol agreement between parties; multidisciplinary planned course of suggested action in relation to specific situations.

proton positively-charged particle forming part of the nucleus of an atom.

protoplasm essential chemical compound of which living cells are made.

provider self-governing trusts, directly-managed units and private institutions that provide health-care services for those wishing to purchase them. *See also* PURCHASER.

proximal in anatomy, nearest that point considered to be the centre of a system; opposite of distal.

pruritus skin irritation; may affect the whole body surface, e.g. as in certain skin and nervous disorders, or be localised. *P. vulvae* localised vulval irritation, associated in pregnancy with glycosuria or THRUSH.

pseudo- prefix meaning 'false'.

pseudocyesis false pregnancy; subjective symptoms in the absence of conception.

pseudohermaphroditism apparently having male and female characteristics; INTERSEX.

pseudomenstruation blood-stained vaginal discharge occurring on about the third day of life in baby girls due to withdrawal of maternal oestrogens.

Pseudomonas Gram-negative, aerobic bacteria, some species of which are pathogenic for plants and vertebrates.

psoas muscle forming part of the posterior abdominal wall.

psoriasis chronic recurrent non-infectious skin disease of unknown cause, characterised by reddish marginated patches with profuse silvery scaling on extensor surfaces such as knees or elbows, but can be more widespread.

psyche conscious and unconscious mind.

psychiatrist doctor who specialises in psychiatry.

psychiatry study of mental disorders and their treatment.

psychologist one who studies normal and abnormal mental processes, development and behaviour.

psychology science of the mind and its functions.

psychomotor pertaining to motor effects of cerebral or psychic activity.

psychopath person with an antisocial personality.

psychoprophylaxis educational method of preparation for labour aimed at preventing pain and modifying the perception of painful sensations associated with normal uncomplicated childbirth.

psychosexual relating to mental aspects of sexual activity.

psychosis severe mental illness affecting the whole personality; of organic or emotional origin and marked by personality derangement, loss of contact with reality, delusions, hallucinations or illusions. adj. *psychotic*.

psychosomatic relating to the mind and the body. *P. disorders* illnesses in which emotional factors have a profound influence.

psychotherapy related techniques for treating mental illness by psychological methods; rely on establishing communication between therapist and patient as a means of understanding and modifying behaviour.

ptosis drooping of the upper eyelid from third nerve paralysis; dropping downwards of an organ or other structure.

ptyalin salivary ENZYME that starts digestion of starches.

ptyalism abnormally increased salivation, often associated in pregnancy with nausea and vomiting and HYPER-EMESIS GRAVIDARUM.

puberty age at which the reproductive organs become functionally active, usually 10–14 years.

pubes region over the pubic bones.

pubic pertaining to the pubes, e.g. *p. arch* bony arch formed by the junction of the *inferior pubic rami*, forming the anterior part of the pelvic outlet.

pubiotomy cutting through the pubic bone to enable birth to take place.

pubis anterior portion of the hip bone; pubic bone.

public health field of medicine concerned with safeguarding and improving physical, mental and social well-being of the community as a whole; environmental aspects are local authority responsibility and communicable disease control is supervised by the medical officer for environmental health; central government formulates national policy and is responsible for international aspects.

pubococcygeus one part of the levator ani muscle extending from the symphysis pubis to the coccyx.

pubovesical pertaining to the pubis and bladder.

pudenda external genitalia.

pudendal pertaining to the external genital organs. *P. block* local analgesia induced by injecting a solution of 0.5% or 1% lidocaine (lignocaine) around the pudendal nerve.

pudendum external genitalia of a woman.

puerperal pertaining to the puerperium. *P. pyrexia* rise of temperature in the puerperium. *P. psychosis* psychosis appearing in the puerperium. *P. sepsis* infection of the genital tract following childbirth.

puerperium 6- to 8-week period following childbirth during which the uterus and other organs and structures are returning to the non-pregnant state.

pulmonary pertaining to or affecting the lungs. *P. circulation see* CIRCULA-TION. *P. embolism see* EMBOLISM. *P. infarction* death of tissue caused by occlusion of a small blood vessel in the lung by a clot. *P. tuberculosis see* TUBERCULOSIS.

pulsation beating or throbbing.

pulse local rhythmic arterial expansion, felt digitally in any artery sufficiently near the surface of the body, corresponding to each contraction of the left ventricle of the heart. Normal rate is about 72 per minute in adults, 130 in infants and 80 in older children. *P. pressure* difference between diastolic and systolic blood pressures, measured by the sphygmomanometer.

puncture to pierce. *Lumbar p.* procedure to remove cerebrospinal fluid from between the third and fourth or fourth and fifth lumbar vertebrae for diagnostic purposes or to relieve cerebral pressure.

pupil opening in the centre of the iris through which light enters the eye.

purchaser health authorities that purchase health-care services from PROVIDERS; responsible for identifying total health needs of the resident population, planning and securing the best and most cost-effective services within the area.

purgative drug that produces evacuation of the bowels.

purine heterocyclic compound that is the nucleus of the purine bases such as adenine and guanine, which occur in DNA and RNA.

purpura haemorrhagica condition characterised by extravasation of blood in skin and mucous membranes, causing purple spots and patches; sometimes associated with deficiency of THROMBOCYTES (THROMBOCYTOPENIA).

purulent containing or resembling pus.

pus thick, semi-liquid substance of dead leucocytes, bacteria, cell debris and tissue fluids, resulting from inflammation caused by invading bacteria, which destroy phagocytes and cause local suppuration.

pustule small, elevated, circumscribed, pus-containing lesion of the skin.

putative supposed, reputed. *P. father* man believed to be the father of an illegitimate child.

pyaemia condition resulting from invasion of the bloodstream by bacteria, which causes blockage of small blood vessels and results in abscess formation, leading to rigors and high fever.

pyelitis inflammation of the renal pelvis; PYELONEPHRITIS.

pyelography radiology of the renal pelvis after the injection of radio-opaque contrast medium. *Intravenous p.* investigative procedure in which water-soluble, iodine-containing contrast medium is injected intravenously and radiographs are taken as the contrast medium is excreted by the kidneys and passes down the ureters into the bladder.

pyelonephritis inflammation of the kidneys and ureters, usually caused by *ESCHERICHIA COLI*; acute symptoms include severe lumbar pain, hyperpyrexia, rigors, tachycardia, vomiting, general malaise; chronic symptoms include backache, vomiting, anaemia; may occur in pregnancy between 18 and 24 weeks' gestation, due to stasis of urine in the dilated and relaxed ureters and pressure from the pregnant uterus, particularly on the right side, which triggers multiplication of bacteria. Asymptomatic bacteriuria may occur in early pregnancy and all women should be screened and treated as necessary. Also occurs in newborn babies, with no obvious signs; the condition may be suspected in any baby who is pale, not feeding well, losing weight and generally not thriving.

pyelonephrosis any disease of the kidney and its pelvis.

pyloric stenosis congenital hypertrophic pyloric stenosis; occurs in 3 in 1000 births. Affected babies have a thickened, strengthened pyloric sphincter, enlarged stomach and palpable pylorus; waves of peristalsis can be seen abdominally during feeding and persistent projectile vomiting occurs; these signs rarely occur before 3–4 weeks of age. Anti-spasmodic drugs (e.g. atropine) may be given with feeds but RAMSTEDT'S OPERATION is often necessary for rapid and complete recovery.

pylorus opening between the stomach and the duodenum.

pyo- prefix meaning 'pus'.

pyogenic producing pus.

pyometra pus in the uterus.

pyosalpinx   pus in the fallopian tube.

pyretic   pertaining to fever.

pyrexia   fever; a rise of body temperature above 37.2°C (99°F).

pyridoxine   vitamin B6; used in the prophylaxis and treatment of vitamin B6 deficiency.

pyrogen   fever-producing substance, possibly of bacterial origin.

pyuria   presence of pus in urine, which becomes cloudy; pus cells will be seen if the urine is examined microscopically.

q

QRS complex group of three distinct waves depicted on an electrocardiogram, created by passage of cardiac electrical impulses through the ventricles. Occurs at the beginning of each contraction of the ventricles; R wave is normally the most prominent.

quadrant one-quarter of the circumference of a circle or of an area such as the abdominal surface.

quadruple test Down's syndrome screening test, the TRIPLE TEST with an additional serum MARKER, INHIBIN A; may be performed as part of the INTEGRATED TEST.

quadruplets four children born at the same labour; more common with the increased use of fertility drugs.

qualitative research systematic subjective research approach, used to describe human life experiences and promote understanding of subjective experiences, e.g. pain, caring, powerlessness, comfort.

quality assurance pledge to the public to work towards optimal achievable degrees of excellence in the (health) services provided, in such a way that standards of care and norms of professional behaviour can be measured according to predefined criteria so that client care can be improved.

Quality Assurance Agency organisation that approves higher education institutions offering courses and awards; has established codes of practice and guidance for programme development, and a Department of Health contract to carry out subject review in England.

quantitative fluorescence polymerase chain reaction (QF-PCR) diagnostic chromosome test used to identify TRISOMY and sex chromosome ANEUPLOIDY; results are usually available within 48 hours of chorionic villus sampling or amniocentesis. The polymerase chain reaction is used to amplify small samples of DNA labelled with fluorescent dyes, which are then analysed; measurements of specific regions on the DNA molecules are displayed in graph form, showing the number of specific chromosomes in each cell. Heavily bloodstained samples may interfere with analysis.

quantitative research formal objective systematic research approach in which numerical data are utilised to obtain information, describe variables, examine relationships among variables, and determine cause and effect interactions between variables; often thought to provide a sounder knowledge base for health-care practice than QUALITATIVE RESEARCH.

quarantine period during which known infected persons, contacts and suspects are isolated to prevent the spread of infection.

Quetelet index body mass index calculated by dividing the weight in kilograms by height in metres squared. The healthy range is considered to be between 20 and 24.9; those below 20 are underweight, those between 25 and 30 are overweight, those over 30 are obese, and those over 40 are severely obese.

'quickening' first perceptible fetal movements, felt by the mother at approximately 18–20 weeks' gestation in primigravidae and between 16 and 18 weeks in multigravidae.

quintuplets five children born at the same labour.

quotient number obtained by division. *Intelligence q. (IQ)* numerical expression of intellectual capacity obtained by multiplying assessed mental age by 100 and dividing by chronological age.

racemose grape-like. *R. cells* those arranged round a central duct. *R. glands* compound, lobulated in structure, e.g. salivary glands, cells of the breasts, glands of the cervix.

rachi(o)- word element meaning 'spine'.

rachitic pelvis bony pelvis with a flat pelvic brim, similar to a platypelloid pelvis, caused by rickets in early childhood.

radial relating to the radius. *R. artery* artery at the wrist. *R. palsy* palsy characterised by wrist drop; seen soon after birth, usually recovers spontaneously over a varying time.

radical dealing with the root or cause of a disease. *R. cure* curing by complete removal of the cause.

radioactive emitting electromagnetic waves, alpha (α), beta (β) or gamma (γ), either naturally, e.g. radium, or artificially by bombardment in an atomic pile, e.g. radioactive iodine (^{131}I).

radiograph picture taken by X-rays.

radiographer professional health-care worker in a diagnostic X-ray department (diagnostic radiographer) or in a radiotherapy department (therapy radiographer).

radiography examination by means of Röntgen or X-rays, rarely performed in pregnancy, except occasionally in the third trimester, because of possible adverse fetal effects.

radioimmunoassay (RIA) sensitive assay method used to measure minute quantities of specific antibodies or any antigen, e.g. hormone or drug, against which specific antibodies can be raised; standard clinical laboratory test for measuring hormones and also used for therapeutic drug monitoring and drug abuse screening.

radioisotope radioactive form of an element consisting of unstable atoms that undergo radioactive decay emitting alpha, beta or gamma radiation, occurring naturally, e.g. radium and uranium, or created artificially.

radio-opaque capable of obstructing the passage of X-rays.

radiotelemetry measurement based on data transmitted by radio waves from the subject to the recording apparatus; radiotelemetry of the fetal heart may be used when the mother is ambulant in labour.

radiotherapy treatment of disease (mainly malignant) with ionising radiation, e.g. X-rays, beta rays, gamma rays, either directed from outside the patient's body or by means of an isotope implanted or instilled into an abnormal tissue or body cavity.

radium metallic element, symbol Ra; a naturally occurring RADIOACTIVE metal.

Ramstedt's operation division of a hypertrophied pyloric sphincter to relieve PYLORIC STENOSIS.

ramus branch, as of the pubic bone, which has an upper and lower branch. pl. *rami*.

random blood sugar test blood glucose test undertaken when a pregnant mother presents with unexplained glycosuria; if the result is suspicious a glucose load or glucose tolerance test may be performed.

randomised controlled trial research trial in which subjects to be studied are chosen at random from a suitable group of potential participants with the aim of increasing the extent to which the sample is representative of the target population; usually involves a control and an experimental group; rarely possible to obtain a purely random sample for clinical studies because of informed consent requirements.

ranitidine H_2 receptor antagonist, given to women in labour before general anaesthesia to inhibit hydrochloric acid production, thus reducing the risk of MENDELSON'S SYNDROME.

rape sexual assault or abuse; criminal forcible sexual intercourse.

raphe seam or ridge of tissue indicating the juncture of two equal parts, e.g. median raphe of the perineal body, anococcygeal raphe.

rash temporary skin eruption. *Heat r.* miliaria. *Napkin r.* cutaneous localised reaction of the baby's buttocks, caused by irritants such as ammonia in decomposed urine and improperly washed nappies, etc. *Nettle r.* urticaria.

raspberry leaf tea herbal preparation sometimes taken in pregnancy to tone and prepare the uterus for labour, facilitating cervical ripening and enhancing uterine efficiency; should be commenced at about 30 weeks' gestation, increased gradually to a maximum of 4 cups daily, but decreased if Braxton Hicks contractions become excessively strong; contraindicated in women with a uterine scar, history of preterm or precipitate labour, multiple pregnancy, antepartum haemorrhage or if elective Caesarean section is indicated.

raspberry mark congenital haemangioma.

Rastelli's operation surgical procedure to treat transposition of the great vessels, in which blood circulation through the heart is diverted to effect adequate oxygenation.

rate speed or frequency with which an event or circumstance occurs per unit of time, population or other standard of comparison. *Basal metabolic r.*

(BMR) rate at which oxygen is utilised in a fasting subject at complete rest expressed as a percentage of a value established as normal for such a subject. *Birth r.* number of live births in a population in a specified period of time (crude birth rate), in the female population (refined birth rate) or in the female population of childbearing age (true birth rate), usually expressed per year per 1000 of the estimated mid-year population. *Death r., mortality r.* number of deaths per stated number of persons (1000 or 10 000, or 100 000) in a certain region in a certain time period (crude death rate); allowances may be made for age and sex distribution in the population (standardised death rate). *Glomerular filtration r.* quantity of glomerular filtrate formed each minute in the kidney nephrons, calculated by measuring the clearance of specific substances, e.g. insulin or creatinine.

ratio expression of the quantity of one substance or entity in relation to that of another; relationship between two quantities expressed as the quotient of one divided by the other. *Lecithin-sphingomyelin r.* ratio of lecithin to sphingomyelin in amniotic fluid.

reabsorption process of absorbing again, e.g. absorption by the kidneys of substances (glucose, proteins, sodium, etc.) already secreted into the renal tubules.

reaction counteraction; response to application of a stimulus; evidence of acidity or alkalinity; pH of a solution.

reagent substance employed to produce a chemical reaction to detect, measure or produce other substances.

real-time scanner ULTRASOUND scanner that gives a moving visual display.

receptor 1. molecule on the surface of or within a cell that recognises and binds to specific molecules, producing some effect in the cell, e.g. the cell-surface receptors of immuno-competent cells that recognise antigens, complement components or lymphokines, or receptors of neurons and target organs that recognise neurotransmitters or hormones. 2. sensory nerve ending that responds to various stimuli.

recession receding or drawing back. *Rib r.* or *sternal r.* inwards movement of the ribs, commonly seen in RESPIRATORY DISTRESS SYNDROME of neonates.

recessive tending to recede; in genetics the opposite of dominant – capable of expression only when carried by both of a pair of homologous chromosomes, i.e. HOMOZYGOUS and not HETEROZYGOUS.

recipient one who receives, e.g. a blood transfusion, tissue or organ graft. *Universal r.* person thought to be able to receive blood of any type without agglutination of the donor cells.

recombinant 1. new cell or individual resulting from genetic recombination. 2. pertaining or relating to such cells or individuals. *R. DNA technology* process of taking a gene from one organism and inserting it into the DNA of another; gene splicing.

rectal relating to the rectum. *R. examination* digital examination of the rectum or adjacent structures.

rectocele hernia of the rectum caused by overstretching of the vaginal wall at childbirth, treated by posterior colporrhaphy.

rectovaginal pertaining to the rectum and vagina. *R. fistula See* FISTULA.

rectovesical pertaining to or communicating with the rectum and bladder.

rectum lower 15 cm (6 in) of the large intestine extending from the pelvic colon to the anal canal.

rectus abdominis pair of muscles running vertically on either side of the midline from symphysis pubis to xiphisternum; in combination with other abdominal muscles they raise

Rectocele

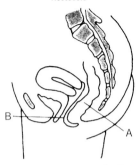

A, rectum; **B**, posterior vaginal wall.

intra-abdominal pressure and assist in flexing the spine; poor muscle tone will adversely affect flexion of the lumbar spine and cause difficulty with pelvic tilting, leading to increased lumbar lordosis and postural problems in pregnancy.

recumbent lying down.

recurrent occurring again.

reduction correction of a fracture, dislocation or hernia.

referred pain pain occurring at a distance from the place of origin, related to distribution of sensory nerves.

reflection process of conscious, systematic thinking about one's actions; review, analysis and synthesis of situations that have occurred, usually after an event; active process by which midwives learn from experience, with a view to improving future practice.

reflex reflected or thrown back. *R. action* involuntary movement resulting from a stimulus, e.g. knee jerk, or from withdrawal of a limb from a pinprick; certain reflexes are present in the term baby, e.g. sucking, swallowing and MORO REFLEXES.

Conditioned r. reflex acquired by regular association of a physiological event with an unrelated outside event, e.g. the draught or milk ejection reflex causes myoepithelial cells in the breast to contract at the sight or sound of a hungry baby, mobilising the milk into the lacteal sinuses where it is immediately available to the baby.

reflexology, reflex zone therapy complementary therapy in which the feet (or hands) represent a map of the rest of the body; by manually working on the feet (or hands) other parts of the body can be influenced and treated; particularly beneficial for stress-related conditions, e.g. hypertension, and mechanical problems, e.g. constipation; in midwifery it may be used to treat urinary retention or to stimulate the pituitary gland in labour or for lactation.

regional anaesthesia epidural, spinal or caudal analgesia.

register epidemiological index of all cases with a particular disease or condition in a defined population.

registered midwife midwife registered to practise in the country in which she resides; she must also be eligible to practise by complying with the mandatory requirements of the RULES FOR MIDWIVES.

registrar of births, marriages and deaths official recorder of births, marriages and deaths in England and Wales, part of the Office for National Statistics, which also regulates and records civil marriages, conducts demographic research and analyses demographic material. Local registry offices are found in most towns; births must be registered within 6 weeks in England (21 days in Scotland).

regulatory body organisation responsible for defining and monitoring preparation and practice of a specific professional group, e.g. Nursing and Midwifery Council, General Medical Council, Health Professions Council.

regurgitation backward flow, e.g. of food into the mouth from the stomach; sometimes occurs in newborn babies, associated with weakness of the cardia of the stomach. *Aortic r.* backward flow of blood into the left ventricle when the aortic valve is incompetent. *Mitral r. see* MITRAL. *Gastro-oesophageal r. see* HEARTBURN.

rehabilitation re-education.

relapse return of a disease following an apparent recovery.

relaxant causing relaxation. *Muscle r.* agent that acts at the neuromuscular junction causing muscle paralysis, such as is used in anaesthesia, or that relieves muscle spasticity and tension by acting directly on muscle or, more commonly, on the central nervous system.

relaxation lessening of tension, e.g. of muscles after they have contracted. Antenatal classes often teach relaxation techniques to prepare the mother for labour. *See also* PSYCHOPROPHYLAXIS.

relaxin hormone thought to cause 'softening' of pelvic tissues and joints in pregnancy, facilitating some increase in pelvic capacity; cause of lumbar lordosis.

releasing factor substance produced in the hypothalamus that causes the anterior pituitary gland to release hormones.

reliability research issue concerned with consistency, dependability, accuracy and comparability of tests or investigations.

renal concerning or affecting the kidney. *R. calculus* kidney stone. *R. disease in pregnancy* rare but serious problem; women already undergoing dialysis have a poor prognosis for successful pregnancy outcome; those who have had a renal transplant have a better prognosis of achieving a live healthy baby. Disease often follows a history of childhood nephritis;

proteinuria is present from early pregnancy; risks include miscarriage, pre-eclampsia, placental abruption, intrauterine growth retardation, fetal death and long-term renal impairment. *R. failure* failure of renal function, giving rise to uraemia. *R. threshold* the level of substances in the blood beyond which they are excreted in the urine; *normal r. threshold* for glucose is 10 mmol/L (180 mg/100 mL): glycosuria results if it exceeds this.

renin enzyme synthesised, stored and secreted by the kidneys that helps to regulate blood pressure by catalysing the conversion of angiotensinogen to angiotensin I, which is in turn converted to angiotensin II, a powerful vasoconstrictor; also stimulates aldosterone secretion, which causes retention of salt and water by the kidneys.

rennin milk-curdling enzyme found in gastric juice of babies; catalyses conversion of casein from a soluble to insoluble form.

reproduction process of producing a new individual of the same kind; creation of a similar object or situation; duplication; replication.

reproductive organs, female ovaries, producing ova or eggs, uterine tubes, uterus, vagina and vulva, comprising the external genitalia; breasts are secondary sexual characteristics, enclosing the mammary glands. *R. o.'s, male* external genitalia (penis, testes and scrotum), accessory glands that secrete special fluids, and ducts through which these organs and glands are connected to each other and through which the spermatozoa are ejaculated during sexual intercourse.

Rescue Remedy liquid Bach flower remedy thought to reduce acute stress, panic, anxiety and hysteria; useful when the mother is especially anxious or nervous; dose: 4 drops neat on the tongue, added to a glass of water or applied neat to temples or wrists;

remedy is preserved in brandy so contraindicated in those with a moral or medical reason to avoid alcohol.

research method of increasing available knowledge through discovery of new information via systematic scientific enquiry.

resection removal of a part.

residential care (for children) care provided by local authority social services departments or registered voluntary organisations for children up to age 18; residential nurseries are provided for under 5 year olds, and community homes and hostels for children between 5 and 18 years; boarding with foster parents is arranged whenever possible.

residual remaining. *R. urine* urine remaining in the bladder after micturition.

resistance power to overcome; natural power of the body to withstand and recover from infection or disease; ability of bacteria to become insensitive to antibiotics, e.g. some staphylococci are resistant to penicillin.

respiration breathing; exchange of OXYGEN and CARBON DIOXIDE between the atmosphere and body cells, including inspiration and expiration, diffusion of oxygen from the pulmonary alveoli to the blood and of carbon dioxide from the blood to the alveoli, and transport of oxygen to and carbon dioxide from the body cells. *Inspiration* involves contraction of external intercostal muscles (which raise the ribs and sternum) and the diaphragm, which descends. *Expiration* involves contraction of internal intercostal muscles, descent of the ribs and relaxation of the diaphragm. The normal respiration rate in adults is 16 breaths per minute at rest; in neonates it is 40–50. *Artificial r.* respiratory movements produced by artificial means.

respiratory distress syndrome (RDS) condition occurring mainly in preterm babies due to lack of SURFACTANT, but also in babies of diabetic mothers or those born by Caesarean section; onset of respiratory difficulty occurs within 4 hours of birth, gradually worsening.

restitution restoration, putting right; movement of the fetal head after delivery in the anteroposterior diameter, to correct its position in relation to the shoulders.

resuscitation restoration from a state of collapse. *Neonatal r.* necessary if the baby fails to breathe after birth; occurs particularly in preterm babies because of immaturity of the lungs, respiratory centre and respiratory muscles. Also required for medullary depression asphyxia, caused by maternal intrapartum drugs that depress the fetal respiratory centre, which can be reversed by antagonist administration; hypoxia from fetal distress; and intracranial intrapartum damage, particularly due to excessive or abnormal moulding. *See* Appendix 7.

retained placenta placenta that fails to be expelled within the expected time limit, dependent on whether the third stage of labour was actively or passively managed. May be caused by placenta accreta, increta or percreta, requiring MANUAL REMOVAL under anaesthetic or, occasionally, hysterectomy. More commonly, the placenta is partially separated as a result of poor uterine action and inadequate uterine contraction following birth of the baby, causing haemorrhage and maternal shock; treated with manual stimulation *per abdomen* or administration of oxytocic drugs to encourage the uterus to contract so that the placenta separates and can be delivered. *See also* POSTPARTUM HAEMORRHAGE, Appendix 6.

retained products of conception tissue retained in the uterus following birth of the baby (*see* RETAINED PLACENTA) or after miscarriage, when evacuation of retained products will be required; uterus will feel 'boggy' when palpated abdominally; abnormal vaginal bleeding may occur. *See also* POSTPARTUM HAEMORRHAGE, Appendix 6.

retardation delay. *Mental r.* subnormal, delayed, intellectual development, leading to impaired learning, social adjustment or maturation.

retching involuntary, spasmodic, ineffectual effort to vomit.

retention holding back. *R. of urine* inability to pass urine, occasionally due to obstruction or, more commonly in obstetrics, neurological damage from overstretching of the urethra and trigone, leading to diminished bladder sensation and perineal discomfort; catheterisation may be necessary but should be avoided if possible, as chronic urinary tract infection can occur as a result, leading to renal failure in severe cases.

reticular resembling a net.

reticuloendothelial system network of tissues and cells found throughout the body, especially in blood, general connective tissue, spleen, liver, lungs, bone marrow and lymph nodes. Large cells are concerned with blood cell formation and destruction, storage of fatty materials, metabolism of iron and pigment, inflammation and immunity; some cells are motile and phagocytic, i.e. they can ingest and destroy unwanted foreign material; spleen cells help to dispose of disintegrated erythrocytes; Küpffer cells in the liver cavities, along with cells of the general connective tissue and bone marrow, are capable of transforming haemoglobin released by disintegrated erythrocytes into bile pigment.

retina inner lining of the eyeball formed of nerve cells and fibres from which the optic nerve leaves the eyeball and passes to the visual area of the cerebral cortex; the impression of the image is focused upon it.

retinopathy general pathological conditions of the retina that may occur with some systemic disorders, e.g. hypertension, severe pre-eclampsia, eclampsia, diabetes. *R. of prematurity* neonatal condition caused by vasoconstriction of retinal capillaries due to very high concentrations of oxygen, which produces overgrowth of blood vessels in the retina; vascular proliferation and exudation of blood and serum detaches the retina, producing scarring and inevitable blindness. Careful monitoring of the oxygen tension level is essential in preterm babies as it is not known what dosage of oxygen will prevent retinal changes.

retraction drawing back; process of permanent progressive shortening of uterine muscle accompanying contractions during labour: dilates the cervix, expels the fetus, separates the placenta and controls bleeding; over-retraction in obstructed labour may cause a *r. ring* to become apparent. See BANDL'S RING.

retractor surgical instrument for drawing apart wound edges to make deeper structures more accessible.

retro- prefix meaning 'behind' or 'backward', e.g. retroversion of the uterus.

retroflexion bent backwards, e.g. when the uterine corpus is bent backwards at an acute angle with the cervix in its normal position.

retrograde going backwards. *R. pyelography* radiography of the kidney and ureter after injection of radio-opaque dye into the renal pelvis.

retrolental behind the lens of the eye. *R. fibroplasia* See RETINOPATHY OF PREMATURITY.

retroplacental behind the placenta. *R. clot* clot of blood behind the placenta.

retrospection morbid dwelling on memories, looking back.

retroversion turning back, as when the uterus is tilted backwards. cf. RETROFLEXION.

Retroversion of uterus

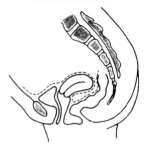

retroverted gravid uterus pregnant uterus tilted backwards; a common occurrence, with the uterus usually spontaneously correcting to an anteverted position; if retroversion persists, INCARCERATION of the retroverted gravid uterus develops, with retention of urine.

retrovirus large group of RNA viruses, including human T-cell leukaemia viruses, lentiviruses and human immunodeficiency virus (HIV).

Rhesus factor three pairs of antigens (Cc, Dd, Ee) in human blood; if present the blood is Rhesus positive, denoted with capital letters (C, D, E), and, if absent, it is Rhesus negative, denoted with lower case letters (c, d, e); about 83% of Caucasians and 99–100% of other races are Rhesus positive. D antigen is responsible for Rhesus immunity in most cases.

rheumatism muscular and joint pains; fibrositis. *Acute r.* acute rheumatic fever associated with streptococcal infection, chorea or acute tonsillitis; causes acute rheumatic ENDOCARDITIS, myocarditis, pericarditis; MITRAL STENOSIS and aortic incompetence may occur later. Any woman with a history of childhood rheumatic fever must be carefully assessed in pregnancy as extra strain is exerted on the heart.

rhinitis inflammation of the nasal mucous membrane, sometimes of staphylococcal origin and occurring in the newborn baby.

rhomboid of Michaelis diamond- or dome-shaped area at the base of the spine marked by dimpling of the skin, with the spinous process of the fifth lumbar vertebra beneath the superior angle; the posterior superior iliac spines are palpable under the lateral angles; inferiorly is the beginning of the gluteal cleft; may be observed in the second stage of labour and represents posterior displacement of the sacrum and coccyx as the fetal occiput moves into the sacral curve; appears to cause the mother to arch her back, push her buttocks forwards and outstretch her arms.

rhythm measured movement; recurrence of an action or function at regular intervals. adj. *rhythmic, rhythmical*. *R. method of family planning* natural method of contraception involving calculation of the 'safe' period during which conception is least likely, daily temperature monitoring and observation of the mucoid discharge from the vagina, i.e. Billings' method.

ribs twelve paired bones extending from the thoracic vertebrae toward the median line on the ventral aspect of the trunk, forming the major part of the thoracic skeleton; costal bones.

riboflavin vitamin B2, required by certain enzymes that catalyse many oxidation–reduction reactions; present in liver, kidney, heart, brewer's yeast, milk, eggs, greens, enriched cereals.

ribonucleic acid (RNA) nucleic acid of a cell, which translates the 'code' of DEOXYRIBONUCLEIC ACID (DNA) into action.

ribosome minute granule in cell cytoplasm concerned with protein synthesis; can be seen with an electron microscope.

rickets rachitis; disease of deficient calcification of bone due to lack of vitamin D, which is necessary for the proper absorption of calcium and phosphorus, leading to bony deformities of skull, ribs, legs and pelvis. Can be prevented by vitamin D administration and exposure to sunlight or ultraviolet light.

rigor sudden shivering attack with rapidly rising temperature, which plateaus then declines following a period of sweating; may occur in severe pyelonephritis in pregnancy or in puerperal SEPTICAEMIA. *R. mortis* body stiffening occurring soon after death, caused by muscle protoplasm coagulation.

risk management structured approach to health care to reduce identifiable risks; helps prevent problems arising and reduces incidence of complaints and consequent litigation costs. Involves agreeing standards of care based on current research to support clinical guidelines; undertaking systematic reviews of clinical records; initiating case discussions and case conferences in the event of adverse outcomes to treatment; undertaking assessments of health and safety; developing training programmes for staff.

ritodrine hydrochloride (Yutopar) beta-2-adrenergic receptor stimulant that decreases uterine activity, prolonging gestation in preterm labour.

Ritter's disease exfoliative dermatitis; rare, severe form of PEMPHIGUS NEONATORUM.

Robert's pelvis abnormal pelvis in which there is bilateral absence of the sacral alae with fusion of the sacrum to the ilium on each side; prevents engagement of the fetal head.

rockerbottom feet prominent heels in babies with chromosomal disorders such as Edward's syndrome (trisomy 18) and Patau's syndrome (trisomy 13).

Rogitine phentolamine; adrenolytic used to test for phaechromocytoma.

Röntgen rays X-RAYS.

rooming-in term used when the baby remains with the mother rather than being cared for in a nursery, which encourages development of the mother–infant relationship.

rooting reflex neonatal reflex elicited by stroking the cheek or side of the mouth: the baby turns to the stimulated side and opens his mouth ready to suckle.

rotation turning of a body on its long axis, as in turning of the fetal head (or presenting part) for proper orientation to the pelvic axis, usually occurring naturally, but occasionally achieved through manual or instrumental manipulation.

rotator muscle that causes rotation of any part.

rotavirus virus that looks like a wheel under the microscope; one of the commonest causes of acute infantile diarrhoea, often preceded by respiratory signs.

Rothera's test test for presence of acetone in urine.

roughage indigestible vegetable fibre; cellulose; gives bulk to the diet and stimulates peristalsis; found in bran, cereals, fruit and vegetable fibres.

round ligaments ligaments extending from the cornua of the uterus to the labia majora.

Royal College of Midwives (RCM) professional body and trade union solely for midwives, concerned with education, standards of professional practice and negotiation of conditions of service and salaries; founded in 1881. *See* Appendix 13.

Royal College of Nursing – Midwifery Society division of the Royal College of Nursing devoted to needs of members who are midwives.

rubella German measles; mild infective disease causing a faint macular body rash and enlargement of the posterior cervical lymph nodes; spread by droplets from an infected person 7 days before the rash appears but is of low infectivity. Uncommon in pregnancy, but the virus crosses the placenta to the fetus and causes abortion, stillbirth, congenital rubella and malformations, e.g. cardiac, ear and eye defects. If infection is acquired in the first 4 weeks of pregnancy the incidence of abnormalities is 50–60%, with multiple defects because of major organogenesis; by 16 weeks' gestation the incidence is 5%. Infection acquired later in pregnancy may cause fetal growth retardation, congenital thrombocytopenic purpura, with the baby having learning difficulties, physical disabilities or deafness; the baby may be a source of infection for up to 2 years. First-trimester exposure to rubella requires that blood be taken to test for immunity; termination may be considered if there is evidence of infection. Vaccination is given [with mumps and measles (MMR)] at 1 year, and is repeated for girls between 11 and 14 years.

Rubin test test for patency of the uterine tubes, made by transuterine inflation with carbon dioxide gas; also called tubal insufflation.

rugae ridges or creases, as in stomach mucosa and squamous epithelium of the vagina.

Rules for Midwives rules produced by the Nursing and Midwifery Council by which all midwives practising in the UK must abide; failure to do so is likely to result in allegations of professional misconduct.

rupture tearing or bursting of a part, e.g. of an aneurysm, of the membranes during labour or of a tubal pregnancy. *Uterine r.* bursting apart of the uterus following obstructed labour, in which the BANDL'S RING, a ridge running obliquely across the abdomen, marks the junction between the grossly thickened upper uterine segment and the dangerously thinned and overstretched lower segment; also, tearing of a uterine scar from a previous Caesarean section during pregnancy or labour – DEHISCENCE may occur insidiously towards term or rapidly during labour as a result of powerful contractions. Shock and blood loss must be treated before attempting to suture the rupture; occasionally, hysterectomy may be required.

Ryle's tube thin rubber tube with a weighted end, introduced via the nose into the stomach, used for withdrawal of gastric contents or administration of fluids.

Sabine vaccine oral vaccine against poliomyelitis consisting of three types of live, attenuated polioviruses given in a capsule, on a lump of sugar or by medicine dropper.

sac pouch-like cavity.

saccharide one of a series of carbohydrates, including the sugars, divided into monosaccharides, disaccharides, trisaccharides and polysaccharides according to the number of saccharide groups.

sacculation of the uterus rare complication of incarceration of the RETROVERTED GRAVID UTERUS; the fundus remains under the sacral promontory and the anterior wall grows to accommodate the fetus.

sacral relating to the sacrum. *S. promontory* upper anterior border of the body of the prominent first sacral vertebra.

sacro- concerning the sacrum. *Sacroanterior* and *sacroposterior* positions in breech presentation, the sacrum being the DENOMINATOR.

sacrococcygeal concerning the sacrum and coccyx. *S. joint* slightly movable pelvic joint between the sacrum and coccyx.

sacrocotyloid concerning the sacrum and acetabulum. *S. diameter* measurement from the sacral promontory to the nearest point of the iliopectineal eminence; measures 9.5 cm (3.75 in).

sacroiliac concerning the sacrum and ilium. *S. joint* or *s. synchondrosis* slightly movable joint between the sacrum and ilium.

sacrum wedge-shaped bone of five united vertebrae between the lowest lumbar vertebra and coccyx; forms the posterior pelvic wall.

Safe Motherhood Initiative World Health Organization campaign to reduce worldwide maternal mortality and morbidity by implementation of simple, appropriate, cost-effective strategies to enable mothers to have access to high-quality, affordable care during pregnancy and childbirth and related events such as fetal loss; aims to improve health, nutrition and general well-being of girls and women of reproductive age before conception and into parenthood, and to reduce long-term sequelae of childbirth, which often result in lifelong disabilities. *See* Appendix 13.

Saf-T-Coil intrauterine contraceptive device.

sagittal arrow-shaped. *S. section* anteroposterior midline section. *S. suture* junction of the parietal bones; a *sagittal* or *third fontanelle* may be noted in the sagittal suture, sometimes associated with DOWN'S SYNDROME.

salbutamol beta-sympathomimetic drug used to suppress preterm labour; contraindicated in pre-eclampsia and antepartum haemorrhage.

salicylate salt or ester of salicylic acid, e.g. aspirin, an analgesic, antipyretic and anti-inflammatory drug; act through inhibition of prostaglandin synthesis, blocking pyretic and inflammatory processes mediated by prostaglandin.

saline containing a salt or salts. *Physiological s.* 0.9% sodium chloride solution, isotonic with blood, given intravenously to replace fluid in shock and haemorrhage; rapidly excreted; formerly *normal s.*

saliva secretion of the salivary glands, which is poured into the mouth when food is eaten; moistens and dissolves certain substances and begins carbohydrate digestion with the action of the enzyme ptyalin, the salivary amylase.

salivation normal flow of saliva; excessive salivation is called PTYAL-ISM, a disorder occurring in some women during pregnancy, particularly those of West African origin.

Salk vaccine preparation of killed polioviruses of three types given in a series of intramuscular injections to immunise against poliomyelitis.

Salmonella genus of bacteria responsible for GASTROENTERITIS.

salpingectomy excision of one or both of the fallopian tubes.

salpingitis fallopian tube inflammation.

salpingogram radiological outline of the fallopian tube interior, used to detect patency and other disorders.

salpingography fallopian tube radiography after intrauterine injection of a radio-opaque medium.

salpingo-oophorectomy removal of a fallopian tube and ovary.

salpingotomy surgical incision of a uterine tube.

salpinx fallopian tube.

salt 1. sodium chloride, common salt, used in solution as a cleansing agent or for infusion into the blood to replace fluid. 2. any compound of an acid with an alkali or base. *S. depletion* loss of salt from the body because of sweating, persistent vomiting or diarrhoea.

sample selected group of a population.

sanguineous pertaining to or containing blood.

saphenous two superficial veins, the long and the short, carrying blood up the leg from the foot.

sarcoma highly malignant tumour developed from connective tissue cells and their stroma. *Kaposi's s.* multifocal, metastasising, malignant viral reticulosis involving skin and visceral lesions, usually starting on the toes or feet as reddish-blue or brownish soft nodules and tumours; frequently seen in ACQUIRED IMMUNE DEFICIENCY SYNDROME.

saturated solution liquid containing the largest amount of a solid that can be dissolved in it without forming a precipitate.

Saving Newborn Lives global initiative led by the Save the Children organisation to ensure that safe motherhood also includes neonatal care strategies.

scalp layer of tissue covering the cranial bones. *S. electrode* small transducer applied *per vaginam* to the fetal scalp during labour to monitor fetal heart rate; the neonate may have small lesions apparent on the scalp at birth at the point where the electrode was sited.

scan image of internal structures and tissues. *See also* COMPUTED TOMOGRAPHY, MAGNETIC RESONANCE IMAGING, ULTRASONOGRAPHY.

scapula large flat triangular bone forming the shoulder blade.

Schilling test test used to confirm diagnosis of pernicious anaemia by estimating absorption of ingested radioactive vitamin B12.

schizophrenia psychosis of unknown cause but showing hereditary links; sufferers feel influenced by external forces, experiencing delusions and hallucinations; pregnancy aggravates the condition.

school health service provision of medical and dental inspection and treatment in local education authority schools.

Schultze expulsion of the placenta normal expulsion of an inverted placenta with the fetal surface appearing first at the vulva; commoner than MATTHEWS DUNCAN EXPULSION with less bleeding.

sciatic relating to the sciatic nerve running down the back of the thigh.

sciatica severe pain down the back of the leg along the course of the sciatic nerve, caused by pressure of the heavy uterus on nearby nerves and ligaments. Advice about body use and posture should be offered; transcutaneous electrical nerve stimulation or complementary therapies such as reflexology or acupuncture may ease it; usually resolves spontaneously following delivery.

sclera tough, white outer coat of the eyeball, covering approximately the posterior five-sixths of its surface, continuous anteriorly with the cornea and posteriorly with the external sheath of the optic nerve. adj. *scleral.*

sclerema uncommon neonatal disease characterised by hardening of the skin and subcutaneous fat; occurs in HYPOTHERMIA.

sclerosis hardening from overgrowth of fibrous and connective tissue, often resulting from chronic inflammation.

scoliosis abnormal curvature of the spine, most commonly applied to a lateral deviation. *See also* LORDOSIS *and* KYPHOSIS.

scopolamine HYOSCINE.

screening means of identifying members of a defined population at higher risk than normal from certain conditions, thus enabling further investigations to be undertaken; e.g. pregnant women are routinely screened for various diseases and fetal anomalies; some tests incorrectly identify a proportion of unaffected individuals as being at higher risk (false positives) and also fail to detect a proportion of affected individuals (false negatives).

Scriver test biological test used for diagnosing inborn errors of metabolism, e.g. PHENYLKETONURIA.

scrotum pouch of skin and soft tissues containing the testicles.

scurvy disease caused by a deficiency of vitamin C, characterised by weakness, anaemia, haemorrhage from mucous membranes, purpuric rash, joint swelling and pain and mouth ulceration; rapidly improves with a diet containing adequate vitamin C.

sebaceous fatty or pertaining to the sebum. *S. glands* sebum-secreting glands in the skin communicating with hair follicles.

sebum fatty secretion of the sebaceous glands.

second-degree perineal lacerations *See* PERINEAL LACERATIONS.

second stage of labour from full dilatation of the uterine cervix to complete birth of the baby.

secondary second in order of time or importance. *S. postpartum haemorrhage* any amount of excessive genital tract bleeding that adversely affects the mother's health, occurring any time from 24 hours up to 6 weeks after delivery; usually caused by retained products of conception and/or infection. Treatment is dependent on the cause but may involve evacuation of retained products, intravenous or oral oxytocics and antibiotics. *See also* POSTPARTUM HAEMORRHAGE.

secretin hormone secreted by the duodenal and jejunal mucosa when acid chyme enters the intestine, which is carried by the blood and stimulates secretion of pancreatic juice, bile and intestinal secretion.

secretion substance produced by a gland.

sedative calming substance, e.g. drug, often facilitating sleep, but not an analgesic.

sedimentation formation of sediment. *S. rate see* ERYTHROCYTE SEDIMENTATION RATE.

segment section or part. *Upper uterine s.* upper three-quarters of the uterus, which contracts and retracts during labour. *Lower uterine s.* lower one-quarter of the uterus, including the cervix, which becomes stretched and dilated in the first stage of labour.

segmentation division of the fertilised ovum into 2 cells, and then 4,

8, 16, etc., as it traverses the fallopian tube.

seizure convulsion or attack of epilepsy.

self-actualisation level of psychological development in which innate potential is realised to the full.

self-governing trust hospitals or other establishments assuming responsibility for ownership and management by 'opting out' of direct NHS control; status is approved by the Secretary of State; each trust has a board of executive and non-executive directors and a chairman approved by the Secretary of State.

Sellick's manoeuvre application of backward pressure on the cricoid cartilage in the throat to occlude the oesophagus and prevent regurgitation of stomach contents into the pharynx with consequent risk of aspiration into the lungs; undertaken during initiation of anaesthesia; pressure is not released until an endotracheal tube has been inserted and the respiratory tract sealed off.

semen male secretion of seminal fluid from the prostate gland and spermatozoa from the testis, produced at ejaculation.

semipermeable property of a membrane, permitting passage of some molecules and hindering others.

semi-prone lying face down with knees turned to one side.

senna (Senokot) laxative from cassia plant; may be too purgative for some women in pregnancy.

sense faculty of perception, e.g. hunger, thirst, pain, equilibrium or well-being, and other senses. The five major senses are vision, hearing, smell, taste and touch.

sensitive reacting to a stimulus.

sensitivity measure of accuracy of a screening test in identifying individuals who have a condition; the proportion of people with the condition found to be positive (high risk) on a screening test; also known as the DETECTION RATE.

sensitisation 1. initial exposure of an individual to a specific antigen, resulting in an immune response. 2. coating of cells with antibody as a preparatory step in eliciting an immune reaction. 3. action of a hormone on a tissue or organ so that it will respond functionally to another hormone.

sensitised rendered sensitive.

sensory pertaining to sensation. *S. nerve* peripheral nerve that conducts impulses from a sense organ to the spinal cord or brain; afferent nerve.

sepsis infection by pathogenic bacteria. *Puerperal s.* genital tract infection occurring during the PUERPERIUM.

septic relating to sepsis.

septicaemia presence and multiplication of pathogenic bacteria in the blood, diagnosed by rapid temperature rise, later becoming fluctuating, rigors, sweating and signs of acute fever. *See also* ENDOTOXIC SHOCK, PUERPERAL SEPSIS.

septum division or partition, e.g. between right and left ventricles of the heart.

septuplet one of seven offspring produced at one birth.

sequela morbid long-term condition following a disease and resulting from it. pl. *sequelae*.

serology study of antigen–antibody reactions *in vitro*. adj. *serological*.

serotonin amine present in blood platelets, the intestine and central nervous system, derived from the amino acid tryptophan and inactivated by monoamine oxidase; acts as a vasoconstrictor.

serrated with a saw-like edge, e.g. fetal skull bones.

serum clear straw-coloured fluid left after blood has clotted; clear residue of blood from which the corpuscles and fibrin have been removed. Serum from blood of a person recovering from a disease may be used to protect another person from the same disease. e.g. diphtheria, tetanus.

service provider clinical institutions providing student midwife/nurse placement experiences, staff to support students and evidence of good practice from clinical audit.

sex 1. fundamental distinction based on the type of gametes produced by the individual. Ova – macrogametes – are produced by females; spermatozoa – microgametes – by males; union of these distinctive germ cells produces a new individual. 2. to determine the sex of an organism.

sex-linked gene gene on the sex chromosome, usually the X or female chromosome.

sextuplet one of six offspring produced at the same birth.

sexual intercourse coitus. *S. i. in pregnancy* libido in pregnancy may be reduced or increased, depending on a variety of factors; some couples may require information and suggestions about changing coital positions or using alternative means of sharing intimacy. *Resumption of s. i. following delivery* mothers should be encouraged to attempt coitus within 6 weeks of delivery, before the postnatal examination, as, occasionally, difficulties with penetration may highlight inadequate perineal or vaginal wound healing or other pathological problems resulting from delivery.

sexually transmitted infection (STI) infection transmitted through heterosexual or homosexual sexual intercourse or intimate contact with the genitals, mouth or rectum; STIs in pregnancy must be identified and treated early to avoid complications, e.g. preterm labour or neonatal death due to vertical transmission from mother to baby. Routine screening in pregnancy is performed to detect SYPHILIS, HEPATITIS B and HUMAN IMMUNODEFICIENCY VIRUS and, in some areas, women under 25 years are screened for CHLAMYDIA infection.

shaken baby syndrome presence of unexplained fractures in a baby's long bones plus evidence of subdural haematoma; caused by violent shaking, which produces a whiplash effect, and rotational head movement, resulting in vomiting, convulsions, irritability, coma and death.

shared care antenatal care shared between a midwife and obstetrician or general practitioner.

sheath tubular case or envelope; condom, worn over the erect penis during intercourse to trap the seminal fluid: a means of contraception; used with a spermicidal preparation reliability is about 97%; also used to prevent transmission of sexually transmitted diseases and HUMAN IMMUNODEFICIENCY VIRUS (HIV) from one partner to another.

Sheehan's syndrome hypopituitarism; uncommon complication following severe prolonged shock after ABRUPTIO PLACENTAE or POSTPARTUM HAEMORRHAGE, with anterior pituitary gland necrosis leading to AMENORRHOEA, genital atrophy and premature senility.

shiatsu complementary therapy similar to ACUPUNCTURE, developed in Japan in the 1950s, involving pressure of the practitioner's fingers, hands, elbows, heels or feet applied to specific points on the client's body; useful for gestational sickness, facilitating uterine action in labour and easing pain, colic and fractiousness in babies.

shingles HERPES ZOSTER.

Shirodkar operation cervical cerclage; operation to prevent abortion resulting from cervical incompetence in which the internal cervical os is closed with a nylon suture, which is then removed shortly before term or earlier if labour should begin.

shock collapse resulting from acute peripheral circulatory failure caused by ante- or postpartum haemorrhage, uterine rupture or inversion, acid aspiration syndrome, pulmonary or amniotic fluid embolism, severe hypotension or endotoxic shock as a result of septicaemia. Signs are hypotension, tachycardia and fluctuating central venous pressure; the woman appears cold, clammy, white and searching for air. Urgent resuscitation is required before the condition becomes irreversible: the airway must be maintained; oxygen is administered if dyspnoea is present; intravenous fluids are administered to combat dehydration; and plasma substitutes are given, the amount dependent on the central venous pressure reading. The foot of the bed can be raised if the baby has been delivered and the mother may be positioned on her left side to prevent inferior vena cava pressure. Sedatives may be given, the mother kept as quiet as possible, and overheating must be avoided. *Endotoxic s.* occurs in serious infection by Gram-negative organisms, e.g. *Escherichia coli*, *Clostridium welchii*; there is widespread arteriole dilatation, venous return is diminished and shock occurs; signs are similar to hypovolaemic shock but rigors may also occur; the infection must be treated urgently with appropriate antibiotics.

shoulder dystocia rare complication occurring after delivery of the fetal head; the shoulders fail to rotate, descend and deliver, usually due to a large baby or contracted pelvic outlet. The mother should be turned into the left lateral position or asked to squat in an attempt to enlarge the outlet and deliver the baby. McRobert's manoeuvre may be performed, in which the woman lies on her back and assumes an exaggerated knee-chest position with the thighs abducted, to enlarge the pelvic outlet. External or internal rotation of the shoulders may be necessary as with WOOD'S

MANOEUVRE; occasionally symphysiotomy is performed or, in extreme cases, the fetal shoulders are fractured to permit delivery of a live baby and prevent serious maternal complication. Alternatively, the Zavanelli manoeuvre, i.e. cephalic replacement followed by Caesarean section, is performed.

shoulder presentation situation that develops if labour commences with the fetus in an incorrected oblique lie: one fetal shoulder is driven down into the maternal pelvis and labour becomes obstructed; may occur in the second stage of a twin labour, after delivery of the first baby. On examination the uterus appears broad and the fundal height is less than expected for the gestation; on vaginal examination the fetal ribs may be felt and an arm may prolapse into the vagina. Caesarean section is required or, if not possible, internal podalic version and a breech extraction are carried out if the baby is alive or, possibly, a destructive operation if the baby is dead, although the maternal risk of a ruptured uterus is extremely high.

'show' blood-stained discharge prior to and at the onset of labour, which comes from the cervical canal plug, the operculum.

shunt 1. to turn to one side; to divert; to bypass. 2. passage or anastomosis between two natural channels, especially blood vessels, either by natural means or operation.

SI units units of measurement used for scientific and technical purposes, constituting the International System of Units or Système International d'Unités (French). *See* Appendix 9.

Siamese twins colloquial term for CONJOINED TWINS.

sibling one of two or more children having the same parents.

sickle cell disease recessively inherited HAEMOGLOBINOPATHY occurring most commonly in people of African

Caribbean and sub-Saharan African origin. Multisystem disorder in which red blood cells become deoxygenated forming rigid sickle-shaped structures that are unable to pass through small capillaries; this causes pain and ischaemic damage, known as a vaso-occlusive crisis; aplastic crisis occurs when erythrocyte production is suppressed; haemolytic crisis occurs when there is a rapidly increased rate of HAEMOLYSIS. Sickled haemoglobin carries less oxygen than adult haemoglobin and deteriorates more rapidly, resulting in chronic anaemia and increased susceptibility to infection. If an individual carries one sickle haemoglobin (HbS) gene and one normal adult haemoglobin (HbA) gene (heterozygous), this is known as sickle cell trait (healthy carrier); if both genes are abnormal (homozygous), the disease is present. Pregnant women who have sickle cell trait should be offered partner testing: if both parents are carriers there is a 25% chance of having an affected baby; neonates are also screened via the NEWBORN BLOOD-SPOT SCREENING PROGRAMME.

sign objective evidence or manifestation of changes in physiology or pathology; signs of pregnancy include abdominal growth and palpation of fetal parts, but the subjective experience of nausea is a SYMPTOM.

silver nitrate $AgNO_3$. Crystalline salt used in solid form as a caustic to reduce excessive granulation tissue.

Silverman–Anderson score system to evaluate breathing performance of preterm babies by assessing five categories, graded as 0, 1 or 2: chest retraction compared with abdominal retraction during inspiration; retraction of the lower intercostal muscles; xiphoid retraction; flaring of the nares with inspiration; expiratory grunt. A score of 0 indicates adequate ventilation; 10 indicates severe respiratory distress.

Simmonds' disease underactivity of the whole PITUITARY GLAND (HYPOPITUITARISM), affecting the total endocrine system; may follow SHEEHAN'S SYNDROME.

Sims' position similar to left lateral position but almost on the face, semi-prone, with the right knee and thigh drawn up and resting on the bed in front of the left leg.

Sims' speculum See Appendix 3.

sinciput brow; part of the skull between the coronal suture and orbital ridges.

Singer's test blood test used to distinguish fetal from maternal blood.

sinoatrial node collection of specialised muscle fibres in the wall of the right atrium where the rhythm of cardiac contraction is usually established; pacemaker of the heart.

sinus cavity; general anatomical term for all cavities in the cranial bones or the dilated channels for venous blood also found in the cranium. See INTRACRANIAL MEMBRANES.

skeleton bone structure of the body, which supports and protects the organs and soft tissues.

Skene's duct largest female urethral gland, opening within the urethral orifice; homologous with the prostate.

skull bony structure of the head enclosing and protecting the brain, divided into three parts, the vault, the base and the face. The base and face bones are firmly united and incompressible. The vault consists of two frontal bones, two parietal bones, two temporal bones and one occipital bone; at birth it is not fully ossified, with membranous spaces between the bones called sutures; three or more sutures meeting together form a fontanelle. During labour, pressure on the fetal skull causes moulding so that the bones overlap the sutures. See also FETAL SKULL.

slapped cheek syndrome See PARVOVIRUS B19.

sleeping position, neonate current research indicates that, to reduce the risk of sudden infant death, the safest position in which to place a sleeping baby is supine (on the back).

slough mass of dead tissue either in or which separates from the adjacent tissue.

small for gestational age baby baby below the 10th centile when ultrasound scan measurements are plotted on a growth chart; if the measurements decrease by a centile, medical review is needed, as growth-restricted babies are more susceptible to HYPOXIA because of poor placental function.

smear specimen of superficial cells, e.g. from vagina or cervix, for microscopical examination, which may reveal hormone levels or early malignant disease.

smegma secretion of sebaceous glands of clitoris and prepuce.

smoking in pregnancy antenatal smoking is harmful as carbon monoxide reduces oxygen transport and nicotine causes vasoconstriction of arterioles, leading to a diminished food and oxygen supply to the fetus and resulting in poor fetal growth and development; continued parental smoking predisposes babies to asthma and other allergenic and respiratory conditions.

snuffles noisy breathing and nasal catarrh in infants with congenital SYPHILIS.

social class Registrar General's classification of individuals according to occupation: I – professionals; II – intermediate; III – skilled workers; IV – semi-skilled; V – unskilled.

social services not-for-profit community services provided to meet certain individual needs.

social services department local authority department that coordinates social services; has a responsibility to children and young persons,

the elderly, physically disabled, those with learning disabilities, the socially inadequate and unsupported parents; some provision may be delegated to voluntary organisations; may also act as an adoption agency.

social worker specially qualified professional who assesses social need and provides necessary resources.

sociology scientific study of relationships and phenomena.

sodium metallic element that is an important constituent of animal tissues; major cation, i.e. positively charged ion, of the extracellular fluid (ECF), thus determining the osmolality of the ECF. The serum sodium level is normally about 140 mEq/L; if this falls, osmoreceptors in the hypothalamus are stimulated, causing decrease of antidiuretic hormone (ADH) from the posterior pituitary gland, which decreases water absorption in the collecting ducts of the kidneys so that water is excreted. If the sodium level and osmolality rise, neurons in the thirst centre of the hypothalamus are stimulated, prompting the person to drink enough fluid to restore osmolality to normal. A serum sodium concentration below normal levels occurs in conditions associated with fluid volume deficit, e.g. diarrhoea and vomiting, acute or chronic renal failure and in diuretic therapy. Excess serum sodium concentration (HYPERNATRAEMIA) occurs when insensible water loss is not replaced by drinking and, in the newborn, when artificial feeds are made up incorrectly with too high a concentration of milk powder. *S. bicarbonate* used, in varying strengths (8.4% or 5%), to reverse metabolic ACIDAEMIA following hypoxia to the tissues. *S. citrate* added to donor blood to prevent clotting. Symbol Na.

soft chancre non-syphilitic venereal ulcer caused by *Haemophilus ducreyi* (Ducrey's bacillus).

soft palate fleshy structure at the back of the mouth, which, with the hard palate, forms the roof of the mouth; in swallowing the soft palate is drawn upwards against the back of the pharynx, preventing food and fluids from entering the nasal passage while they pass through the throat.

solar plexus network of sympathetic nerve ganglia in the abdomen; nerve supply to abdominal organs below the diaphragm.

solute substance dissolved in a solution.

solvent a liquid that dissolves, or has the power to dissolve.

somatic relating to the body as opposed to the mind.

somatome 1. appliance for cutting the body of a fetus. 2. somite.

somatotrophin growth hormone. adj. *somatotrophic.*

somite one of the paired segments along the neural tube of the vertebrate embryo, formed by transverse subdivision of the thickened mesoderm next to the mid-plane, which develop into the vertebral column and muscles.

sonar (SOund Navigation And Ranging) technique using the transmission of sound pulses and pulse echoes under water to locate and track objects; the basis of ULTRASONOGRAPHY.

sonogram image obtained through the use of ULTRASONOGRAPHY.

sonography *See* ULTRASONOGRAPHY.

soporific causing sleep.

sordes brown crusts forming on the teeth and lips of unconscious patients or those suffering from acute or prolonged fevers; caused by poor mouth hygiene.

sore buttocks usually refers to perianal excoriation commonly associated with frequent loose stools, most likely in artificially fed babies, but also occurs with infrequent nappy changing, poor hygiene, incorrect laundering of napkins, diet (extra sugar) and infection such as candidiasis. Treatment includes good hygiene, exposure of the buttocks to the air and investigations of feeding, laundering of napkins and infection. *See* NAPKIN RASH.

souffle soft blowing sound heard on auscultation of the pregnant abdomen. *Uterine s.* due to blood passing through the uterine arteries, particularly over the placental site; synchronous with the maternal pulse.

soya milk milk substitute for babies unable to tolerate breast or cows' milk constituents such as lactose; contains only vegetable fats.

Spalding's sign gross overlapping of the fetal cranial bones, seen on abdominal radiograph, indicating that intrauterine death occurred several days previously.

Spalding's sign

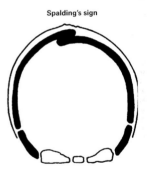

spasm sudden involuntary muscle contraction.

spastic pertaining to spasm; increased muscle tone resulting from brain or spinal cord injury; also used as a term for CEREBRAL PALSY.

specific gravity weight of a substance compared with that of an equal volume of another substance, e.g.

specific gravity of water is 1000, of urine is 1010–1020 and of blood is 1055.

specificity measure of accuracy of a screening test in identifying people who do not have a condition; the proportion of people not affected by a disorder who will be found to be negative (low risk) on a screening test for that disorder; linked to the true positive rate.

specular reflection reflecting from a surface; in ULTRASOUND an interface giving a strong reflection or echo, e.g fetal skull.

speculum instrument used to open up a cavity, normally not visible, to enable inspection. pl. *specula. See* Appendix 3.

Spencer Wells type of artery forceps. *See* Appendix 3.

sperm male reproductive cell; spermatozoon. *S. count* method of determining the concentration of spermatozoa in a semen sample. *S. donation* seminal fluid provided by donors to enable women whose partners are sterile to conceive.

spermatic pertaining to spermatozoa or semen. *S. cord* structure extending from the abdominal inguinal ring to the testis, comprising the pampiniform plexus, nerves, ductus deferens, testicular artery and other vessels.

spermatogenesis development of mature spermatozoa from spermatogenia.

spermatozoa (pl.) male generative cells forming the essential part of semen; normally 50 million cells per mL. sing. *spermatozoon.*

spermicide agent that destroys spermatozoa; often a cream, foam or paste applied to vaginal or cervical caps for contraceptive purposes.

sphenoid wedge-shaped. *S. bone* bone forming part of the base of the skull.

spherocyte small, globular, completely haemoglobinated erythrocyte without the usual central pallor; characteristically found in hereditary spherocytosis but also in acquired haemolytic anaemia.

spherocytosis presence of spherocytes in the blood.

sphincter ring-shaped muscle that contracts to close a natural orifice.

sphingomyelin complex molecule of protein and fatty acid used to measure the ratio of LECITHIN in amniotic fluid.

sphygmomanometer instrument used to measure arterial blood pressure.

spigot small peg or bung to close the opening of a tube.

spina bifida congenital condition in which the arches at the back of the spine are incomplete; sometimes there is only a bony gap (*spina bifida occulta*) but sometimes the spinal cord may be exposed. The presence of a sac over the spinal cord is called a MENINGOCELE; if nerves are exposed or involved in the sac it is called a MENINGOMYELOCELE.

spinal relating to the spine. *S. cord see* CORD. *S. anaesthesia* technique in which the dura is pierced and single-dose local anaesthetic is injected directly into the cerebrospinal fluid to provide fast-acting (but short-lived) reliable analgesia in labour; uses smaller doses of anaesthetic than for epidural analgesia; risks include dramatic hypotension, nausea and vomiting, post-spinal headache and infection.

spine 1. vertebral column. 2. sharp process of bone.

spinnbarkeit thread of mucus secreted by cervix uteri; used to determine ovulation, which usually coincides with the time when the mucus can be drawn out on a glass slide to its maximum length.

spirit alcoholic solution of a volatile substance, or an alcohol itself.

spirochaetae micro-organisms with a flexible, spiral filament, e.g. *Treponema pallidum*, cause of SYPHILIS.

spirograph apparatus for measuring and recording respiratory movements.

spirometer instrument for measuring air taken into and expelled from the lungs.

splanchnic pertaining to viscera. *S. nerves* three nerves from the thoracic sympathetic ganglia distributed to the viscera.

spleen vascular lymphoid organ in the left hypochondrium under the border of the stomach, having a framework of fibrous trabeculae with pulp in the spaces. It assists in the formation of erythrocytes in fetal life only; the production of lymphocytes throughout life; control of red cell breakdown and excretion of the resulting products; and formation of ANTIBODIES.

splenomegaly enlargement of the spleen.

splint piece of wood or metal used to support and immobilise an injured limb.

spondylolisthesis forward displacement of the fifth lumbar vertebra on the first sacral segment, which narrows the true conjugate by the formation of a false promontory; rare cause of DYSTOCIA.

spondylosis ankylosis of a vertebral joint; general term for degenerative changes in the spine.

spontaneous occurring naturally with no external aid. *S. evolution see* EVOLUTION. *S. version* change of the fetus from one lie to another with no obstetrical interference.

sporadic scattered or discontinuous, as in isolated cases of disease occurring in various scattered places.

spore reproductive element of certain plants, fungi and bacteria. Tetanus bacilli are spore-bearing, with the spores being resistant to high temperatures and strong antiseptics meaning that they can remain dormant for years.

spurious labour false labour. *See* LABOUR.

squamous scaly or plate-like. *S. bone* thin part of the temporal skull bone articulating with the parietal bone. *S.epithelium* thin-celled skin, e.g. lining of the vagina.

squatting position with the hips and knees flexed, buttocks resting on the heels; partial or full squatting may facilitate delivery, both by the effects of gravity and by slightly enlarging the pelvic outlet.

standard deviation (σ) measure of the dispersion of a random variable: the square root of the average squared deviation from the mean. For data that have a normal distribution about 68% of the data points fall within one standard deviation from the mean and about 95% fall within two standard deviations.

Staphylococcus genus of pyogenic bacteria, which, microscopically, appear grouped together in small masses like bunches of grapes; cause skin infections, including PEMPHIGUS NEONATORUM, MASTITIS, PUERPERAL SEPSIS. *S. aureus* or *S. pyogenes* coagulase-positive, causes severe infections and may be resistant to antibiotics. *S. albus* skin COMMENSAL that may cause urinary tract infection.

stasis stagnation or stoppage. *Intestinal s.* sluggish movement of the bowel wall muscle causing constipation. *S. of urine* occurs naturally in pregnancy but may lead to urinary tract infection. *See* PYELONEPHRITIS.

stat *statim* (immediately).

station location of the presenting fetal part in the birth canal, designated between −5 and −1 according to the number of centimetres the part is above an imaginary plane passing through the ischial spines, 0 when at the plane and between +1 and +5 according to the number of centimetres the part is below the plane.

statistical significance research conclusion that the results achieved have little probability of occurring by chance; below 1 in 20 or the 0.05 probability level, something other than chance produced the result.

statistics 1. numerical facts pertaining to a particular subject or body of objects. 2. science dealing with the collection, tabulation and analysis of numerical facts.

status condition, state. *S. epilepticus* rapid succession of epileptic spasms without intervals of consciousness; brain damage may result.

statutory bodies organisations that control practice by law, e.g. control of the practice of midwives is the responsibility of the NURSING AND MIDWIFERY COUNCIL.

Statutory Maternity Pay payment made by employer to all working pregnant women to enable them to take time off work before and after the birth. *See* Appendix 12.

Stein–Leventhal syndrome condition of either AMENORRHOEA or OLIGOMEN-ORRHOEA, hirsutism, infertility and enlarged cystic ovaries from which excessive male hormones may be produced.

Stemetil *See* PROCHLORPERAZINE.

stenosis narrowing or contraction of a channel or opening. *Aortic s.* narrowing of the aortic valve of the heart due to scar tissue resulting from inflammation. *Mitral s.* of the mitral orifice from the same cause. *Pyloric s.* generally caused by congenital hypertrophy.

stercobilin bile pigment derivative formed by air oxidation of stercobilinogen; brown/orange/red pigmentation contributing to the colour of faeces and urine.

sterile 1. barren; incapable of producing young. 2. free from micro-organisms.

sterilise 1. to make sterile by operation, e.g. ligation of the fallopian tubes. 2. to render sterile dressings, instruments, etc.

steriliser apparatus in which objects can be sterilised.

sternum plate of bone forming the middle of the anterior thoracic wall and articulating with the clavicles and cartilages of the first seven ribs; by 36 weeks' gestation the uterine fundus normally reaches the xiphoid process at the lower end of the body of the sternum.

steroids substances containing carbon and hydrogen and having a particular chemical structure, including sex hormones, adrenocortical hormones, cholesterol and bile acids.

stethoscope instrument used to auscultate sounds within the body, e.g. of heart, lungs. *Binaural s.* branches into two flexible tubes, one for each ear of the examiner. *Fetal* or *monaural s.* metal trumpet-shaped instrument placed on the abdomen over the fetal shoulders to hear the heart sounds; Pinard's stethoscope.

stilbestrol *See* DIETHYLSTILBESTROL.

stilette wire for keeping clear the lumen of hollow structures such as needles; fine probe.

stillbirth baby delivered after the 24th week of pregnancy who has not, at any time after being completely expelled from the mother, breathed or shown any sign of life. adj. *stillborn*. The midwife must by law ensure notification, certification and registration of the stillbirth and notify the supervisor of midwives.

stillbirth certificate certificate issued by a registered medical practitioner (or midwife if no medical practitioner was involved in antenatal care) who was present at delivery of the dead baby or who examined the body; must legally be given to the qualified informant (usually the father or mother) so that the birth can be registered and a certificate of burial or cremation issued; if there is an inquest the coroner issues the order for burial.

stomach dilated portion of the alimentary canal between the oesophagus and duodenum, just below the diaphragm; the wall consists of serous, muscular, submucous and mucous coats; gastric juice contains HYDROCHLORIC ACID and the enzymes PEPSIN and RENNIN.

stomatitis inflammation of the lining of the mouth.

stool bowel motion or discharge; in the newborn baby this is first meconium, gradually changing to brown, then to a soft bright yellow stool.

strabismus squint; deviation of the eye. The visual axes assume a position relative to each other which is different from that required by the physiological conditions.

straight sinus venous sinus in the fetal skull at the junction of the falx cerebri and tentorium cerebelli, which may rupture and cause intracranial haemorrhage if excessive or abnormal fetal head moulding occurs during delivery.

strawberry mark congenital haemangioma.

Streptococcus genus of bacteria occurring in a chain-like formation; may be haemolytic or non-haemolytic, aerobic or anaerobic. The beta-haemolytic streptococcus of Lancefield group A (*Streptococcus pyogenes*) causes scarlet fever and severe tonsillitis; PUERPERAL SEPSIS may be caused by aerobic or anaerobic streptococci.

streptokinase enzyme produced by streptococci that catalyses the conversion of plasminogen to plasmin; when administered as a thrombolytic it requires careful usage to avoid haemorrhage; may also trigger severe antigenic reactions upon readministration.

stress undue strain of mind or body, liable to cause impaired mental or physical function. The body's reaction to acute stress is triggered by the adrenal medulla, which pours adrenaline (epinephrine) into the bloodstream causing increased heart rate, blood pressure and blood glucose and dilatation of the blood vessels in the muscles to give them immediate use of this energy; in continuing stress the glands continue to produce a steady supply of hormones, apparently increasing the body's resistance. Diseases commonly resulting from prolonged stress include coronary artery disease, high blood pressure and cancer. *S. incontinence* involuntary leakage of urine in pregnancy, caused by hormonal laxity of pelvic floor muscles, relaxation of the internal urethral sphincter and reduced bladder capacity, and in the puerperium, caused by overstretching of the pelvic floor muscles. Women in whom the problem persists, despite performing pelvic floor muscle exercises in the puerperium, should be encouraged to seek specialist medical and physiotherapy help.

striae gravidarum skin marks caused by stretching, often appearing on the abdomen, breasts and thighs during and after pregnancy, first as reddish marks and later fading to a silvery white colour.

sub- prefix meaning 'under' or 'below'.

subacute moderately acute; disease that progresses moderately rapidly but does not become acute.

subarachnoid below the arachnoid. *S. space* space between the arachnoid and pia mater, in which the cerebrospinal fluid circulates. *S. haemorrhage* haemorrhage into this space.

subclavian beneath the clavicle. *S. artery* main artery to the arm.

subcutaneous beneath the skin, e.g. subcutaneous injection.

subdural under the dura mater. *S. haemorrhage* intracranial bleeding under the dura mater; seen in the neonate following traumatic delivery; subdural tap may be used to withdraw blood to relieve the pressure.

subfertility less than normal fertility.

subinvolution incomplete or delayed return of the uterus to its non-pregnant size during the puerperium, usually due to retained products of conception and infection.

subluxation partial dislocation.

submucous beneath the mucous membrane.

subnormal below normal.

subtotal hysterectomy *See* HYSTEREC-TOMY.

succenturiate additional or accessory. *S. placenta see* PLACENTA.

sudden infant death syndrome (SIDS) sudden unexpected death of an apparently healthy asymptomatic infant or one who has had only a slight cold, typically occurring between the age of 3 weeks and 5 months with an incidence of about 6 cases per 1000 live births and not explained by post-mortem examination; more common in preterm babies, less common in breastfed babies. The baby may be found dead in the cot, hence 'cot death'. Predisposing factors include lying the baby in the prone position, tobacco smoke and overheating.

sugar carbohydrates including mono-saccharides, e.g. glucose, fructose and galactose, and disaccharides, e.g. sucrose (cane sugar) and lactose (milk sugar).

sulcus groove or furrow, as between the cotyledons of a placenta. pl. *sulcii*.

sulphonamides group of chemothera-peutic drugs used orally to treat bacterial infections, e.g. streptococci, gonococci, *Escherichia coli* and other bacteria, although some of these organisms are now resistant.

super- prefix meaning 'over' or 'above'.

superfecundation fertilisation of two ova from the same ovulation by sperm-atozoa from two different individuals.

superfetation fertilisation of an ovum occurring during the course of pregnancy.

superior 1. higher than, above. 2. better than. 3. one in charge of others. *S. longitudinal sinus* upper venous sinus between the layers of the falx cerebri, which separates the two hemispheres of the brain.

supervisor of midwives practising midwife with a minimum of 3 years' experience, at least 1 year of which must have been in the immediate past 2 years, appointed by the LOCAL SUPERVISING AUTHORITY (LSA) in accordance with the Nurses, Midwives and Health Visitors (Midwives Amendment) Rules and specially trained to exercise supervision over midwives in its area. Responsible for receipt and monitoring of notification of intention to practise forms from all midwives working in the area and submitting them to the LSA; monitoring standards of midwifery practice and providing professional, clinical and educational support and guidance; issuing supply orders for controlled drugs, witnessing the destruction of controlled drugs where appropriate and ensuring that midwives are competent to administer medicines; monitoring and storing written records from all midwives in the area; investigating allegations of malpractice, negligence or misconduct; referring midwives to the Health Committee of the Nursing and Midwifery Council and notifying the LSA of midwives liable to be a source of infection.

supination turning upwards. *S. of hand* the palm is upward. cf. PRONATION.

supine lying on the back. *S. hypotensive syndrome* hypotension due to pressure of the gravid uterus on the inferior vena cava, reducing venous return, cardiac output and blood pressure, making the woman feel faint and adversely affecting OXYGEN flow to the fetus; may occur in late pregnancy if the woman lies in the dorsal position and can be aggravated by EPIDURAL ANALGESIA. Treatment is to sit the woman upright.

supplement something added to supply a deficiency.

supplementary of the nature of a supplement. *S. feed* feed given to a baby instead of or in addition to a breast-feed. cf. COMPLEMENTARY.

supply of controlled drugs community midwives obtain supplies of controlled drugs such as pethidine by applying to the supervisor of midwives who issues a supply order form. The midwife then goes to the approved pharmacist who issues the new stock, with the midwife and pharmacist entering the details in the midwife's personal register and drug book. All controlled drugs supplied to the midwife must be kept in a fixed locked cupboard to which only she has access.

supply order form official authorisation provided by the supervisor of midwives to a practising midwife to enable her to obtain a supply of PETHIDINE or other permitted controlled drugs.

suppository solid cone-shaped medicated compound introduced into the rectum, either to cause a bowel action (e.g. glycerine or bisacodyl suppositories) or to administer drugs, particularly analgesics (e.g. Anusol suppository for painful haemorrhoids).

suppression complete cessation of a secretion. If the mother is unable or unwilling to breastfeed lactation is suppressed, either naturally, i.e. by not removing the milk, or with drugs such as bromocriptine, which inhibits prolactin release from the pituitary gland.

suppuration formation or discharge of pus.

supra- prefix meaning 'above'.

suprapubic above the pubic bones.

suprarenal above the kidney. *S. glands* two small triangular endocrine glands, one above each kidney, which secrete ADRENALINE (epinephrine) and NORADRENALINE (norepinephrine) from the medulla and several hormones from the cortex.

surfactant LECITHIN in the lungs, which helps the alveoli to remain open; deficient in RESPIRATORY DISTRESS SYNDROME, which may be predicted by estimating the LECITHIN–SPHINGOMYELIN RATIO before delivery.

Sure Start government programme aiming to deliver the best start in life for every child in the UK, through provision of early education, childcare, health and family support, especially for those in disadvantaged areas.

surrender of controlled drugs unwanted controlled drugs may be surrendered by the midwife to an 'authorised' person, e.g. pharmacist from whom the drugs were originally obtained or medical officer, but not to the supervisor of midwives. *See also* DESTRUCTION OF CONTROLLED DRUGS.

surrogate substitute. *S. mother* woman who bears a baby for another with the intention that the child be handed over after birth.

survey systematic collection of information, not forming part of a scientific epidemiological study.

suture 1. stitch or series of stitches to close a wound. 2. fibrous joint in which the opposed bony surfaces are very closely united by thin connective tissue, permitting movement only in the neonate. *See* FETAL SKULL.

symmetrical cortical necrosis rare complication of severe concealed ABRUPTIO PLACENTAE with destruction of large areas of the cortex of both kidneys resulting from internal spasm of the renal cortical arteries. Impaired renal function or death from renal failure may follow. *See also* TUBULAR NECROSIS.

sympathetic exhibiting sympathy.

sympathetic nervous system part of the autonomic system, which, when stimulated, prepares the body for emergency or flight; the pulse rate increases, blood pressure rises, pupils become dilated and peristalsis slows.

symphysiotomy division of the symphysis pubis to facilitate delivery in cases of disproportion; used when Caesarean section is not possible, to avoid delivering a woman too many times by Caesarean section and in regions where midwifery services are inadequate, to avoid leaving a woman with a uterine scar.

symphysis joint in which the bone surfaces are joined by fibrocartilage and movement is very slight. *S. fundal* *height* measurement (in centimetres) taken between the upper border of the symphysis pubis and the uterine fundus; sequential measurements, plotted on a growth chart, facilitate identification of changes in uterine or fetal growth rates. *S. pubis* fibrocartilaginous junction of the two pubic bones. *S. pubis diastasis* slight separation of the fibrocartilaginous junction from the two pubic bones, caused by the hormones progesterone and relaxin in pregnancy, resulting in discomfort, pain and difficulty in walking; physiotherapy, osteopathy or chiropractic may help.

symptom evidence of a disease or condition observed by the woman herself, e.g. AMENORRHOEA and certain breast changes are symptoms of pregnancy. *See also* SIGN.

syn- prefix meaning 'together'.

synapse junction between the processes of two neurons or between a neuron and an effector organ, where neural impulses are transmitted by chemical means, causing release of a neurotransmitter, e.g. acetylcholine or noradrenaline (norepinephrine), from the presynaptic membrane of the axon terminal.

synclitism state when the fetal head enters the pelvic brim with both parietal eminences at the same level. *See* ASYNCLITISM.

syncope fainting; loss of consciousness caused by diminished cerebral blood flow.

syncytium, syncytiotrophoblast outer layer of the TROPHOBLAST, which does not have cell boundaries but scattered nuclei in the protoplasm; persists throughout pregnancy, covering the CHORIONIC VILLI, unlike the CYTOTROPHOBLAST cells.

syndactyly webbed fingers or toes.

syndrome group of symptoms and signs typical of a distinctive disease.

synthesis joining together of substances, either naturally or artificially.

synthetic chemical; artificially formed compound.

Syntocinon *See* OXYTOCIN.

Syntometrine oxytocic drug containing 0.5 mg of ergometrine and 5 units of Syntocinon in 1 mL, commonly administered intramuscularly to the mother with the birth of the anterior fetal shoulder to manage the third stage of labour actively; causes rapid sustained uterine contraction and separation of the placenta from the uterine wall.

syphilis SEXUALLY TRANSMITTED INFECTION caused by the spirochaete *Treponema pallidum*; the incidence is currently rising significantly. Primary syphilis, in which a small painless ulcer (chancre), usually on the vulva, can easily be missed. Secondary syphilis occurs from 3 weeks to 3 months after primary infection, with pyrexia, general malaise, rash and lymphadenopathy. Tertiary syphilis occurs after a latent period, which can last for several years; gummatous tumours develop and there is neurological and cardiac involvement. Syphilis can be vertically transmitted from mother to fetus from 9 weeks' gestation, causing miscarriage, stillbirth, neonatal death and long-term morbidity. All pregnant women are offered serological screening, initially with the Venereal Disease Research Laboratory (VDRL) and rapid plasma reagin (RPR) tests; if results are positive, diagnosis is confirmed by syphilis-specific tests, e.g. FLUORESCENT TREPONEMAL ANTIBODY-ABSORBED TEST (FTA-ABS). Treatment with penicillin is effective.

syringocele cavity containing herniation of the spinal cord through the bony defect in spina bifida.

syringomyelocele hernial protrusion of the spinal cord through the bony defect in a spina bifida, the mass containing a cavity connected with the central canal of the spinal cord.

Système International d'Unités (SI units) international system of measurement used in science and industry and for general use; agreed in 1960, it is now illegal in the UK to prescribe or dispense drugs in any other units.

systemic pertaining to or affecting the body as a whole. *S.lupus erythematosus (SLE)* autoimmune connective tissue disease, commonly presenting as arthritis but also affecting the skin, kidneys and neurological system. Diagnosis is made on clinical features and the presence of autoantibodies, which increase the risk of pregnancy complications and fetal loss, e.g. ANTIPHOSPHOLIPID ANTIBODIES may cause abnormal clotting and thrombolysis.

systole contraction of the heart. cf. DIASTOLE. *Ventricular s.* contraction of the ventricles, by which the blood is pumped into the aorta and pulmonary arteries.

systolic pertaining to systole. *S. murmur* abnormal sound produced during systole in heart affections. *S. pressure see* BLOOD PRESSURE. *S. sound* dull sound of the heart in ventricular systole, caused by its movement against the chest wall.

T cell lymphocyte derived from the thymus, responsible for cell-mediated immunity.

TAB vaccine against typhoid, paratyphoid A and paratyphoid B. *TABT* protects, in addition, against tetanus.

taboo negative traditions and behaviours regarded as harmful to social welfare and health.

tachycardia abnormally rapid heart and pulse rate.

tachypnoea abnormally rapid respiration, sometimes seen in neonatal RESPIRATORY DISTRESS SYNDROME.

tactile pertaining to touch.

t'ai chi Chinese martial art involving very gentle exercise and movement, breathing and concentration, now used to promote and maintain general health and well-being.

taking up of cervix effacement of the cervical canal early in labour. *See* DILATATION.

talipes clubfoot; congenital deformity of uncertain cause, usually detected on first paediatric examination, in which the foot develops at an abnormal angle to the leg. Mild positional talipes may occur in babies of women with OLIGOHYDRAMNIOS in pregnancy when the fetus becomes cramped *in utero*; may be an equinovarus or calcaneovalgus combination. Physiotherapy commenced immediately may correct mild talipes, but stretching, massage, splinting or operative treatment may be needed if the condition is severe. *See diagram.*

talipomanus clubhand.

talus ankle bone; the highest of the tarsal bones.

tamoxifen non-steroidal oral anti-oestrogen used palliatively in postmenopausal women with breast cancer and to stimulate ovulation in infertility.

tampon gauze plug with a long tape introduced into the vagina during repair of episiotomy or perineal laceration.

tapotement manual technique used in massage, involving gentle finger tapping to stimulate the circulation.

tarsus 1. bones composing the articulation between the foot and leg: talus, calcaneus, navicular, medial, intermediate and lateral cuneiform, and cuboid; the ankle or instep. 2. cartilaginous plate forming the framework of either (upper or lower) eyelid.

taurine crystallised acid from bile; found also in small quantities in lung and muscle tissue; present in high quantities in breast milk; necessary for conjugation of bile acids in the first week of life until glycine takes over the function and for nervous system development.

Taussig–Bing syndrome transposition of the great vessels of the heart with a ventricular septal defect straddled by a large pulmonary artery.

taxonomy orderly classification of organisms into appropriate categories (taxa) with application of suitable and correct names.

Tay–Sachs disease infantile form of amaurotic familial idiocy, inherited as an autosomal recessive trait and affecting chiefly Ashkenazic Jews; progressive disorder marked by a degeneration of brain tissue and maculas (with formation of a cherry red spot on the retinas), dementia, blindness and death. Antenatal diagnosis at 14 weeks' gestation reveals absence

Talipes

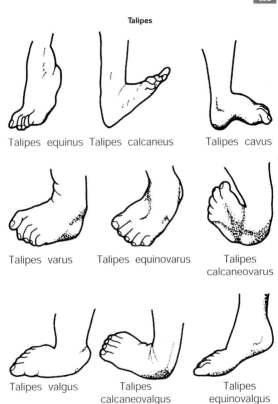

Talipes equinus Talipes calcaneus Talipes cavus

Talipes varus Talipes equinovarus Talipes calcaneovarus

Talipes valgus Talipes calcaneovalgus Talipes equinovalgus

of the enzyme hexosaminidase A, which indicates conclusively that the fetus has Tay–Sachs disease. Carriers of the trait have a lower level of the enzyme in their blood.

tea tree oil aromatherapy essential oil; highly anti-infective, being antibacterial, antifungal, antiviral and antimicrobial; has been found to be useful for vaginal thrush and herpes lesions;

also used for MRSA and those with HIV-related infections.

team midwifery system of midwifery management with midwives divided into teams to care for identified groups of women; aims to improve communication and continuity of care by reducing the number of midwives whom an individual mother sees for maternity care. *See also* CASELOAD MIDWIFERY.

teat 1. nipple of the breast. 2. manufactured nipple used on infants' feeding bottles.

teething eruption of the teeth through the gums; the first tooth usually erupts between 6 and 9 months, with the full set of 20 baby teeth fully erupted by about 30 months.

telemeter to transmit readings of an instrument by radio waves.

telemetry remote control record of fetal heart and uterine contractions, enabling ambulation during labour.

temazepam hypnotic drug; should be avoided in the first trimester.

temperature degree of heat measured by a thermometer, taken via the mouth, rectum, axilla or groin, or via mechanical apparatus. *Normal t.* of the human body is 36–37°C (97–98.4°F); varies slightly during the day; in women it is higher during the second half of the menstrual cycle. *See* PYREXIA *and* FEVER.

temporal pertaining to the side of the head. *T. bone* irregular skull bone with the squamous part forming part of the vault.

tendon cord or band of strong white fibrous tissue connecting muscle to bone; when the muscle contracts it pulls the tendon, which moves the bone.

tension 1. act of stretching. 2. pressure or concentration of a gas; *see* Po_2. *Premenstrual t.* symptoms occurring as a result of hormonal changes in the 5–7 days before a menstrual period, e.g. abdominal distension, headaches, emotional lability,

poor coordination, fluid retention and others.

tentorium cerebelli septum of dura mater, separating the cerebral hemispheres from the cerebellum. *See* INTRACRANIAL MEMBRANES.

tepid slightly warm; 32–37°C.

teras malformed fetus or infant. adj. *teratic*.

teratogen agent causing physical defects in the developing embryo. adj. *teratogenic*.

teratoma congenital tumour containing teeth, hair and cells of other tissues not normally found in the place where it is situated.

term end of pregnancy, normally calculated as 280 days or 40 weeks from the first day of the last normal menstrual period but considered to be any time after the 37th week of pregnancy.

termination of pregnancy (TOP) abortion that is induced, legally or illegally.

tertiary third. *T. syphilis see* SYPHILIS.

testicles, testes two glands in the scrotum that produce spermatozoa and male sex hormones. *Undescended t.* condition in which the organ remains in the pelvis or inguinal canal.

testosterone hormone produced by the testes that stimulates development of male characteristics.

tetanic relating to tetanus. *T. spasms* occur in strychnine poisoning.

tetanus disease caused by *Clostridium tetani*, an anaerobe found in cultivated soil and manure; in those exposed to infection, tetanus antitoxin will confer passive immunity.

tetany condition caused by calcium deficiency, alkalaemia or impaired parathyroid gland function; tonic contraction of hand and feet muscles (carpopedal spasm) with hypersensitivity of other muscles occurs; sometimes seen in artificially-fed neonates who have low serum calcium concentrations. *See also* HYPOCALCAEMIA.

tetracycline antibiotic substance effective against many different micro-organisms; should be used only with caution during pregnancy as may cause yellow discoloration and subsequent premature degeneration of the baby's first teeth.

tetradactyly four digits on the hand or foot.

tetralogy group or series of four. *Fallot's t.* congenital heart defect involving pulmonary stenosis; ventricular septal defect; dextroposition of the aorta, in which the aortic opening overrides the septum and receives blood from both the right and left ventricles; and right ventricular hypertrophy; surgical correction is required.

thalamus part of the brain at the base of the cerebrum; most sensory impulses pass from the body to the thalamus and are transmitted to the cortex and forebrain.

thalassaemia RECESSIVELY inherited HAEMOGLOBINOPATHY preventing normal haemoglobin production; an individual with one thalassaemia gene and one normal adult haemoglobin (HbA) gene (heterozygous) has a thalassaemia trait (healthy carrier); when both genes are abnormal (homozygous) the disease is present. Alpha thalassaemia (abnormal production of alpha globin chains) occurs mainly in Chinese, South-east Asian and Mediterranean racial groups and those with a trait have no symptoms; carrier status is confirmed by specialist DNA testing; alpha thalassaemia major is incompatible with life and causes intrauterine hydrops (Bart's hydrops). Beta thalassaemia (abnormal production of beta globin chains) occurs mainly in Mediterranean and some Asian racial groups; those with beta thalassaemia trait have no clinical symptoms, but carrier status is suspected if erythrocytes are small and anaemia is present; beta thalassaemia major is not clinically apparent at birth because fetal haemoglobin has a compensatory effect but, as fetal haemoglobin levels decline, the baby becomes anaemic and blood transfusions are required every 4–6 weeks for life, with risk of transfusion reactions, infection and iron overload; iron chelation therapy is given from the age of 2 to prevent toxic accumulation of iron. Pregnant women are screened for beta thalassaemia carrier status and offered partner testing if appropriate; if both parents are carriers there is a 25% chance of having an affected baby.

thalidomide sedative hypnotic drug; causes serious developmental deformities of the fetus if taken in pregnancy, mainly absence or foreshortening of one or more limbs.

theophylline respiratory stimulant with no known long-term side effects; reduces the incidence of apnoeic attacks in small preterm babies.

therapeutic abortion legally induced abortion performed when the fetus is grossly malformed or in cases when the mother's physical or mental health is in jeopardy if the pregnancy continues.

therapy treatment. *Chemotherapy* treatment with chemical drugs.

thermometer instrument for measuring temperature. *Clinical t.* special thermometer used to measure and record body temperature.

thermoregulation balance between heat production and heat loss.

thiamine vitamin B1; component of the B complex group of vitamins, found in various foods; present in plasma and cerebrospinal fluid; deficiency causes neurological symptoms, cardiovascular dysfunction, oedema and reduced intestinal motility.

thiazole group of benzothiadiazine sulphonamide derivatives, e.g. chlorothiazide; act as diuretics by inhibiting reabsorption of sodium in the proximal renal tubule and stimulating chloride excretion, with a resultant increase in water excretion.

thiopental barbiturate, given intravenously to induce general anaesthesia.

third-degree perineal laceration complete tear of the whole perineal body extending through the anal sphincter and into the rectum.

third stage of labour from birth of the baby to complete expulsion of placenta and membranes, involving separation and expulsion of the placenta and membranes and control of haemorrhage; may be managed *physiologically* (duration 5 minutes to 2 hours with an average of 20–30 minutes) or *actively*, in which case an oxytocic drug is administered to expedite placental separation and to control haemorrhage (duration 5–10 minutes). Active delivery of placenta and membranes with CONTROLLED CORD TRACTION may also be undertaken.

thoracic relating to the thorax. *T. duct* large lymphatic vessel situated in the thorax along the spine, opening into the left subclavian vein.

thorax chest; cavity containing the heart, lungs, bronchi and oesophagus, bounded by the diaphragm below, sternum in front and dorsal vertebrae behind; enclosed by the ribs as a protective framework.

threatened abortion vaginal bleeding, usually slight, sometimes accompanied by abdominal pain but with no dilatation of the cervix; usually resolves spontaneously but if cervical dilatation begins abortion becomes INEVITABLE. *See also* ABORTION.

threshold level that must be reached for an effect to be produced; the degree of intensity of stimulus that just produces a sensation.

thrill tremor or vibration elicited by tapping the wall of a cavity containing fluid, e.g. pregnant uterus with POLYHYDRAMNIOS.

thrombectomy surgical removal of a clot from a blood vessel.

thrombin substance formed in the blood by the action of thromboplastin on PROTHROMBIN in the presence of calcium; thrombin then converts the plasma protein fibrinogen into fibrin, which forms a clot.

thrombocyte blood platelet.

thrombocythaemia increase in the number of circulating blood platelets.

thrombocytopenia uncommon deficiency of PLATELETS, sometimes seen in neonates, especially of mothers with purpura; characterised by purpuric haemorrhages; usually resolves spontaneously; also occurs in congenital RUBELLA.

thromboembolism obstruction of a blood vessel with thrombotic material carried by the blood from the site of origin to plug another vessel; major cause of maternal death in Britain.

thrombokinase activated clotting factor X.

thrombolysis dissolution of a thrombus.

thrombophilia screen six to eight tests used to identify familial or acquired disorders that increase thrombosis risk, e.g. antithrombin, protein C, protein S, activated protein C resistance, factor V Leiden and factor II variant lupus type inhibitor. Women with a personal or family history of venous thromboembolism (deep vein thrombosis or pulmonary embolus) should be offered the test to identify those at increased risk of INTRAUTERINE GROWTH RESTRICTION, PRE-ECLAMPSIA and fetal loss.

thrombophlebitis inflammation of a vein with clot formation, usually adherent to the vein wall; rarely separates so danger of EMBOLISM is small. *Femoral t.* may occur postnatally following pelvic infection. cf. PHLEBOTHROMBOSIS.

thromboplastin substance liberated by injured tissue and platelets. *See* THROMBIN *and* PROTHROMBIN.

thrombosis formation of a thrombus. *Coronary t.* formation of a clot in a coronary vessel, thus heart muscle is deprived of blood according to the size of the vessel blocked; if the thrombus detaches itself from the wall and is carried along by the bloodstream, the clot or embolus leads to EMBOLISM.

thrombus stationary blood clot produced by coagulation of blood, usually in a vein, often due to PHLEBITIS.

thrush whitish spots on the mucous membrane of the mouth due to fungal infection with *Candida albicans*; babies may acquire it during delivery as they pass through the maternal vulva. An erythmatous napkin rash with small, white-headed pustules is usually due to *Candida albicans*; spreads quickly in bottle-fed babies as it is killed only by autoclaving and not by other methods of sterilisation; antibiotics and fungicidal drugs, e.g. nystatin, are given or TEA TREE OIL may be effective.

thymus gland between the lungs and above the heart, which grows until puberty, then gradually involutes; the cortex contains many small T lymphocytes, which play a part in the immunological reactions of the body.

thyroid function test (TFT) test to screen for or diagnose thyroid disorder; measures thyroid-stimulating hormone (TSH), which is produced in the pituitary gland and stimulates thyroxin production in the thyroid gland. High TSH levels indicate hypothyroidism; low levels indicate hyperthyroidism although levels may be low in the first trimester. Pregnant women with thyroid disease require specialist monitoring and medication; the baby should also be carefully observed.

thyroid gland endocrine gland in the neck in front of the trachea; secretes thyroxine and triiodothyronine, which control metabolism; overactivity causes thyrotoxicosis, underactivity causes myxoedema; babies with inadequate thyroid function suffer from cretinism.

thyrotoxic toxic (excessive) activity of the thyroid.

thyrotrophin anterior pituitary gland hormone that stimulates the thyroid gland; thyroid-stimulating hormone (TSH).

thyroxine thyroid gland hormone containing iodine, a derivative of the amino acid TYROSINE; affects metabolic rate (oxygen consumption); growth and development; metabolism of carbohydrates, fats, proteins, electrolytes and water; vitamin requirements; reproduction; and resistance to infection. Can be extracted from animals or produced synthetically; prescribed for HYPOTHYROIDISM and GOITRE.

tidal volume amount of gas passing into and out of the lungs in each respiratory cycle.

tissue mass of cells or fibres uniting to perform a particular function in the body. *Connective t.* tissue that connects, e.g. adipose (fatty), areolar (elastic supporting), bone, blood and cartilage. *Brown adipose t., brown fat t.* thermogenic adipose tissue containing a dark pigment, arising in embryonic life in specific areas, e.g. between the shoulder blades, behind the sternum, in the neck and around the kidneys and suprarenal glands; utilised by the neonate to produce heat. *Epithelial t.* covers all inner and outer body surfaces, may be ciliated (e.g. lining of the fallopian tubes), some columnar (e.g. lining of the cervical canal) and some squamous (e.g. lining of the vagina). *Erectile t.* spongy tissue that expands and becomes hard when filled with blood. *Granulation t.* material formed in repair of wounds and soft tissue, consisting of connective tissue cells and ingrowing young capillaries; ultimately forms fibrous tissue; a scar. *Muscular t.* striated (skeletal or voluntary), unstriated (plain or involuntary) and cardiac (striated but involuntary). *Nervous t.* consists of nerve cells and their processes. *Subcutaneous t.* layer of loose connective tissue directly under the skin.

tissue fluid fluid in the tissue spaces between cells; extracellular fluid; excess constitutes OEDEMA.

titre amount of a substance, e.g. antibody, in the blood, estimated by finding the amount needed to correspond with a known amount of another substance.

toco-, toko- word element meaning 'childbirth', 'labour'.

tocograph instrument for measuring the pattern and pressure of uterine contraction.

tocolytics drugs used to arrest threatened preterm labour; ritodrine hydrochloride (Yutopar), salbutamol (Ventolin).

tocopherol vitamin E, present in wheatgerm, green leaves and milk.

tomography method of producing images of single tissue planes. *Computed t.* (CT) radiological imaging modality using computer processing of X-ray photons detected by a detector bank after passing through the patient; image generated represents tissue densities within a 'slice', 1–10 mm thick, through the patient's body; computed axial tomography (CAT). *Ultrasonic t.* ultrasonographic visualisation of a cross-section of a predetermined plane of the body.

tone normal degree of tension, e.g. muscle tone.

tongue tie shortening of the frenulum that anchors the tongue to the floor of the mouth; does not usually interfere with feeding.

tonic contraction of the uterus sustained abnormal uterine contraction, either generalised, which may lead to fetal anoxia, or localised, i.e. *constriction ring*, which forms most commonly round the fetal neck,

adversely affecting labour progress; deep anaesthesia may be required for relaxation, although inhaling amyl nitrite may sometimes help.

tonus muscle tone.

'topping up' epidural anaesthesia repeat administration of the bupivicaine used for epidural anaesthesia following insertion of the cannula and administration of the first dose of analgesic by the anaesthetist; appropriately trained and assessed midwives are permitted by the Nursing and Midwifery Council to perform this technique, subject to cross-checking with a colleague and written instructions from the anaesthetist. Maternal blood pressure must be recorded every 5 minutes for a period of 30 minutes and every 15 minutes thereafter.

torsion twisting; may occur as a complication of ovarian cyst in which the pedicle produces venous congestion and consequent gangrene.

torticollis contracted state of the cervical muscles, producing neck torsion; may be congenital, hysterical or due to accessory nerve pressure, inflammation or muscle spasm.

tourniquet instrument applied to a limb to arrest bleeding or to make a vein more prominent.

toxaemia blood poisoning by the absorption of toxins, once thought to be responsible for PRE-ECLAMPSIA.

toxic poisonous, relating to a poison.

toxin poison, usually bacterial; does not produce symptoms until after a period of incubation, during which time the microbes multiply sufficiently to overwhelm the leucocytes and other types of antibodies; cause antitoxins to form, providing a means of establishing immunity to certain diseases.

toxoid toxin rendered non-toxic but which retains its protective qualities, e.g. APT (alum-precipitated toxoid), used in diphtheria immunisation.

Toxoplasma parasitic protozoa that cause TOXOPLASMOSIS.

toxoplasmosis an infection with *Toxoplasma* causing a glandular fever-like syndrome; if the fetus becomes infected it may cause hydrocephalus, intracranial calcification, splenomegaly, anaemia, jaundice and retinal damage.

trachea windpipe; cartilaginous tube lined with ciliated epithelium, extending from the lower part of the larynx to the bronchi.

tracheo-oesophageal fistula congenital defect with an opening between the trachea and lower oesophagus. *See also* OESOPHAGEAL ATRESIA.

tracheostomy emergency creation of an opening into the trachea through the neck, with insertion of an indwelling tube, used to restore the airway in acute obstruction or improve the airway and aspirate secretions.

traditional birth attendant unqualified women, usually mothers themselves, who traditionally help other women to deliver their babies, found in developing countries where midwifery or obstetric help may not be available; indigenous midwife, hilot, dunken, dai.

trait characteristic behaviour pattern. ***Sickle cell t.*** tendency for red blood cells to sickle, without accompanying anaemia, in someone who is HETEROZYGOUS for the condition.

tranquillisers drugs, e.g. chlorpromazine and promethazine, used to allay anxiety and calm the patient, e.g. in labour.

transcervical ligaments *See* CARDINAL LIGAMENTS.

transcutaneous blood gas monitor measures neonatal PO_2 and PCO_2 via a skin probe heated to 44°C; accuracy depends on peripheral circulation and it is usually used in conjunction with intermittent arterial sampling.

transcutaneous electrical nerve stimulation (TENS) mild electrical stimulation applied by electrodes in contact with the skin over a painful area; stimulates the large myelinated nerve fibres and relieves pain in line with the GATE CONTROL THEORY; also causes release of endogenous opiates or endorphins in cerebrospinal fluid, which reduces pain perception. In labour four electrodes are placed parallel and close to the spine between T10 and T11 and in the sacral area between S2 and S4; pain relief is controlled by the mother by increasing the degree of stimulation during a contraction; enables her to be ambulant; approved by Nursing and Midwifery Council for use by midwives.

transducer device that transforms one form of energy into another, e.g. in ULTRASOUND ceramic crystal is moulded into a disc and used to transform vibrations from electrical charges into waves of ultrasound of a certain frequency.

Positions of TENS electrodes for pain relief in labour

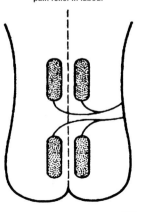

transferase enzyme that catalyses the transfer of a chemical group, which does not exist in free state during the transfer, from one molecule to another.

transferrin serum globulin that binds and transports iron.

transfusion direct administration into the bloodstream of blood or other solutions to increase blood volume. *Exchange t.* repeated small withdrawals and replacement of blood to alter the constituents but not blood volume, e.g. in haemolytic disease of the newborn to decrease the amount of bilirubin; replacement transfusion. *Feto-maternal t.* from fetus to mother via the placenta; transplacental transfusion (TPT).

transient temporary. *T. tachypnoea of newborn* condition of neonate, common after Caesarean, characterised by rapid respirations of up to 120 per minute for up to 5 days and cyanosis but with mostly normal blood gases; there is little rib recession or expiratory grunt. Oxygen therapy is administered; other causes of respiratory distress must be eliminated, e.g. infection, respiratory distress syndrome.

transillumination passage of a strong light through a body structure to permit inspection by an observer on the opposite side.

translocation in GENETICS, the shifting of part of one CHROMOSOME on to another.

transmigration wandering. *External t.* passage of an ovum from its ovary to the fallopian tube on the opposite side.

transplacental through the placenta.

transport movement of materials in biological systems, particularly into and out of cells and across epithelial layers. *Active t.* movement of materials across cell membranes and epithelial layers resulting directly from expenditure of metabolic energy.

transposition cross-placement. *T. of the great vessels* the pulmonary artery arises from the left ventricle instead of the right, so that poorly oxygenated blood leaves the right ventricle by the aorta; a patent ductus or creation of an atrioseptal shunt are the only ways to maintain life.

transudate fluid passing through a membrane, having a high fluid content and low protein and cellular content, e.g. vaginal fluid. opp. *exudate*.

transvaginal (TV) scan ultrasound scan using a probe inserted into the vagina, commonly performed in the first trimester of pregnancy as intrauterine detail is often much clearer than via the abdominal route. It is recommended that first-trimester non-viability is confirmed by TV scan. Also used to visualise fetal parts in the pelvic cavity in late pregnancy.

transverse arrest deflexed fetal head is caught above the level of the ischial spines with the sagittal suture in the transverse diameter of the pelvis; causes cephalopelvic disproportion and OBSTRUCTED LABOUR. *See* DEEP TRANSVERSE ARREST.

transverse lie longitudinal fetal axis lies across that of the maternal uterus; if uncorrected it may cause SHOULDER PRESENTATION and obstructed labour; due to lax abdominal and uterine muscles, as in grande multiparae, multiple pregnancy, placenta praevia or contracted pelvic outlet. On examination the uterus usually appears broad, asymmetrical with a low fundus and the fetal head is felt in the flank or iliac fossa. After 30 weeks' gestation a persistent transverse lie may require external cephalic version and, towards term, controlled membrane rupture/induction of labour if appropriate or elective Caesarean section.

transverse sinuses venous sinuses in the tentorium cerebelli by which blood is drained from the head.

transvestite person, usually male, who has an habitual, persistent desire to dress as a member of the opposite sex.

trauma injury.

traumatic caused by injury. *T. haemorrhage* vaginal bleeding, commencing immediately after delivery of the baby, which continues despite good uterine contractions, caused by cervical, vaginal or perineal body lacerations; treatment involves applying direct pressure to the bleeding point with artery or sponge-holding forceps or with digital pressure until the lacerations can be sutured.

travail labour, childbirth.

travel in pregnancy mothers should be advised how to ensure their comfort and safety when travelling, e.g. postural and back-care advice, frequent stops for the lavatory, avoiding unnecessary travel in late pregnancy; if wearing car seatbelts is too uncomfortable the mother should obtain a medical certificate to allow her not to use them; airlines usually require a medical certificate or letter if a woman wishes to fly in late pregnancy, although many refuse to accept pregnant passengers who are near term.

travellers generic term used to describe nomadic families; may suffer prejudice and are often marginalised by conventional health- and social-care services; some health authorities now have specially designated services for these families in an attempt to provide maternity care in which there is some element of continuity.

treatment mode of dealing with a patient or disease. *Active t.* specific medical or surgical intervention is given. *Conservative t.* employs natural means, e.g. rest, fluid replacement, rather than active or radical treatment. *Palliative t.* relieves distressing symptoms but not the disease. *Prophylactic t.* aims to prevent disease or pathology.

Trendelenburg position *See* POSITION.

Treponema pallidum SPIROCHAETE causing syphilis.

trial labour conducted in consultant obstetric unit when the fetal head is not engaged as a result of slight cephalopelvic disproportion to see if normal vaginal delivery is possible; if good contractions occur the head may flex and descend with moulding through the pelvic brim, facilitating normal delivery; if there is lack of progress in descent of the head and dilatation of the cervix despite good contractions, or signs of fetal or maternal distress, Caesarean section can be performed.

trial of scar controlled, often induced labour to observe the mother's condition and progress when she has a uterine scar from a previous Caesarean or other uterine surgery; increased risk of scar dehiscence particularly in multigravidae, which requires labour to be carefully monitored in a consultant unit so that emergency measures can be implemented if necessary.

trichomoniasis, *Trichomonas vaginalis* sexually transmitted disease caused by *Trichomonas vaginalis*, a flagellate protozoon; causes thin and watery or yellow-green frothy vaginal discharge, vulval pruritus and inflammation; treatment is with metronidazole 200 mg daily for 10 days for both mother and her partner.

triglyceride compound consisting of three molecules of fatty acid bound with one molecule of glycerol; neutral fat that is the usual storage form of lipids in animals.

trigone triangular area. *T. of the bladder* triangular non-elastic area forming the base of the bladder, between the ureteric openings and urethral orifice; embedded in the anterior vaginal wall, which, if distended in labour, may adversely affect bladder function.

trimester period of 3 months.

trimethoprim oral or intravenous antibiotic for urinary and respiratory tract infections; contraindicated in pregnancy and neonates.

tripartite placenta placenta divided into three lobes, each with a cord leaving it that join to form one cord a short distance from the lobes.

triple test biochemical Down's syndrome screening test conducted on maternal blood taken between 15 and 20 weeks' gestation. ALPHA FETO-PROTEIN (AFP), HUMAN CHORIONIC GONADOTROPHIN (hCG) and UNCONJUGATED OESTRIOL (UE₃) levels are measured and compared with the median value for that gestational age; higher than average hCG and lower than average AFP and UE₃ levels are associated with increased risk of Down's syndrome. Maternal age, gestation and biochemical marker levels are calculated together to give a *combined* Down's syndrome risk; if this is higher than 1 in 250 at term (e.g. 1 in 100, 1 in 249), the mother is in the higher risk range and is offered diagnostic AMNIOCENTESIS or CHORIONIC VILLUS SAMPLING.

triple vaccine combined dose of diphtheria, tetanus and pertussis vaccines.

triplets three children born at one labour; incidence formerly 1 in 6400 births, now more common because of infertility treatments.

triploidy (69XXX, 69XXY) syndrome in which three HAPLOID sets of chromosomes are present; may occur when two sperm fertilise one egg. The normal human karyotype contains 46 chromosomes (23 from each parent). Many triploidy pregnancies miscarry spontaneously and liveborn babies may have craniofacial abnormalities, eye defects and other anomalies, as well as developmental delay.

trisomy additional chromosome with one particular pair. *Trisomy 21* extra chromosome with the 21st pair; DOWN'S SYNDROME. *Trisomy 18*

EDWARD'S SYNDROME; *trisomy 13* PATAU'S SYNDROME.

trizygotic formed from three separate zygotes.

trocar sharply pointed surgical instrument in a metal cannula for aspiration or removal of fluids from cavities.

trochanter one of two prominences below the neck of the femur. *Greater t.* on the outer side; *lesser t.* on the inner side.

trophoblast outer covering of the blastocyst from which the placenta and chorion develop.

trophoblastic tissue SYNCYTIOTROPHOBLAST and CYTOTROPHOBLAST.

true conjugate *See* CONJUGATE.

trypsin powerful pancreatic enzyme that continues protein digestion to form amino acids.

tubal insufflation test to assess fallopian tube patency by transuterine inflation with carbon dioxide gas.

tubal ligation method of sterilisation in which the fallopian tubes are tied, either by laparoscopy and diathermy or with potentially removable clips applied to the tubes.

tubal mole mass of blood clot retained in the fallopian tube after a tubal pregnancy.

tubal pregnancy pregnancy embedded in the lining of the fallopian tube.

tube feeding administration of liquid (and for adults semi-solid foods) through a nasogastric, gastrostomy or enterostomy tube; common method of feeding preterm babies who tire easily when suckling and have immature swallowing and gag reflexes.

tuberculosis infection caused by *Mycobacterium tuberculosis*, commonly in the lung but any part of the body may be affected. Treatment is usually with streptomycin, isoniazid, para-aminosalicyclic acid or ethambutol; rifampicin is contraindicated in the first trimester. Antenatal care is shared between obstetrician and chest physician; if the mother has positive sputum, hospital admission and isolation are necessary, and care will be provided by staff immune to the infection. Epidural anaesthesia, forceps delivery and intravenous ergometrine to limit blood loss are used in labour to endure delivery is as easy as possible; if maternal sputum is positive lactation is suppressed and the baby is segregated until the mother is Mantoux test positive. The baby is given bacille Calmette–Guérin (BCG) vaccination as soon as possible after birth and entered on the 'at risk' register.

tuberosity expanded portion of bone or a protuberance; the transverse diameter of the pelvic outlet is measured between the *ischial tuberosities*.

tubular necrosis (acute) 1. when protein is deposited in the collecting and distal convoluted renal tubules, as with an incompatible blood transfusion or septic abortion, the epithelium is damaged and urine dammed back, thus preventing further activity of the GLOMERULUS; usually clears in 7–14 days. 2. if the proximal convoluted tubule becomes ischaemic or bacterial toxins are released the epithelium may necrose with death of the tubule; kidney function may recover in 10–30 days if there is only partial necrosis.

tubule microscopic tube forming one part of the nephron.

tumescence swelling or enlargement of a part; penile erection.

tumour growth or swelling.

tunica coat. *T. albuginea* dense layer of connective tissue below the germinal epithelium of the ovary.

tunnel passageway through a solid body with open ends. *Carpal t.* osseofibrous tunnel for the median nerve and the flexor tendons; carpal tunnel syndrome occurs if the median nerve becomes compressed, causing pain and tingling paraesthesia in the fingers and hand, sometimes extending to the elbow because of oedema.

Tuohy needle cannula and needle used to site a catheter in the epidural space; usually 16 or 18 gauge.

Turner's syndrome (XO, monosomy X, 45X) chromosome disorder caused by absence of one copy of the X chromosome, occurring in approximately 1 in 2500 female births. Affected individuals are of short stature with neck webbing, normal vagina, uterus and fallopian tubes, non-functional ovaries, no pubertal development and infertility; aortic narrowing may also occur and there may be some learning difficulties, e.g. impaired spatial awareness and mathematical skills. Fetal Turner's syndrome may be suspected from abnormal ultrasound findings, e.g. CYSTIC HYGROMA, heart defects, ascites, renal abnormalities; diagnosis is confirmed with karyotyping. There is no increased recurrence risk within families.

twins two babies developing in the uterus together. Genetically identical (monozygous) twins arise from division of a single fertilised egg; if this occurs in the MORULA within 4 days of fertilisation, twins will be dichorionic and diamniotic (DC-DA) with separate placentae, although they may fuse; if the BLASTOCYST divides between 4 and 8 days after fertilisation, monochorionic (one placenta) diamniotic twins (MC-DA) result. Vascular connections in the common placenta may result in TWIN-TO-TWIN TRANSFUSION SYNDROME. Very occasionally the blastocyst divides between 8 and 13 days after fertilisation giving rise to monochorionic monoamniotic twins (MC-MA), the shared amniotic cavity causing high fetal mortality and morbidity. Dizygotic non-identical twins occur when two separate eggs are fertilised, and have two placentae and two amniotic sacs (DC-DA). *See also* MULTIPLE PREGNANCY.

twin-to-twin transfusion syndrome haemodynamic imbalance between

MONOCHORIONIC twins, with chronic interfetal transfusion resulting in discordant growth; in severe cases the larger twin develops POLYCYTHAEMIA and POLYHYDRMANIOS and the smaller twin becomes anaemic with OLIGOHYDRAMNIOS. Previously untreatable, contemporary management now includes methods to reduce amniotic fluid volume in the larger sac, septostomy to allow free passage of amniotic fluid between the two sacs or laser ablation of the interlinked placental vessels. Pregnancies with monochorionic twins should be monitored closely between 14 and 26 weeks' gestation to ensure early detection and treatment of the syndrome.

tympanic pertaining to the tympanum. *T. membrane* thin, semi-transparent membrane stretching across the ear canal separating the tympanum (middle ear) from the external meatus (outer ear); eardrum.

typing method of measuring the degree of organ, solid tissue or blood compatibility between two individuals, in which specific histocompatibility antigens, e.g. those present on leucocytes or erythrocytes, are detected by means of suitable isoimmune antisera.

tyramine enzyme present in cheese, game, yeast extracts, wine, beer and broad bean pods having adrenaline-like effects; should be avoided by those taking monoamine oxidase inhibitor (MAOI) drugs.

tyrosine naturally occurring amino acid present in most proteins; product of phenylalanine metabolism and a precursor of melanin, catecholamines and thyroid hormones.

ulcer skin or mucous membrane lesion resulting from trauma, infection, pressure or nerve injury.

ultrasonic beyond audible range; relates to sound waves with a frequency of over 20 000 cycles per second.

ultrasonogram echo picture obtained using ULTRASOUND.

ultrasonography radiological technique that enables deep body structures to be visualised by recording reflections (echoes) of ultrasonic waves directed into the tissues; widely used in obstetrics to confirm gestation, locate the placenta, estimate fetal size, weight and maturity, estimate liquor volume, identify fetal abnormalities, examine uterine contents in abortion, ectopic or multiple pregnancy or hydatidiform mole, measure fetal and uteroplacental blood flow and observe fetal movements, e.g. sucking, swallowing, breathing, eye movement, filling and emptying of stomach and bladder; may be used during invasive procedures, e.g. amniocentesis and chorionic villus biopsy to avoid fetal or placental damage. *See* GREY-SCALE DISPLAY.

ultrasound sound at frequencies above the upper limit of normal hearing, i.e. greater than 20 000 cycles per second; used in the technique of ULTRASONOGRAPHY.

umbilical relating to the umbilicus. *U. catheterisation* insertion of a catheter into the baby's umbilical vein or artery to administer drugs or fluids or for continuous monitoring of blood gases, exchange transfusion or obtaining blood samples *U. hernia* protrusion of intestine through the umbilicus. *See* EXOMPHALOS.

umbilical cord cord connecting fetus and placenta, usually 50–60 cm (20–24 in) long with a spiral twist, consisting of two umbilical arteries carrying deoxygenated blood and one umbilical vein carrying oxygenated blood, surrounded by Wharton's jelly and covered by amnion. Soon after birth the cord is clamped and cut, leaving a stump about 2.5 cm long attached to the baby's umbilicus; this separates naturally through dry, aseptic necrosis within 5–7 days. *U. c. presentation* cord lying below the presenting part with intact membranes. *U. c. prolapse* cord lying below the presenting part with ruptured membranes, resulting in danger of pressure on cord vessels leading to fetal anoxia; usually results from a

Prolapse of the umbilical cord

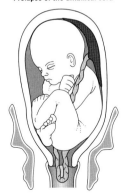

233

high or ill-fitting presenting part, allowing a loop of cord to slip past; treatment involves maintenance of fetal oxygenation and delivery of the baby as quickly as possible.

umbilicus navel; abdominal point at which the umbilical cord was attached.

unconjugated oestriol (UE₃) biochemical MARKER used in second-trimester serum screening for Down's syndrome, levels being reduced in affected pregnancies. UE$_3$ is produced by the placenta and fetal adrenals. *See also* QUADRUPLE TEST and TRIPLE TEST.

unconscious 1. insensible; incapable of responding to sensory stimuli. 2. part of mental activity including primitive or repressed wishes, concealed from consciousness.

uni- prefix meaning 'one'.

unicellular consisting of one cell.

unilateral on one side only.

uniovular from one ovum. *See* MONOZYGOTIC.

universal donor *See* ABO BLOOD GROUPS.

universal recipient *See* ABO BLOOD GROUPS.

unstable lie condition in which the fetal lie keeps changing after 36 weeks' gestation, predisposing the mother and baby to life-threatening complications; the mother may be admitted to hospital before the onset of labour for external fetal version, controlled membrane rupture and induction of labour or Caesarean section.

unsupported mother one-parent family; the mother may be unmarried, separated, divorced or widowed.

urachal pertaining to the urachus. *U. cyst* congenital abnormality in which a small cyst persists along the course of the urachus. *U. fistula* fistula forming when the urachus fails to close, causing urine to leak from the umbilicus.

urachus fibrous band uniting the apex of the bladder to the umbilicus; remnant of a canal present in the fetus.

uraemia renal failure with very high blood urea, characterised by headache, vertigo, vomiting, convulsions and coma; may complicate nephritis, concealed ABRUPTIO PLACENTAE or ECLAMPSIA.

urea end product of protein metabolism, excreted in the urine. *Blood u.* amount of urea present in blood; normally 2.5–5.8 mmol/L (15–35 mg/100 mL) but, in pregnancy, usually 2.3–5.0 mmol/l (14–30 mg/100 mL).

ureters two fibromuscular tubes conveying urine from kidneys to bladder; dilatation occurs during pregnancy because of relaxation of smooth muscle by PROGESTERONE, leading to stasis of urine and multiplication of micro-organisms. *See* PYELONEPHRITIS.

ureteric relating to the ureter. *U. catheter* fine catheter for insertion via the ureter into the renal pelvis, either for drainage or retrograde PYELOGRAPHY.

ureterovesical pertaining to a ureter and the vagina. *U. fistula* abnormal passage between ureter and vagina; rare complication of prolonged or obstructed labour when ureteric tissue becomes devitalised because of prolonged pressure from the fetal head.

urethra canal through which urine is discharged from the bladder; the male urethra is 20–22.5 cm long, the female urethra 3.7 cm.

urethral relating to the urethra.

urethritis inflammation of the urethra. *Non-specific u.* male sexually transmitted disease of unknown origin.

urethrocele prolapse of female urethral wall, which may result from intrapartum pelvic floor damage.

uric pertaining to urine. *U. acid* end product of purine metabolism or oxidation, present in blood in a concentration of about 0.13–0.42 mmol/L and excreted in urine in amounts of slightly less than 1 g per day.

urinalysis physical and/or chemical examination of urine to detect disorders or investigate symptoms. Visual examination may reveal dark urine, indicating dehydration, or cloudy urine, indicating infection. Reagent dipsticks are used to detect protein, glucose, ketones and pH: normal pH is between 4.8 and 8; regular antenatal urine tests for protein are used to diagnose urinary tract infection or PRE-ECLAMPSIA; ketones test for dehydration, especially in labour or HYPEREMESIS GRAVIDARUM; glucose tests for gestational diabetes mellitus (GDM), although this is unreliable because increased glomerular filtration in pregnancy often leads to glycosuria and absence of glucose in the urine may conceal a diagnosis of gestational diabetes. Urine may be examined microbiologically or molecularly to identify bacteria, blood cells and other micro-organisms.

urinary relating to urine.

urination micturition.

urine fluid secreted by the kidneys, excreted by the bladder in micturition; normal pH is about 6; consists of 96% water containing dissolved waste products, e.g. UREA and CREATININE, sodium chloride and phosphates.

urinometer glass instrument to measure urinary specific gravity.

urodynamics dynamics of the propulsion and flow of urine in the urinary tract.

urticaria vascular skin reaction marked by transient appearance of slightly elevated patches, redder or paler than surrounding skin, often accompanied by severe itching; caused by food intolerance, infection or stress.

uterine pertaining to the uterus. *U. apoplexy see* COUVELAIRE UTERUS. *U. souffle see* SOUFFLE. *U. tubes* FALLOPIAN TUBES.

uteroplacental pertaining to the uterus and placenta.

uterosacral pertaining to the uterus and sacrum. *U. ligaments* two

ligaments passing backwards from the cervix to sacrum, encircling the rectum, which help to maintain the uterus in a position of anteversion.

uterosalpingography radiography of the uterus and uterine tubes; hysterosalpingography.

uterotomy hysterotomy; incision of the uterus.

uterotonics drugs that stimulate the smooth myometrium, e.g. Syntometrine, Syntocinon, ergometrine, prostaglandins.

uterovesical referring to the uterus and bladder. *U. pouch* fold of peritoneum between uterus and bladder.

uterus pear-shaped, hollow, muscular organ in the pelvic cavity between the bladder and rectum, supported by parametrium; 7.5 cm long, 5 cm at the widest part, 2.5 cm thick; divided into the upper two-thirds, the corpus with the fundus at the top between the cornua, and the lower one-third, the cervix or neck. The uterine cavity communicates at the cornua with the fallopian tubes and at the internal os with the cervix, and has a mucous membrane lining of ENDOMETRIUM into which the fertilised ovum embeds; if there is no pregnancy it is shed about

Uterus and appendages

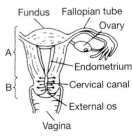

A, body of uterus; **B,** cervix.

235

every 28 days. The MYOMETRIUM has interlacing spiral muscle fibres, which expand to accommodate the fetus. The outer covering of PERIMETRIUM hangs loosely over the fundus to form the UTEROVESICAL POUCH anteriorly and the POUCH OF DOUGLAS posteriorly. *Bicornuate u*. congenital malformation in which the uterus has two horns. *U. didelphys* double uterus caused by failure of the two sides to unite during development. *U. unicornus* uterus with only one horn, the other being underdeveloped.

uvula small, fleshy mass hanging from the soft palate above the root of the tongue.

vaccinate to inoculate with a vaccine to procure immunity to a disease. *See* IMMUNITY.

vaccination injection of a particular bacterial vaccine. *See* BACILLE CAL-METTE-GUÉRIN.

vaccine suspension of killed organisms in normal saline. *Attenuated v.* prepared from living organisms that, through long cultivation, have lost their virulence. *Bacille Calmette-Guérin v.* attenuated bovine bacillus used to protect against tuberculosis. *Salk v.* prepared from a strain of poliomyelitis virus.

vacuum aspiration method used to perform abortions during the first 3 months of pregnancy or to remove a hydatidiform mole.

vacuum extractor apparatus used as an alternative to obstetric forceps; metal cup is attached by suction to the fetal scalp and gentle traction, synchronised with uterine contractions, is exerted. *See* Appendix 3 (Figure 5).

vagal pertaining to the vagus nerve.

vagina squamous epithelium-lined canal leading from the vulva to the cervix; part of the birth canal, having an anterior wall of 6.5–7.5 cm in length with the urethra and bladder base embedded in it, and a posterior wall of 9–10 cm, in contact with the perineal body, rectum and pouch of Douglas; lateral walls are in contact with the levator ani muscles.

vaginal pertaining to or through the vagina. *V. bleeding see* ANTEPARTUM HAEMORRHAGE. *V. discharge see* DISCHARGE. *V. examination* or *examination per vaginam* means of assessing aspects of obstetric and gynaecological conditions by palpation with one or two fingers in the vagina.

vaginismus painful spasms of the muscles of the vagina.

vaginitis vaginal inflammation, often due to *Candida albicans* infection, which causes irritation, or to *Trichomonas vaginalis*, characterised by frothy, intensely irritant, greenish discharge.

vagus 10th cranial nerve; parasympathetic nerve with wide distribution in the body, supplying the heart, lungs, liver and part of the alimentary tract.

validation process of approval, e.g. of an academic course such as nursing and midwifery: all preregistration programmes are approved by the NURSING AND MIDWIFERY COUNCIL to ensure consistent standards.

validity research term used to determine the extent to which a process actually reflects the construct being examined when used for a specific group or purpose.

Valium *See* DIAZEPAM.

Valsalva manoeuvre increase of intrathoracic pressure by forcible exhalation against the closed glottis. Babies with respiratory distress adopt a partial Valsalva manoeuvre by grunting, thereby maintaining a positive pressure in the chest even during exhalation, i.e. POSITIVE END-EXPIRATORY PRESSURE (PEEP).

value measure of worth or efficiency; quantitative measurement of activity, concentration, etc., of specific substances. *Normal v.'s* range in concentration of specific substances found in normal healthy tissues, e.g. secretions.

valve membranous fold in a canal or passage that prevents backward flow of material passing through it.

valvotomy surgical operation to increase the lumen of a narrowed valve, e.g. mitral valvotomy to relieve MITRAL STENOSIS.

valvuloplasty plastic repair of a valve, especially a valve of the heart.

vanillylmandelic acid (VMA) excretory catecholamine product, used to test for adrenaline (epinephrine) metabolism; raised levels occur in adrenal tumours, e.g. PHAEOCHROMO-CYTOMA, assessed from a 24-hour urine sample.

variable in epidemiology any measurement that can have different values. *Dependent v.* variable dependent on the effect of other variables in an epidemiological study. *Independent v.* variable not influenced by other variables in an epidemiological study but which may cause alterations in these variables.

variance measure of the variation seen in a set of data.

varicella-zoster virus (VZV, chickenpox) viral infection commonly acquired during childhood, spread via upper respiratory tract droplets, causing non-specific malaise followed by abdominal and facial rash of vesicles that rupture, forming a crust. The person is infective from 2 days before the appearance of the rash until the last vesicle crusts over (or 6 days after the rash appears, if later). The virus remains latent in the dorsal root ganglia, reactivation leading to shingles; previous infection usually confers lifelong immunity to chickenpox. Pregnant women who have not had primary infection are advised to avoid contact with infected people; delivery should be delayed as long as possible if primary infection occurs after 36 weeks' gestation, allowing the fetus to develop passive immunity from maternal antibodies. Maternal complications from primary infection include encephalitis, hepatitis and pneumonia; congenital varicella syndrome from infection before 20 weeks' gestation can affect development of fetal skin, eyes, limbs and brain; infection after 36 weeks causes severe neonatal varicella; immunoglobulin can be given to reduce the severity of the illness.

varicose swollen or dilated. *V. veins* abnormally distended and tortuous veins, usually of the leg, caused by inefficient valves permitting back- or cross-flow of blood, particularly between superficial and deep veins; high progesterone levels in pregnancy relax vein walls causing stasis and inefficient venous return; may also develop in the vulva or rectum as HAEMORRHOIDS.

variola smallpox.

varix enlarged tortuous vein, artery or lymphatic vessel. pl. *varices*.

vas vessel. pl. *vasa*. *V. deferens* tube through which spermatozoa pass from the testis to be stored in the seminal vesicle to become part of the semen.

vasa praevia presentation, in front of the fetal head during labour, of the blood vessels of the umbilical cord where they enter the placenta in a velamentous insertion of the cord; when the membranes rupture, bleeding may occur leading to fetal distress.

vascular relating to, or consisting largely of, vessels.

vasectomy male sterilisation method involving removal of a portion of the VAS DEFERENS through a small scrotal incision.

vasoconstrictor causing contraction of blood vessels.

vasodepressor 1. lowers blood pressure through reduction in peripheral resistance. 2. agent causing vasodepression.

vasodilator causing dilatation of blood vessels.

vasomotor controlling the muscles of blood vessels, both dilator and constrictor.

vasopressin pressor agent produced in the pituitary gland; antidiuretic hormone.

vasopressor 1. stimulating contraction of capillary and arterial muscular tissue. 2. vasopressor agent.

vault part of the fetal skull (excluding the base and face) containing the cerebral hemispheres, consisting of two frontal, two parietal, two temporal and one occipital bones separated by membranous sutures, which allow skull moulding in labour and brain growth. *V. cap* contraceptive device; bowl-shaped cap attached to the vaginal vault by suction to prevent spermatozoa entering the cervix; best used with a spermicidal agent to increase effectiveness. *V. of the vagina* upper part of the vagina into which the cervix protrudes.

vegan vegetarian who excludes all foods of animal origin from the diet.

vegetarian person who eats only food of vegetable origin. *V. diet* one in which no meat is eaten. *Lacto-vegetarian diet* prohibits intake of meat, poultry, fish and eggs.

vein vessel carrying blood from capillaries back to the heart; has thin walls and a lining endothelium from which the venous valves are formed.

velamentous like a veil. *V. insertion of the umbilical cord* placenta in which the umbilical cord vessels divide before reaching the placenta. *See also* VASA PRAEVIA.

vena cava one of the two trunk veins returning venous blood to the right atrium of the heart.

venepuncture puncture of a vein, usually to obtain blood or administer a drug.

venereal concerning or resulting from sexual intercourse. *V. diseases* syphilis, gonorrhoea and soft chancre. *V. Disease Research Laboratory (VDRL) test* blood test for SYPHILIS performed at booking. False-negative results can occur in the early stages and the test

Velamentous insertion of cord

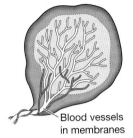

Blood vessels
in membranes

may be positive in the absence of syphilis. Other causes of a positive result include infectious mononucleosis, antiphospholipid antibody syndrome, lupus, hepatitis A, leprosy and malaria. Diagnosis should therefore be confirmed by a syphilis-specific test, such as the FLUORESCENT TREPONEMAL ANTIBODY-ABSORBED TEST (FTA-ABS).

venesection opening a vein and withdrawing blood to relieve congestion.

ventilation 1. providing fresh air in a room or building. 2. process of exchange of air between the lungs and ambient air. *Pulmonary v.* total exchange of air. *Alveolar v.* ventilation of the alveoli where gas exchange with the blood takes place. *Intermittent positive-pressure v. (IPPV)* mechanical ventilation by a machine designed to deliver breathing gas until equilibrium is established between the lungs and the VENTILATOR.

ventilator apparatus designed to qualify the air breathed through it or to intermittently or continuously control pulmonary ventilation; respirator.

Ventolin *See* SALBUTAMOL.

ventouse *See* VACUUM EXTRACTOR.

ventricle small pouch or cavity, especially the lower chambers of the heart and the four cavities of the brain.

ventricular septal defect congenital heart defect with persistent patency of the ventricular septum, which allows a flow of blood directly from one ventricle to the other, thereby bypassing the pulmonary circulation and causing cyanosis due to OXYGEN deficiency.

ventrosuspension an operation to shorten the round ligaments to help antevert a RETROVERTED UTERUS.

venule minute vein.

vernix caseosa greasy substance covering the fetus *in utero*; sebaceous gland secretion with desquamated cells; appears at about 30–32 weeks and remains until, or even past, full term.

version turning the fetus *in utero* to alter a lie or presentation to a more favourable one. *Cephalic v.* turning the fetus to make the head present. *External v.* turning the fetus by manipulation via the abdominal wall. *External cephalic v.* is often performed about 34 weeks' gestation to turn breech presentation. *Internal v.* inserting the hand into the uterus, turning the fetus with one hand in the uterus and the other on the abdomen. *Podalic v.* turning the fetus to make the breech present; occasionally, internal podalic version (followed by breech extraction) may be performed when a multipara is in labour with an oblique fetal lie or in the event of an oblique lie of a second twin.

vertebrae irregular bones forming the spinal column: seven cervical, 12 thoracic, five lumbar, five sacral (sacrum) and four coccygeal (coccyx) bones. sing. *vertebra*.

vertex area of the head bounded by the anterior and posterior fontanelles, and laterally by the parietal eminences. *V. presentation* the vertex lies over the internal os, the fetal head is well flexed; the most favourable presentation for delivery.

vertigo giddiness, temporary dizzy sensation with loss of equilibrium.

vesica bladder, usually urinary bladder; *see* ECTOPIA VESICAE.

vesical relating to the bladder.

vesicle blister or small sac usually containing fluid.

vesicoureteric reflux ureteric shortening and change of angle to the perpendicular caused by displacement by the enlarging uterus, leading to loss of efficiency at the junction of the ureter and bladder; reflux occurs in approximately 3% of women towards term, but it is not certain if this is a cause of ascending urinary tract infection.

vesicovaginal pertaining to bladder and vagina. *V. fistula* abnormal opening between bladder and vagina; rare complication of prolonged or obstructed labour when the tissues of the bladder are devitalised by prolonged pressure of the fetal head.

vesicular relating to, or containing, vesicles. *V. mole* HYDATIDIFORM MOLE.

vestibule entrance; part of the vulva lying between the labia minora.

vestige remnant of a structure that functioned in a previous stage of species or individual development. adj. *vestigial*.

viable, viability capable of life; pregnancy is viable when fetal heart pulsations are seen on ultrasound scan; also describes gestational age at which a baby would be capable of independent existence; legal age of viability is 24 weeks' gestation, but babies of 22–23 weeks' gestation may sometimes be successfully resuscitated after delivery.

Viagra (sildenafil citrate) oral drug used to treat erectile dysfunction; increases ability to achieve and maintain penile erection during sexual stimulation.

vicarious substituted for another. *V. liability* employer is vicariously liable for the torts of the employee during the course of his/her employment, e.g. health authority is vicariously liable for the torts of a midwife during the course of her employment.

villi fine hair-like processes projecting from a surface. *Chorionic v.* branched processes that develop on the trophoblast and which dip into the maternal blood of the placental site. *See* PLACENTA *and* CHORIONIC VILLI. *Intestinal v.* minute projections on the intestinal mucosa, each having a blood capillary and a lacteal; sites of absorption of fluids and nutrients. sing. *villus.*

viraemia presence of viruses in the blood.

viral caused by or having the nature of a virus.

virgin someone who has not had sexual intercourse.

virility 1. possessing masculine qualities. 2. male sexual potency.

virus small complex infective agent that can only grow and reproduce in living cells, only visible with an electron microscope. Viruses cause smallpox, poliomyelitis, influenza, measles, rubella and many more infections; they can cross the placenta and cause fetal abnormalities, especially in the first trimester.

viscera internal organs in the body cavities, e.g. heart, liver, uterus.

viscid sticky and glutinous.

visual analogue scale method of quantifying subjective feelings such as pain, sedation, etc. using a line, one end of which indicates absence of the feeling and the other extreme sensation; the subject marks a point along the line representing the sensation experienced at that time; distance from the left-hand end of the line to the point is measured and represents a numerical assessment of the sensation.

visual disturbances during pregnancy may occur in women with severe PRE-ECLAMPSIA or impending ECLAMPSIA because of retinal and optic nerve oedema.

visualisation technique that uses imagination and relaxation to create any desired changes in a person's life.

vital relating to or necessary to life. *V.statistics* records of births and deaths among the population, including causes of death and factors that seem to influence their rise and fall.

vitamins food substances, minute quantities of which are essential to nutrition and health; vitamins A, D, E and K are fat soluble, and B and C are water soluble. *Vitamin A* is found in fish liver oils, cream, milk, egg yolk, carrots, spinach, watercress; deficiency causes night blindness, growth retardation, lack of resistance to infection. *Vitamin B* group: thiamine (aneurine, vitamin B1), found in cereal husks and yeasts; deficiency causes neurological symptoms, cardiovascular dysfunction, oedema, reduced intestinal motility; nicotinic acid (niacin), found in liver, kidney, yeast; deficiency causes pellagra, including gastrointestinal, skin and mental disturbances; riboflavin (B2), found in liver, kidney, heart, brewer's yeast, milk, eggs, greens, enriched cereals; deficiency causes tongue inflammation, seborrhoeic dermatitis; cyanocobalamin (B12) and folic acid, both essential for red cell formation; deficiency causes megaloblastic or macrocytic ANAEMIA; pantothenic acid, pyridoxine (B6) and biotin are also part of the B complex. *Vitamin C* (ascorbic acid) is found in citrus fruit, blackcurrants, tomatoes, rosehips; deficiency causes scurvy and delays wound healing. *Vitamin D* is found in similar animal sources to vitamin A but also manufactured by skin exposed to sunlight; essential for absorption of calcium and phosphorus; deficiency causes rickets, osteomalacia, neonatal HYPOCALCAEMIA. *Vitamin E* deficiency leads to sterility in rats, but function in humans is not known. *Vitamin K* is necessary for the formation of PROTHROMBIN; found in spinach, cabbage, cauliflower, oats and synthesised in intestine by bacteria; deficiency rarely occurs except when the gut is sterile, i.e. when taking a broad-spectrum antibiotic or if HAEMORRHAGIC DISEASE occurs in the first days of life.

volvulus torsion of a loop of intestine, causing obstruction with or without strangulation.

vomiting expulsion of stomach contents through the mouth. *V. of blood* HAEMATEMESIS. *V. in the newborn* (a) Bile-stained vomit without passage of meconium indicates intestinal obstruction; the sooner after delivery the higher the site. (b) Blood-stained vomit may be due to maternal blood swallowed at delivery or ingested from cracked nipples, or to the baby's own blood in cases of HAEMORRHAGIC DISEASE. (c) Milk may be vomited owing to infections of the urinary tract, GASTROENTERITIS and MENINGITIS, relaxed cardia, feeding problems,

raised intracranial pressure. *V.in pregnancy* occurs in up to 90% of pregnancies, most commonly in the first 3 months but may persist throughout pregnancy; characterised by nausea, vomiting, heartburn; occurs at any time of day or night; severe vomiting leads to HYPEREMESIS GRAVIDARUM. Intercurrent vomiting may be due to PYELONEPHRITIS, other gastrointestinal tract conditions or severe illness. Vomiting with hypertension, oedema and proteinuria in late pregnancy may be a serious sign of severe PRE-ECLAMPSIA or impending ECLAMPSIA caused by liver oedema and/or haemorrhage. *Projectile v.* occurs in hypertrophic PYLORIC STENOSIS.

vomitus material vomited.

vulsellum *See* FORCEPS *and* Appendix 3.

vulva external female genital organs.

vulvectomy excision of the vulva.

vulvitis inflammation of the vulva.

'waiter's tip' characteristic position of forearm and hand in ERB'S PARALYSIS.

warfarin anticoagulant drug given to control the prothrombin time to 2.5–3.5 times above normal; crosses the placenta so should only be used from gestational weeks 16 to 36.

wart epidermal tumour of viral origin. *Genital w.* spread in pregnancy to vulva, perineum and anal regions; treated with local podophyllin.

water birth labour care in which the mother chooses to labour, and may deliver, in water for relaxation and pain relief; midwives should receive adequate training before taking responsibility for this type of care.

weaning detaching from an accustomed habit, e.g. change of infant feeding from breast to bottle or cup feeding, from bottle to cup feeding or, more commonly, from any type of milk feed to solid food.

webbed connected by a membrane or strand of tissue. *W. hands* or *feet* congenital abnormality in which the digits are not separated from each other; syndactyly. *W. neck* folds of skin in the neck giving a webbed appearance, as in some congenital conditions, e.g. Turner's syndrome.

weight gain during pregnancy normal weight gain is usually about 10–12 kg, approximately 2.5 kg in the first 20 weeks and 0.5 kg per week thereafter; accounted for by fetus at term (3.4 kg), placenta (0.7 kg), amniotic fluid (1 kg), uterus (1 kg), blood (1.4 kg) and breasts (1 kg), plus tissue fluid, fat and protein deposition. Excess weight gain may be due to OEDEMA, as in PRE-ECLAMPSIA, multiple pregnancy or large baby; poor weight gain may indicate INTRAUTERINE GROWTH RETARDATION. *W. g. in babies* a neonate loses up to 10% of their birthweight in the first few days of life because of passage of meconium but should have regained this by 10–14 days; weight gain is then approximately 200 g per week.

Weil's disease spirochaetal jaundice caused by *Leptospira icterohaemorrhagiae*, transmitted in rat urine; acquired through the skin or from infected food or water.

well woman clinic clinic to screen women early for breast and cervical cancer, anaemia, diabetes, hypertension and other conditions.

Wernicke's encephalopathy acute haemorrhagic encephalitis, occurring occasionally in severe HYPEREMESIS GRAVIDARUM as a result of vitamin B1 deficiency.

Wertheim's operation *See* HYSTERECTOMY.

Wharton's jelly connective tissue of the umbilical cord.

whey fluid part of milk, separated from the curd after the addition of rennet; easily digested as the casein and fat have been removed.

white blood cell *See* LEUCOCYTE.

white leg *See* PHLEGMASIA ALBA DOLENS.

white matter, white substance white nervous tissue, consisting of myelinated nerve fibres; constitutes the conducting portion of the brain and spinal cord. Grey matter or substance is used to describe unmyelinated fibres.

WHO International Code of Marketing of Breast Milk Substitutes World Health Organization and UNICEF code to protect and promote breastfeeding and control marketing of products for artificial feeding, especially in developing countries. Recommends prohibition of advertising/promotion direct to the public; no free breast milk substitute samples or other free gifts, special offers and discounts for mothers; no financial or other rewards for health workers for the purpose of promoting breast milk substitutes; professional information on breast milk substitutes should contain only scientific factual data, in no way implying superiority over human breast milk.

whooping cough   *See* PERTUSSIS.

Widal reaction   blood test used in the diagnosis of typhoid and paratyphoid fevers.

Wilson–Mikity syndrome   BRONCHOPULMONARY DYSPLASIA, a condition occurring in babies who have been ventilated for long periods or who have needed prolonged OXYGEN therapy.

wolffian bodies   two small organs in the embryo, the primitive kidneys.

womb   uterus.

Wood's manoeuvre   method of facilitating delivery of the baby in shoulder dystocia by inserting a hand into the vagina to identify the fetal chest, then exerting pressure on the posterior fetal shoulder to rotate it, enabling delivery to be completed.

World Health Organization (WHO)   specialised United Nations agency concerned with international health; campaigns include Safe Motherhood For All by 2000, an attempt to reduce high maternal mortality rates in developing countries.

wound   physically-induced bodily injury that causes disruption of the normal function of local structures. *W. healing* in healing by first intention, restoration of tissue function occurs directly without granulation; in healing by second intention, wound repair is accomplished by closure of the wound with granulation tissue; healing by third intention occurs when closure of a contaminated wound is delayed until 4–5 days after the injury.

Wrigley's forceps   obstetric forceps used for very low forceps deliveries, assisting delivery of the aftercoming head of the breech or at Caesarean section. *See* Appendix 3.

X chromosome sex chromosome. Female cells carry two X chromosomes (XX) and male cells one X and one Y chromosome (XY). During maturation of the ovum and spermatozoon, one of the two chromosomes is cast off; at fertilisation the two remaining chromosomes determine the baby's sex: two X chromosomes produce a girl, whereas an X and a Y chromosome produces a boy. *See also* TURNER'S SYNDROME *and* KLINE-FELTER'S SYNDROME.

X-linked transmitted by genes on the X chromosome; sex-linked.

X-rays RÖNTGEN RAYS; electromagnetic waves capable of penetrating many substances, e.g. paper, wood, flesh, but absorbed by lead, platinum and bone.

xiphisternum XIPHOID PROCESS; base of the sternum.

xiphoid process small cartilaginous process at the lower end of the sternum; also called xiphisternum and ensiform cartilage. Landmark to which the uterine fundus is related in later pregnancy to assess gestation.

XO *See* TURNER'S SYNDROME.

Xylocaine *See* LIDOCAINE (LIGNOCAINE) HYDROCHLORIDE.

XYY syndrome (47XYY) genetic condition, occurring in approximately 1 in 1000 men, in which an additional Y chromosome is inherited; those affected tend to be taller than the norm, but physical development is otherwise normal; mental maturity and speech development may be delayed and they may also exhibit excessive violent criminal tendencies although increased levels of early structured activity such as sport can limit this.

Y

Y chromosome sex chromosome; male cells carry one Y and one X chromosome.

yaws non-venereal, tropical, treponemal infection; local lesions are similar to those of SYPHILIS and serological tests for syphilis are positive.

yeast fungus that produces fermentation; THRUSH is due to infection with the yeast-like fungus *Candida albicans*.

yin and yang two opposing yet complementary principles in Chinese philosophy; yin indicates the feminine, dark, negative or passive side; yang indicates the masculine, bright, positive, assertive side. Each person should ideally have a balance of both yin and yang; harmony denotes optimum health and well-being.

yoga Indian philosophical approach to health and well-being, involving breathing, relaxation and exercise; may be suitable for pregnant women.

yolk sac one of two spaces in the inner cell mass of the trophoblast, surrounded by entodermal cells; the other space, the amniotic cavity, is surrounded by ectodermal cells and between the two is an intervening layer of mesoderm. The embryo is formed from the area where the three tissues, ectoderm, mesoderm and entoderm, lie in apposition.

Yutopar *See* RITODRINE HYDROCHLORIDE.

zero nought; symbol 0. In the Celsius thermometer, 0 °C is the melting point of ice; in the Fahrenheit thermometer, 0°F is 32° below the melting point of ice. *See* FAHRENHEIT *and* CELSIUS.

zidovudine antiviral drug used to slow the progress of AIDS; also known as azidothymidine or AZT.

zinc trace element, a component of several enzymes, found in red meat, shellfish, liver, peas, lentils, beans and rice; severe deficiency causes a low sperm count in men, miscarriage, growth retardation and slow wound healing.

zona pellucida transparent, non-cellular, secreted layer surrounding an OVUM. SPERM release enzymes that allow penetration of the zona pellucida; only one sperm enters the ovum at the time of fertilisation.

Zovirax *See* ACICLOVIR.

zygote fertilised ovum before SEGMENTATION. *Z. intrafallopian transfer (ZIFT)* infertility treatment in which ovulation is stimulated artificially, oocytes are harvested using ultrasound-directed follicle aspiration (UDFA), transvaginally or at laparoscopy, and, once fertilisation has occurred, the resulting zygote is transferred at laparoscopy into the midampullary section of the fallopian tube.

APPENDICES

Apgar score

SIGN	SCORE		
	0	1	2
Colour	Blue to pale	Body pink, limbs blue	Pink
Respiratory	Absent	Irregular gasps	Strong cry effort
Heart rate	Absent	Less than 100/minute	Over 100/minute
Muscle tone	Limp	Some flexion of limbs	Strong active movements
Reflex	Nil	Grimace or sneeze	Cry irritability

Apgar score 8–10: normal.
Apgar score 5–8: mild asphyxia.
Apgar score 4 or below: severe asphyxia.
See also Appendix 7.

APPENDIX 2

Normal blood and urine values and tests

Values should be used as a guide only as those for normal or reference ranges will vary between laboratories although national and international standardisation has limited this. However, certain parameters, particularly enzymes, may vary considerably depending on assay conditions and units of measurement. Some laboratories may use 'traditional' units as opposed to SI units, which may have a very significant effect on the numeric value of a result. Before taking samples for laboratory analysis it is advisable to check whether any preparations of the patient or special timing or conditions for handling the sample are necessary as these may vary between laboratories. It is *essential* that the reference ranges for the laboratory providing the analysis are used to evaluate results of tests. Specimens should be collected into the correct containers at appropriate times and under appropriate conditions.

Specimens and request forms must be adequately labelled with patient's name, number or date of birth, location, date and time of specimen. *Failure to comply* may result in serious errors in diagnosis and management. Colour coding of blood sample bottles is not standardised 'and care should be taken to use the correct specimen preservatives. Be careful to avoid contamination of samples with preservatives from other bottles. Pathology departments usually contain different laboratories: *B*iochemistry (may be called *C*hemical *P*athology), *H*aematology, Blood *T*ransfusion, *M*icrobiology, *H*istopathology.

LABORATORY	NOTE	TEST/REASON	MOTHER		BABY	
			Sample	Size	Sample	Size
T/H		ABO group + Rh factor	Clotted/EDTA	6 mL	Clotted/EDTA	1 mL
B		Abuse drug screen (urine)	MSU	20 mL	MSU	2 mL
B	1	AFP/Bart's/Leeds	Clotted	6 mL	-	-
T/H		Antibodies	Clotted/EDTA	6 mL	Clotted/EDTA	1 mL
B		Blood sugar	Fluoride oxalate	2 mL	Fluoride oxalate	1 mL
H/B		Chromosomes	Heparinised	4 mL	Heparinised	2 mL
H		Clotting studies	Citrate	3 mL	Citrate	1 mL
H		Ferritin	Clotted	6 mL	Clotted	2 mL
H		Folate (RBC)	EDTA	3 mL	-	-
H	1	Folate (serum)	Clotted	6 mL	-	-
T/H	2	Fragile X	-	-	EDTA	2 mL
H		Full blood count (FBC)	EDTA	3 mL	EDTA	1 mL
H		Genotype/electrophoresis	EDTA	3 mL	EDTA	1 mL
H		Haemoglobin (Hb)	EDTA	3 mL	EDTA	1 mL
B	4	HbA$_{1c}$	EDTA	2 mL	-	-
M		HBsAg	Clotted	6 mL	Clotted	2 mL
M	4	HIV	Clotted	6 mL	Clotted	2 mL

(Table continued on following page)

251

LABORATORY	NOTE	TEST/REASON	MOTHER			BABY		
			Sample	Size		Sample	Size	
B	3	Liver function test	Clotted	6 mL		Heparinised	2 mL	
B		Pregnancy test (blood)	Clotted	2 mL		-	-	
M		Pregnancy test (urine)	MSU	20 mL		-	-	
M		Rubella immunity	Clotted	6 mL		Clotted	2 mL	
B	3	Thyroid function test	Clotted	6 mL		Heparinised	2 mL	
M		Toxoplasmosis	Clotted	6 mL		Clotted	2 mL	
M		TPHA	Clotted	6 mL		Clotted	2 mL	
B	5	U & E	Clotted	6 mL		Heparinised	2 mL	
B		Urate	Clotted	6 mL		Heparinised	2 mL	
M		VDRL	Clotted	6 mL		Clotted	2 mL	
H	6	Vitamin B12	Clotted	6 mL		-	-	

Notes
1. May not be routinely available or subject to local practice – check with laboratory.
2. Sample must go to laboratory immediately.
3. Note local reference ranges.
4. May need preliminary patient counselling.
5. Sample should reach laboratory in <3 hours for potassium.
6. Vitamin B12 falls throughout pregnancy.

	UNITS	MOTHER		BABY	BABY AGE	COMMENTS
		Non-pregnant	Pregnant			
BLOOD						
Red cells (erythrocytes/RBC)	×10¹²/L	4–5		6–6.5 4–5	Birth 4 weeks	
Glucose (fasting)	mmol/L	3.3–5.3	3.3–6.1	1.0–6.0		
Haemoglobin	g/dL	12–15		12.2–24 12.2–22	Birth 1 week	Check local units
Packed cell volume (PCV haematocrit)	L/L	0.42–0.50		0.52–0.58 0.46–0.54	Day 1 2 weeks	Check local units
Reticulocytes	×10⁹/L	20–100		100–300		
Leucocytes	×10⁹/L	4.0–11.0	4.0–15.0	5–23 5–19	Day 1 Day 7	
Neutrophils	×10⁹/L	2.5–7.5				
Lymphocytes	×10⁹/L	1.8–3.5				
Monocytes	×10⁹/L	0.2–0.8				
Eosinophils	×10⁹/L	0.04–0.4				
Basophils	×10⁹L	0.0–0.1				
Platelets	×10⁹/L	150–400				
pH		7.35–7.45		7.35–7.45		

(Table continued on following page)

253

	UNITS	MOTHER		BABY	BABY AGE	COMMENTS
		Non-pregnant	Pregnant			
P_{CO_2}	kPa	4.7–6.0				Check local units
Standard bicarbonate	mmol/L	24.0–32.0				
PLASMA/SERUM						
Albumin	g/L	36–52	22–44	28–40		
Alanine aminotransferase (ALT/SGPT)	IU/L	5–35				Check local ranges
Aspartate aminotransferase (AST/SGOT)	IU/L	5–35				Check local ranges
Bilirubin	µmol/L	<17	<17	<200	<10 days	See charts below
				<40	>10 days	
Calcium	mmol/L	2.1–2.6	2.2–2.4	1.9–2.9		
Chloride	mmol/L	95–105		96–106		
Cholesterol	mmol/L	3.6–6.7	5.4–7.8	2.1–4.1		
Creatinine	µmol/L	60–120		9–62		
Ferritin	µg/L	14–40		90–640	2 weeks to 6 months	
Folate	µg/L	1.7–10				
Magnesium	mmol/L	0.8–1.0		0.6–1.6		

	UNITS	MOTHER Non-pregnant	MOTHER Pregnant	BABY	BABY AGE	COMMENTS
Osmolality	mOsm/kg	285–295		280–305		
Phosphate	mmol/L	0.8–1.4	0.8–1.5	1.3–2.7		
Potassium	mmol/L	3.8–5.0		4.0–6.0		Elevated by haemolysis
Protein (total)	g/L	62–75	50–70	50–65		
Sodium	mmol/L	135–145		136–143		
Thyroid-binding globulin (TBG)	Variable	Variable	Elevated			Check local units
Thyroid-stimulating hormone (TSH)	mU/L	0.5–4.7		<0.5–8.0		
Thyroxine (free) FT4	pmol/L	9–25		15–30		
Thyroxine (total) TT4	nmol/L	50–140	72–206	140–300	1–3 days	
				125–200	1–4 weeks	
Triiodothyronine (free) FT3	pmol/L	3–9		3–9		
Triiodothyronine (total) TT3	nmol/L	0.9–3.0				
TT4/TBG ratio			Reduced			
Urate	mmol/L	0.09–0.36	0.15–0.52	0.12–0.34		Check local units

(Table continued on following page)

| | UNITS | MOTHER | | BABY | BABY AGE | COMMENTS |
		Non-pregnant	Pregnant			
Urea	mmol/L	2.5–5.8	2.3–5.0	3.4–8.4		
Vitamin B12	ng/L	179–1132	Reduced			Falls until term
RED CELL						
Folate	μg/L	125–800				
Glucose-6-phosphate dehydrogenase (G6PD)	IU/g Hb	4.6–13.5		4.6–13.5		Elevated by reticulocytosis
URINE						
Calcium	mmol/24 h	2.5–7.5				
Creatinine	mmol/24 h	9–17				
Calcium–creatinine ratio				<1.2		
Creatinine clearance	mL/min	80–130	80–140			
Osmolality	mOsm/kg	>600		40–1400		Consider with serum
Potassium	mmol/24 h	25–125		25–125		
Protein	g/24 h	<0.15				
Protein	g/L			<0.05		

	UNITS	MOTHER		BABY	BABY AGE	COMMENTS
		Non-pregnant	Pregnant			
Reducing substances		Negative		Negative		Must be fresh sample
Sodium	mmol/24 h	27–290		40–210		Diet dependent
CSF						
Glucose	mmol/L	2.5–4.5		2.5–5.0		Relates to blood glucose
Protein	g/L	0.15–0.40		0.15–0.50		
STOOL						
Reducing substances				Negative		Must be fresh sample

Values given are intended as a guide only. Local units and reference ranges should always be used in preference to those shown. Where ranges are not shown the same values as given for *non-pregnant mother* apply.

Obstetric instruments

FIGURE 1 Copeland fetal skin electrode.

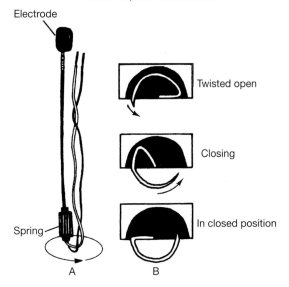

A, Copeland electrode; B, cross-section of a Copeland electrode.

FIGURE 2 Instruments for artificial rupture of the membranes.

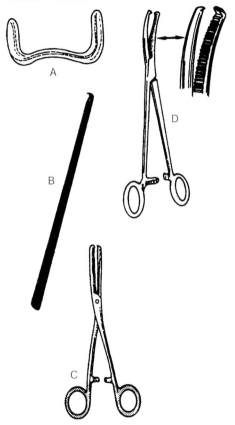

A, Sims' speculum; **B,** Amnihook; **C,** straight Kocher forceps; **D,** curved Kocher forceps.

FIGURE 3 Instruments for perineal repair.

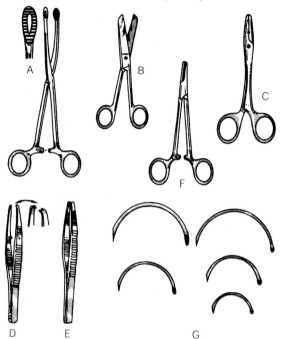

A, Sponge-holding forceps; **B,** blunt-ended scissors; **C,** needle holder; **D,** toothed dissecting forceps; **E,** non-toothed dissecting forceps; **F,** small Spencer Wells artery forceps; **G,** needles: left, round-bodied, Nos 8 and 12; right, cutting, Nos 6, 8 and 12; atraumatic needle 40 mm on Dexon suture now commonly used.

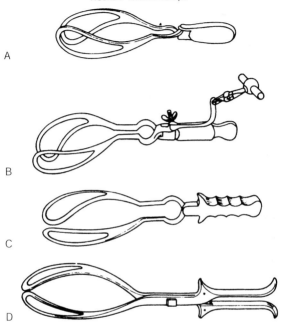

FIGURE 4 Obstetric forceps.

A, Wrigley's; **B,** axis-traction; **C,** Anderson's; **D,** Kielland's.

FIGURE 5 Malmström vacuum extractor, showing the vacuum pump and three sizes of cup; chain and handle, and components of the extraction pump.

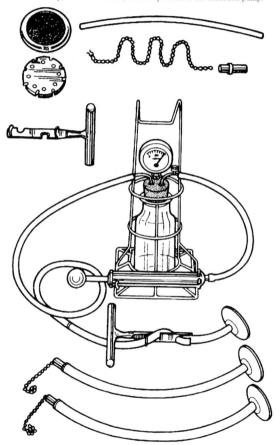

FIGURE 6 Various specula.

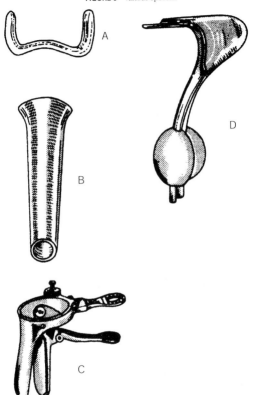

A, Sims'; **B,** Fergusson's; **C,** Cusco's; **D,** Auvard's.

FIGURE 7A–C Instruments for Caesarean section.

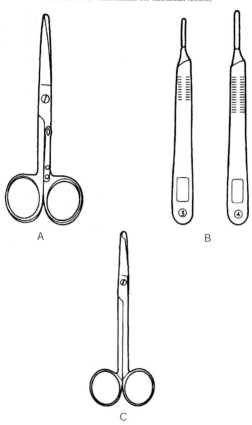

A, Nurse's scissors; **B,** blade handles; **C,** Spencer stitch scissors.

FIGURE 7D–F

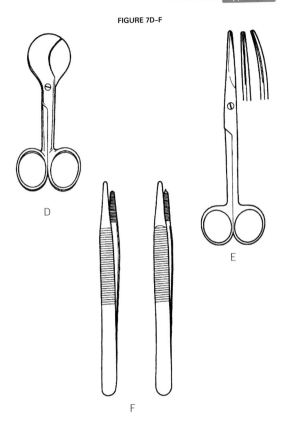

D, umbilical scissors; **E,** Mayo scissors; **F,** plain and toothed Bonney dissecting forceps.

(*Illustration continued on following page*)

FIGURE 7G–J (*Continued*) Instruments for Caesarean section.

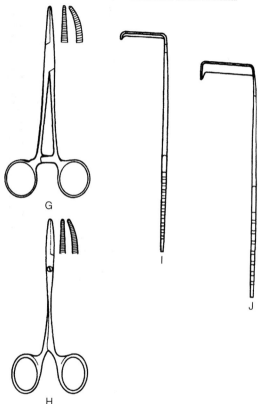

G, Moynihan artery forceps; **H,** Spencer Wells forceps; **I,** Langenbeck retractor;
J, Morris retractor.

FIGURE 7K–N

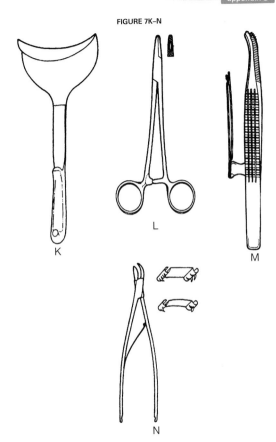

K, Doyen retractor; **L,** Mayo needle holder; **M,** Childe approximating forceps; **N,** Michel clips.

(*Illustration continued on following page*)

FIGURE 70-Q (*Continued*)   Instruments for Caesarean section.

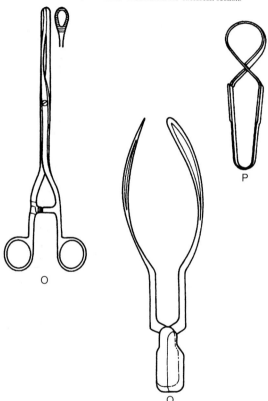

O, Rampley sponge-holding forceps; **P,** Backhaus H cross action towel clips; **Q,** Wrigley's forceps.

FIGURE 7R–S

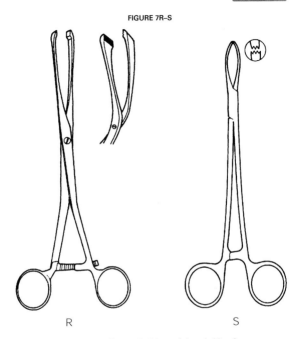

R

S

R, Green Armytage forceps; **S,** Littlewood tissue-holding forceps.

(Illustration continued on following page)

FIGURE 7T (*Continued*)   Instruments for Caesarean section.

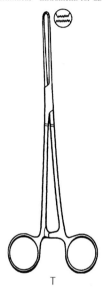

T

T, Stiles forceps.

Identification of fetal position on examination *per vaginam*

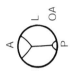

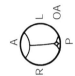

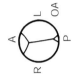

Occipitoanterior positions viewed from the pelvic outlet.

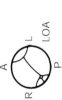

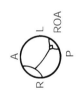

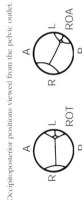

Occipitoposterior positions viewed from the pelvic outlet.

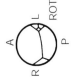

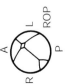

Identifying the position of the fetus on vaginal examination by identifying the position of the sutures and fontanelles in relation to the pelvis.

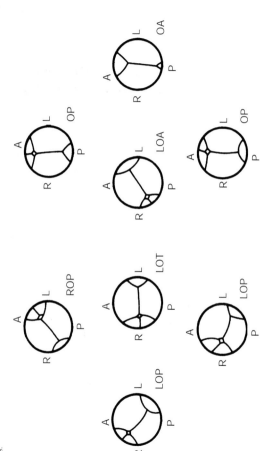

272

Normal labour: cervicogram; partogram; cardiotocograph recordings

FIGURE 1

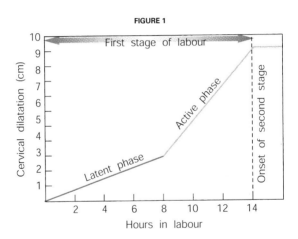

A cervicogram [reproduced from Sweet BR (ed.) *Mayes' Midwifery – a Textbook for Midwives*. Edinburgh: Churchill Livingstone, 1997, with permission].

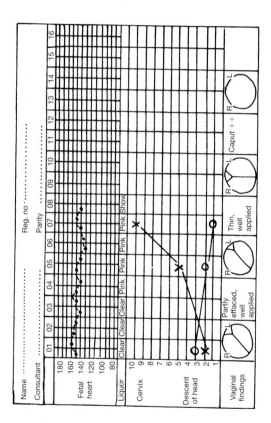

FIGURE 2 Diagram of a partogram.

FIGURE 2 (*Continued*) Diagram of a partogram.

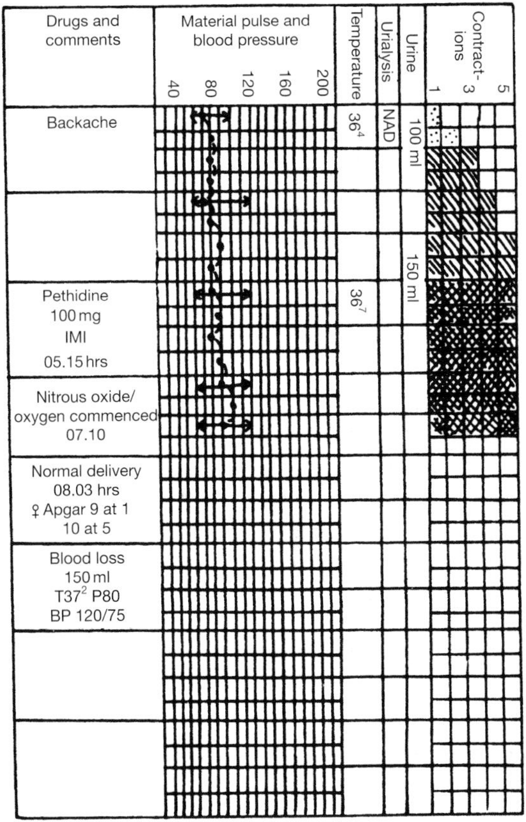

FIGURE 3 Cardiograph recordings.

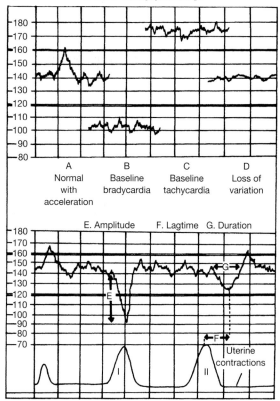

I. Early deceleratin (type 1 dip); II. late deceleration (type 2 dip).

Management of postpartum haemorrhage

(*See also* POSTPARTUM HAEMORRHAGE.)

Aims of management:

1. to help the uterus to contract firmly;
2. to deliver the placenta if still *in situ*;
3. to arrest haemorrhage as soon as possible and reduce shock.

Action:

- Call skilled obstetrician or emergency obstetric unit if available.
- If bleeding is uterine give oxytocic drug, e.g. ergometrine 0.5 mg intravenously or Syntometrine 1 mL intramuscularly.
- Massage uterine fundus via abdomen to encourage contraction.
- Empty bladder, catheterise if necessary; examine vagina for lacerations.
- When uterus well contracted attempt controlled cord traction to deliver placenta.
- Prepare equipment for oxytocic intravenous infusion and manual removal of placenta; take blood for cross-matching.
- In rare cases bimanual compression of non-contracted uterus can save life.
- In isolated areas midwife may have to perform MANUAL REMOVAL OF PLACENTA.

Neonatal resuscitation

Asphyxia neonatorum should be anticipated if there are any signs of fetal hypoxia in labour. The midwife should check and prepare resuscitation equipment and alert the paediatrician. At delivery the midwife should:

- note the time;
- aspirate mucus from the baby's naso- and oropharynx;
- cut the cord;
- dry and wrap the baby warmly;
- place the baby under a radiant heater on the equipment, in a supine position with the head slightly lower and extended;
- assess the Apgar score at 1 minute (*see* Appendix 1).

Apgar score 8–10: no further treatment needed.

Apgar score 5–8: mild asphyxia:

- call paediatrician;
- give oxygen by intermittent positive pressure ventilation via bag and mask or by mouth to mouth/nose resuscitation;
- stimulate the baby gently;
- administer naloxone 0.01 mg/kg body weight if mother had pethidine.

Apgar score below 5: severe asphyxia:

- summon paediatrician urgently;
- clear airways gently;
- give oxygen (max. pressure 30 cmH$_2$O) by intermittent positive pressure ventilation at 30 times per minute or intubate with endotracheal tube if trained to do so;
- check heart rate;
- apply cardiac massage if heart rate less than 40 beats per minute at 100–120 times per minute;
- assist with administration of drugs as appropriate.

Conversion charts

CONVERSION OF BABIES' WEIGHTS (lb, oz to g)

oz	0	1	2	3	4	5	6	7	8	9	10	11	12	13	14	15
lb																
0		28	57	85	113	142	170	198	227	255	283	312	340	368	397	425
1	454	482	510	539	567	595	624	652	680	709	737	765	794	822	850	879
2	907	935	964	992	1020	1049	1077	1105	1134	1162	1190	1219	1247	1275	1304	1332
3	1360	1389	1418	1446	1475	1503	1531	1560	1588	1616	1645	1673	1701	1730	1758	1786
4	1815	1843	1871	1900	1928	1956	1985	2013	2041	2070	2098	2126	2155	2183	2211	2240
5	2268	2296	2325	2353	2381	2410	2438	2466	2495	2523	2551	2580	2608	2636	2655	2683
6	2721	2750	2778	2806	2835	2863	2891	2920	2948	2976	3005	3033	3061	3090	3118	3146
7	3175	3203	3231	3260	3258	3316	3345	3373	3401	3430	3458	3486	3515	3543	3571	3600
8	3628	3656	3685	3713	3741	3770	3798	3826	3855	3883	3911	3940	3968	3996	4025	4053
9	4081	4110	4138	4166	4195	4223	4251	4280	4308	4336	4355	4383	4421	4450	4468	4506
10	4535	4563	4591	4620	4648	4676	4705	4733	4761	4790	4818	4846	4875	4903	4931	4960

In making this conversion it is generally sufficient to use the nearest round figure, e.g. 5.5 lb = 2495 g, rounded to 2.5 kg.

FIGURE 1 Weight and height conversion charts for antenatal women.

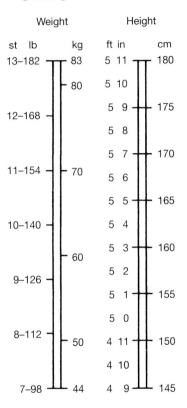

FIGURE 2 Linear equivalents for lengths of babies.

Length

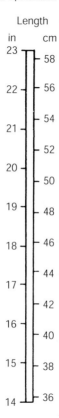

FIGURE 3 Celsius/Fahrenheit equivalents.

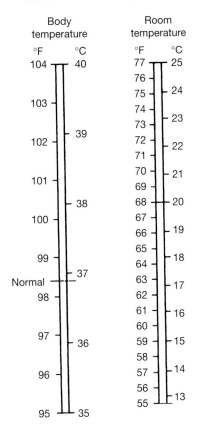

SI Units (Système International d'Unités)

Metric system for scientific measurements. The unit of weight is the gram (g), of length the metre (m) and of capacity the litre (L).

Measurements smaller than a unit

Prefix	Symbol	Meaning	Example
deci	d	One-tenth	dL = one-tenth of a litre
centi	c	One-hundredth	cm = one-hundredth of a metre
milli	m	One-thousandth	mL = one-thousandth of a litre
micro	μ	One-millionth	μg = one-millionth of a gram

Multiples of units

Prefix	Symbol	Meaning	Example
deca	da	10	da L = 10 litres
hecto	h	100	hg = 100 grams
kilo	k	1000	kg = 1000 grams
mega	M	1 million	MJ = 1 million joules

Mass

Calculation of drug doses is vitally important, especially with neonates when the dose is given according to the weight of the baby. The following equivalents may be useful:

1 kilogram (kg)	= 1000 grams (g)
1 gram (g)	= 1000 milligrams (mg)
1 milligram (mg)	= 1000 micrograms (μg)
1 microgram (μg)	= 1000 nanograms (ng)
1 nanogram (ng)	= 1000 picograms

Index notation

If one unit is used for very large or small quantities the numbers may involve many zeros and be clumsy to read or write, with the risk of inaccuracies. The 'index' is a small raised number that can be used to indicate the number of times the quantity must be multiplied by 10. For example:

$100 = 10 \times 10$	= index 10^2
$10\,000 = 10 \times 10 \times 10 \times 10$	= index 10^4

When fractions of a unit are used the index has a minus sign to represent the number of times the quantity should be divided by 10. For example:

$0.1 = 1/10$ = index 10^{-1}
$0.01 = 1/100$ = index 10^{-2}

Index notation is now used in pathology reports. For example:

	Old value	*Index notation*
Total white blood count	$5000–10\,000/mm^3$	$5.0–10.0 \times 10^9/L$
Red cell count	4.5 million$/mm^3$	$4.5 \times 10^{12}/L$

Features of preterm and small for gestational age babies

FEATURE	PRETERM	SMALL FOR GESTATIONAL AGE
Skin	Reddish pink with lanugo	Grey or yellowish from meconium; dry, sometimes cracked
Length	Proportionate to weight	Proportionate to gestation, i.e. long for weight
Head	Cranial bones soft	Cranial bones hard, unyielding
Face	Eyes closed; peaceful expression	Eyes often open; worried expression
Ear pinna	Soft, remains folded	Resistant to folding
Breast size	Tissue <1 cm diameter	Palpable tissue ≥1 cm diameter
Abdomen	May be prominent	Often scaphoid
Behaviour	Weak cry, inactive; no attempt to suck/swallow; flaccid limbs abducted; lies in 'frog' position	Stronger, more mature cry; hungry sucking; swallows; lively, active, good muscle tone

Limits of serum bilirubin levels in neonates

Kernicterus may occur when the levels of unconjugated bilirubin exceed the following levels, depending on gestation:

Under 27 weeks	250 µmol/L
28–30 weeks	280 µmol/L
31–34 weeks	310 µmol/L
35–38 weeks	350 µmol/L
39 + weeks	380 µmol/L

Maternity and other relevant social security benefits

BENEFIT	DETAILS
CHILD BENEFIT	
Weekly payment to primary responsible adult, payable for all children up to age 16 (or 19 if still in full-time education)	Not dependent on income or savings
CHILD TAX CREDIT	
Payment to support families with children under 16 or under 19 if in full-time college (but not university) education	Amount based on household income
DISABILITY LIVING ALLOWANCE	
Benefit for physically or mentally disabled children or adults who need help with personal care or who have walking difficulties	Consists of a care component (if help is needed with daily care) and a mobility component (if physically unable to move or get around). Tax free, not dependent on income or savings
NHS DENTAL CARE AND PRESCRIPTIONS	
Free to all pregnant women and for up to 1 year following delivery; free for all children under 16 or under 19 if in full-time education	
STATUTORY MATERNITY LEAVE AND PAY	
Weekly payment to encourage all women to take time off work before and after delivery. Entitled to	Paid by employer; tax and National Insurance are deducted. Must be employed by same employer for at

BENEFIT	DETAILS
52 weeks' leave from work including 39 weeks on statutory maternity pay	least 26 weeks by the 15th week before EDD; must work until at least the 15th week before EDD; payment commences any time after 11th week before EDD for a continuous period of 39 weeks

STATUTORY PATERNITY LEAVE AND PAY

Financial payments and up to 2 week's leave to encourage fathers to be involved in the early care of their baby	Based on income, paid by employer. Must have responsibility for the child's upbringing, be the biological father or the mother's partner; also payable to adoptive fathers. Must have worked continuously for employer for 26 weeks ending with the 15th week before the baby is due

SURE START MATERNITY GRANT

One-off payment from the Social Fund to help those on very low incomes with the costs of having a new baby	Payable to those receiving Income Support, income-based Jobseeker's Allowance, Pension Credit, Child Tax Credit at a rate higher than the family element or Working Tax Credit when a disability or severe disability element is included in the award. Does not have to be repaid

WORKING TAX CREDIT

Payable to 'top up' the low earnings of employed or self-employed adults, including those without children, to encourage them to remain in work	Includes extra supplements for families with young children requiring child-care and for those with a disability

APPENDIX 13

Useful addresses and websites

Association for Postnatal Illness, 145 Dawes Road, Fulham, London SW6 7EB
www.apni.org

Action on Pre-eclampsia (APEC) www.apec.org.uk

Association for Improvements in Maternity Services (AIMS), 5 Ann's Court, Grove Road, Surbiton, Surrey KT6 4BE chair@aims.org.uk

Association of Medical Research Charities, 61 Gray's Inn Road, London WC1X 8TL
www.armc.org.uk

Association of Radical Midwives, 62 Greetby Hill, Ormskirk, Lancashire L39 2DT
www.radmid.demon.co.uk

Baby Friendly Initiative, 64–78 Kingsway, London WC2B 6NB
www.babyfriendly.org.uk

Bandolier (website that summarises randomised controlled trials)
www.jr2.ox.ac.uk/bandolier

British Association of Counselling, 37a Sheep Street, Rugby, Warwickshire CV21 3BX www.bacp.co.uk

British Medical Association, BMA House, 179 Tavistock Square, London WC1H 9JP
www.bma.org.uk

British National Formulary (drug information) www.bnf.org

British Pregnancy Advisory Service, 4th floor, Amec House, Timothy's Bridge Road, Stratford-upon-Avon CV37 9BF www.bpas.org.uk

Childline, Royal Mail Building, Studd Street, London N1 0QW
www.childline.org.uk

Cochrane Foundation (electronic publication of high-quality professional health research evidence) www.update-software.com

Complementary Maternity Forum, 2 Marigold Way, Shirley Oaks, Croydon CR0 8YD www.c-m-f.co.uk

CRY-SIS, BM Cry-sis, London WC1N 3XX www.cry-sis.org

Department of Health (England), Richmond House, 79 Whitehall, London SW1A 2NS www.doh.gov.uk

Expectancy – Expectant Parents' Complementary Therapies Consultancy
www.expectancy.co.uk

Family Planning Association, 50 Featherstone Street, London EC1Y 8QU
www.fpa.org.uk

Foresight (preconception care) www.foresight.gov.uk

Foundation for the Study of Infant Deaths, Artillery House, 11–19 Artillery Row, London SW1P 1RT www.sids.org.uk

Human Fertilisation and Embryology Authority (HFEA), 21 Bloomsbury Street, London WC1B 3HF www.hfea.gov.uk

Index Medicus (includes full listing of journal abbreviations used for Index Medicus) www.medscape.com

International Confederation of Midwives, Eisenhowerlaan 138 2517 KN, The Hague, Netherlands www.internationalmidwives.org

King's Fund, 11–13 Cavendish Square, London W1M 0AN www.kingsfund.org.uk

Medicines and Healthcare Products Regulatory Agency (MRHA), Market Towers, 1 Nine Elms Lane, London SW8 5NQ www.mhra.gov.uk

MIDIRS (Midwives' Information and Resource Service), 9 Elmdale Road, Clifton, Bristol BS12 2LQ www.midirs.org

MIND (National Association for Mental Health), 15–19 Broadway, London E15 4BQ www.mind.org.uk

MIRIAD (Midwifery Research Database), Manchester Metropolitan University, Cavendish North Building, Cavendish Street, Manchester M15 6BG www.miriad.nmu.ac.uk

Miscarriage Association, c/o Clayton Hospital, Northgate, Wakefield, West Yorkshire WF1 3JS www.miscarriageassociation.org.uk

National Childbirth Trust, Alexandra House, Oldham Terrace, Acton, London W3 6NH www.nct.org.uk

National Council for One Parent Families, 255 Kentish Town Road, London NW5 6NH www.oneparentfamilies.org.uk

National Electronic Library for Health (research website) www.nelh.nhs.uk

National Institute for Clinical Excellence (NICE), 90 Long Acre, London W3 6PH www.nice.org.uk

National Society for Prevention of Cruelty to Children (NSPCC), 67 Curtain Road, London EC2A 3NH www.nspcc.org.uk

Nursing and Midwifery Council (all NMC documents downloadable from the website), 23 Portland Place, London W1N 3AF www.nmc-uk.org

Prince's Foundation for Integrated Health, 33–41 Dallington Street, London EC1V 0BB www.fih.org.uk

PubMed (National Library of Medicine's free search service for contemporary professional research and review papers) www.ncbi.nlm.nih.gov/entrez

Research Council for Complementary Medicine, 1 Harley Street, London W1G 9QD www.rccm.org.uk

Royal College of Midwives, 15 Mansfield Street, London W1G 9NH www.rcm.org.uk

Royal College of Nursing, 20 Cavendish Square, London W1M 0AB www.rcn.org.uk

Royal College of Obstetricians and Gynaecologists, 27 Sussex Place, Regent's Park, London NW1 4RG www.rcog.org.uk

Safe Motherhood Initiative www.safemotherhood.org

Stillbirth and Neonatal Death Society (SANDS), 28 Portland Place, London W1N 4DE www.uk-sands.org

Sure Start, Department for Education and Skills and Department for Work and Pensions, Level 2, Caxton House, Tothill Street, London SW1H 9NA www.surestart.gov.uk

Twins and Multiple Birth Association (TAMBA), 2 The Willows, Gardner Road, Guildford GU1 4PG www.tamba.org.uk

Well-being of Women, 27 Sussex Place, Regent's Park, London NW1 4SP www.well-being.org.uk

Immunisation schedule for children

AGE DUE	IMMUNISATION
2 months	Diphtheria, tetanus, pertussis (whooping cough), polio and *Haemophilus influenzae* type b (Hib) Pneumococcal infection (PCV)
3 months	Diphtheria, tetanus, pertussis (whooping cough), polio and *Haemophilus influenzae* type b (Hib) Meningitis C
4 months	Diphtheria, tetanus, pertussis (whooping cough), polio and *Haemophilus influenzae* type b (Hib) Meningitis C Pneumococcal infection (PCV)
12 months	*Haemophilus influenzae* type b (Hib) Meningitis C
13 months	Measles, mumps and rubella (MMR)
3 years 4 months to 5 years	Pneumococcal infection (PCV) Diphtheria, tetanus, pertussis (whooping cough) and polio Measles, mumps and rubella (MMR)
13–18 years	Diphtheria, tetanus, polio (booster)

Abbreviations

AABR	automated auditory brainstem response
ACA	anticardiolipin antibody
ACH	aftercoming head (of breech)
ACTH	adrenocorticotrophic hormone
ADH	antidiuretic hormone
AF	artificial feeding
AFI	amniotic fluid index
AFLP	acute fatty liver of pregnancy
AFP	alpha fetoprotein
AID	artificial insemination by donor
AIDS	acquired immune deficiency syndrome
AIH	artificial insemination by husband
AN(C)	antenatal (clinic)
AP	anteroposterior
AP(E)L	accreditation of prior (experiential) learning
APH	antepartum haemorrhage
ARM	artificial rupture of membranes
ART	antiretroviral therapy
ASD	atrial septal defect
BBA	born before arrival (of the midwife)
BCG	bacille Calmette–Guérin
b.d.	twice daily
BF	breastfeeding
BFI	Baby Friendly Initiative
BLISS	Baby Life Support System
BMA	British Medical Association
BMI	body mass index
BMR	basal metabolic rate
BP	1. blood pressure. 2. British Pharmacopoeia
BPD	biparietal diameter
BSD	bisacromial diameter
BV	bacterial vaginosis
C	Celsius
Ca	calcium
CAH	congenital adrenal hyperplasia
CAM	complementary and alternative medicine
CAT	computed axial tomography

CATS	credit accumulation and transfer system
CCT	controlled cord traction
CDH	congenital dislocation of the hip
CEMD	Confidential Enquiry into Maternal Deaths
CESDI	Confidential Enquiry into Stillbirth and Deaths in Infancy
CF	cystic fibrosis
CHAI	Commission for Healthcare Audit and Inspection
CHD	congenital heart disease
CHT	congenital hypothyroidism
CIP	continuous inflating pressure
CMV	1. controlled mechanical ventilation. 2. cytomegalovirus
CNP	continuous negative pressure
CNS	central nervous system
CNST	Clinical Negligence Scheme for Trusts
COC	combined oral contraceptive
COSHH	Control of Substances Hazardous to Health
CNEEP	continuous negative end-expiratory pressure
CPAP	continuous positive airway pressure
CPD	1. cephalopelvic disproportion. 2. continuing professional development
CPR	cardiopulmonary resuscitation
CRB	Criminal Records Bureau
CRL	crown–rump length
CRP	C-reactive protein
CRIES	pain assessment tool
CSF	cerebrospinal fluid
CSM	Committee on Safety of Medicines
CSU	catheter specimen of urine
CT	computed tomography
CTG	cardiotocograph
CVP	central venous pressure
CVS	1. chorionic villus sampling. 2. cardiovascular system
Cx	cervix
D&C	dilatation and curettage
D&V	diarrhoea and vomiting
DARE	Database of Abstracts of Reviews of Effectiveness
DAT	direct antiglobulin test
DH	Department of Health
DHA	district health authority
DIC	disseminated intravascular coagulation
Dip	Diploma
DMPA	depot, medroxyprogesterone acetate
DMU	directly managed unit
DNA	1. did not attend. 2. deoxyribonucleic acid
DSS	Department of Social Security
DTA	deep transverse arrest
DVT	deep venous thrombosis
E_1	estrone (oestrone)
E_2	estradiol-17β (oestradiol)

E₃	estriol (oestriol)
EBM	expressed breast milk
ECG	electrocardiogram
ECMO	extracorporeal membrane oxygenation
ECT	electroconvulsive treatment/therapy
ECV	external cephalic version
EDD	expected date of delivery
EEG	electroencephalogram
EPA	examination *per abdomen*
EPAU	early pregnancy assessment unit
EPDS	Edinburgh postnatal depression scale
EPV	examination *per vaginam*
ERPC	evacuation of retained products of conception
ESR	erythrocyte sedimentation rate
EUA	examination under anaesthetic
F	Fahrenheit
FAS	fetal alcohol syndrome
FBS	fetal blood sampling
FDPs	fibrin degradation products
Fe	iron
FH (HR)	fetal heart (heard and regular)
FIGO	International Federation of Gynaecology and Obstetrics
FIH	Prince's Foundation for Integrated Health
FISH	fluorescent *in situ* hybridisation
FMH	fetomaternal haemorrhage
FRCGP	Fellow of the Royal College of General Practitioners
FRCOG	Fellow of the Royal College of Obstetricians and Gynaecologists
FSH (RF)	follicle-stimulating hormone (releasing factor)
FSID	Foundation for Study of Infant Deaths
FTA-ABS	fluorescent treponemal antibody-absorbed test
g	gram
G	gravida
GBS	group B streptococcus
GIFT	gamete intrafallopian transfer
GIT	gastrointestinal tract
GMC	General Medical Council
GP (O)	general practitioner (obstetrician)
G6PD	glucose-6-phosphate dehydrogenase
GTT	glucose tolerance test
H	hydrogen
HAART	highly active antiretroviral therapy
HAI	hospital-acquired infection
Hb	haemoglobin
hCG	human chorionic gonadotrophin
HCl	hydrochloric acid
HDN	haemolytic disease of the newborn
HEA	Health Education Authority

HELLP	haemolysis, elevated liver proteins and low platelets
HFEA	Human Fertilisation and Embryology Authority
HFOV	high frequency oscillation ventilation
Hg	mercury
HIV	human immunodeficiency virus
hPL	human placental lactogen
HPV	human papilloma virus
HSV	herpes simplex virus
HTA	health technology assessment
HV(A)	Health Visitor (s' Association)
HVS	high vaginal swab
HWY	hundred women-years
IAT	indirect antiglobulin test
ICM	International Confederation of Midwives
ICN	International Council of Nurses
ICP	1. intracranial pressure. 2. intrahepatic cholestasis of pregnancy
ICSH	interstitial cell-stimulating hormone
ICSI	intracytoplasmic sperm injection
ICU/ITU	intensive care unit/intensive therapy unit
IEM	inborn errors of metabolism
Ig	immunoglobulin
IGT	impaired glucose tolerance
IHD	ischaemic heart disease
IM	intramuscular
IMV	intermittent mandatory ventilation
IPPV	intermittent positive pressure ventilation
IRT	immune-reactive trypsin
IUCD	intrauterine contraceptive device
IUD	intrauterine death
IUGR	intrauterine growth restriction
IUT	intrauterine fetal transfer
IV (I)	intravenous (infusion)
IVF	*in vitro* fertilisation
IVH	intraventricular haemorrhage
IVP/IVU	intravenous pyelogram/urogram
J	joule
K	potassium
k	kilo
KC	kangaroo care
kcal	kilocalorie
kJ	kilojoule
LA	local authority
LAM	lactational amenorrhoea method (of contraception)
LBW	low birthweight
LFD	light for dates
LFT	liver function tests

LH	luteinising hormone
LMA	left mentoanterior
LML	left mentolateral
LMP	1. left mentoposterior. 2. last menstrual period
LOA	left occipitoanterior
LOL	left occipitolateral
LOP	left occipitoposterior
LOT	left occipitotransverse
LP	lumbar puncture
LSA	1. local supervising authority. 2. left sacroanterior
LSCS	lower segment Caesarean section
LSL	left sacrolateral
LSP	left sacroposterior
L/S	lecithin–sphingomyelin ratio

m	milli, meta
M	mega
MAOI	monoamine oxidase inhibitor
MCA	1. maternity care assistant. 2. middle cerebral artery
MCADD	medium-chain acyl-coenzyme A dehydrogenase deficiency
MCH	mean corpuscular haemoglobin
MCHC	mean corpuscular haemoglobin concentration
MCV	mean corpuscular volume
mL	millilitre
mm	millimetre
mmol	millimole
MOH	Medical Officer of Health
MOM	multiple of the median
MRC	Medical Research Council
MRCOG	Member of the Royal College of Obstetricians and Gynaecologists
MRI	magnetic resonance imaging
MRSA	methicillin-resistant Staphylococcus aureus
MSAC	Maternity Services Advisory Committee
MSH	melanocyte-stimulating hormone
MSU	midstream specimen of urine
MV	mentovertical

Na	sodium
NAD	nothing abnormal detected
NAI	non-accidental injury
NBFD	Neville Barnes forceps delivery
ND	normal delivery
NCT	National Childbirth Trust
NEC	necrotising enterocolitis
NFP	natural family planning
NHS	NHS
NICE	National Institute for Health and Clinical Excellence
NICU	neonatal intensive care unit
NMC	Nursing and Midwifery Council
NMR	nuclear magnetic resonance

NND	neonatal death
NNU	neonatal unit
NSAID	non-steroidal anti-inflammatory drug
NSC	National Screening Committee
NSF	National Service Framework
NSU	non-specific urethritis
NT	nuchal translucency
NTD	neural tube defect
NTE	neutral thermal environment
O	oxygen
OA	occipitoanterior
OAE	otoacoustic emissions (test)
OAPR	odds of being affected given a positive result
OCD	obsessive compulsive disorder
ODA	operating department assistant
OHSS	ovarian hyperstimulation syndrome
OL	occipitolateral
OP	occipitoposterior
OPD	outpatient department
OT	occipitotransverse
OTC	over-the-counter (drugs)
P	1. phosphorus. 2. para, parity
P	probability
Pa	pascal
PA	*per abdomen*
P_aO_2	partial pressure of oxygen in arterial blood
PAP	Papanicolau (smear)
PAPP-A	pregnancy-associated plasma protein-A
PCC	postcoital contraception
PCG	primary care group
PCO_2	partial pressure of carbon dioxide
PCOS	polycystic ovary syndrome
PCR	polymerase chain reaction
PCT	primary care trust
PCV	1. packed cell volume. 2. pneumococcal conjugate vaccine
PDA	patent ductus arteriosus
PEEP	positive end-expiratory pressure
PG	prostaglandin
pg	picogram
PGCE(A)	Postgraduate Certificate in Education (of Adults)
PGD	pre-implantation genetic diagnosis
pH	acid–alkali balance
PID	pelvic inflammatory disease
PIH	pregnancy-induced hypertension
PKU	phenylketonuria
PM	post mortem
PMR	perinatal mortality rate
PO_2	partial pressure of oxygen

POP	persistent occipitoposterior
PPH	postpartum haemorrhage
PPR	Price precipitation reaction
PR	*per rectum*
PREP	post-registration education and practice
prn	as required, when necessary
PTSD	post-traumatic stress disorder
PUBS	percutaneous umbilical cord blood sampling
PUO	pyrexia of unknown origin
PV	*per vaginam*

Q	quadrant
q.d.	every day
q.d.s.	four times a day
QF-PCR	quantitative fluorescence polymerase chain reaction
q.h.	every hour
q.i.d.	four times daily
q.q.h.	every 4 hours

RBC	1. red blood cells. 2. red blood count
RCGP	Royal College of General Practitioners
RCM	Royal College of Midwives
RCN	Royal College of Nurses
RCOG	Royal College of Obstetricians and Gynaecologists
RCT	randomised controlled trial
RDS	respiratory distress syndrome
R(G)N	Registered (General) Nurse
Rh	Rhesus (factor)
RIA	radioimmunoassay
RM	Registered Midwife
RMA	right mentoanterior
RML	right mentolateral
RMP	right mentoposterior
RNA	ribonucleic acid
ROA	right occipitoanterior
ROL	right occipitolateral
ROP	right occipitoposterior
RPCF	Reiter's protein complement fixation
RPR	rapid plasma reagin
RSA	right sacroanterior
RSL	right sacrolateral
RSP	right sacroposterior
Rx	treatment

S	sulphur
SB	stillbirth
SBR	serum bilirubin
SC	subcutaneous
SCBU	special care baby unit
SCD	sickle cell disease

SFD	small for dates
SGOT	serum glutamate oxaloacetate transaminase
SGPT	serum glutamate pyruvate transaminase
SI	Système International d'Unités
SIDS	sudden infant death syndrome
SLE	systemic lupus erythematosus
SMP	Statutory Maternity Pay
SPD	symphysis pubis diastasis/discomfort
SRM	spontaneous rupture of membranes
SSP	Statutory Sick Pay
STI/STD	sexually transmitted infection/disease
SVD	spontaneous vaginal delivery
TBA	1. traditional birth attendant. 2. to be advised
TBC	to be confirmed
TBG	thyroid-binding globulin
TCM	traditional Chinese medicine
t.d.s.	three times daily
TENS	transcutaneous electrical nerve stimulation
TFT	thyroid function test
TOP	termination of pregnancy
TORCH	toxoplasmosis, rubella, cytomegalovirus, herpes
TPHA	*Treponema pallidum* haemagglutination
TPN	total parenteral nutrition
TPT	transplacental transfusion
TRAP	twin reversed arterial perfusion
TSH	thyroid-stimulating hormone
TTA/TTO	to take away/to take out
TTN	transient tachypnoea of the newborn
TTTS	twin-to-twin transfusion syndrome
TV	transvaginal
U&E	urea and electrolyte (estimations)
UDFA	ultrasound-directed follicle aspiration
UNICEF	United Nations International Childrenís Emergency Fund
URTI	upper respiratory tract infection
US (S)	ultrasound (scan)
UTI	urinary tract infection
VDRL	Venereal Disease Research Laboratory
VE	vaginal examination
VLBW	very-low-birthweight
VMA	vanillylmandelic acid
VZV	varicella-zoster virus
WBC	white blood cell/count
WHO	World Health Organization
WR	Wassermann reaction
ZIFT	zygote intrafallopian transfer